Temporomandibular Disorders

Manual therapy, exercise, and needling

Temporomandibular Disorders

Manual therapy, exercise, and needling

Edited by

César Fernández-de-las-Peñas
and
Juan Mesa-Jiménez

Forewords
Leon Chaitow
Thomas List
Jeffrey P. Okeson

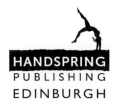

HANDSPRING
PUBLISHING
EDINBURGH

HANDSPRING PUBLISHING LIMITED
The Old Manse, Fountainhall,
Pencaitland, East Lothian
EH34 5EY, Scotland
Tel: +44 1875 341 859
Website: www.handspringpublishing.com

First published 2018 in the United Kingdom by Handspring Publishing
Reprinted 2018, 2019

ISBN 978-1-909141-80-3

British Library Cataloguing in Publication Data
A catalogue record for this book is available from the British Library

Library of Congress Cataloguing in Publication Data
A catalog record for this book is available from the Library of Congress

Notice
Neither the Publisher nor the Authors assume any responsibility for any loss or injury and/or damage to persons or property arising out of or relating to any use of the material contained in this book. It is the responsibility of the treating practitioner, relying on independent expertise and knowledge of the patient, to determine
the best treatment and method of application for the patient.

Commissioning Editor Mary Law
Project Manager Morven Dean
Copy editor Sally Davies
Designer Bruce Hogarth
Cover designer Bruce Hogarth
Indexer Aptara
Typesetter DSM Soft, India
Printer Replika Press Pvt. Ltd., India

The
Publisher's
policy is to use
paper manufactured
from sustainable forests

CONTENTS

FOREWORD by Leon Chaitow

What emerges from the pages of this absorbing book is a revelation. There is a proverb, attributed to various cultures, that states 'It takes a village to raise a child' and, as this textbook illustrates, it takes a large team to comprehensively describe temporomandibular disorders (TMDs) and to accurately and safely examine, identify, understand, treat, and manage these extremely widespread musculoskeletal pain conditions, that are (depending on the diagnostic criteria) second only to nonspecific low back pain in prevalence worldwide, affecting approximately 10 per cent of the adult population.

The opening chapters set the scene by clearly outlining and detailing the examination, classification, including trigeminal nociceptive processing, pathophysiology, sensory testing, and referred pain associated with TMDs (and orofacial pain). Now, it might be thought that defining TMDs would be straightforward. However, as is forensically explained in the first chapter – Definition, epidemiology and etiology of painful temporomandibular disorders – in order to manage these conditions effectively, it is vital that clinicians understand and appreciate the multiple factors that can influence the evolution and maintenance of the dysfunction and pain associated with TMDs.

Before the chapters that detail the effective examination and manual therapy treatment and management of TMDs, it becomes apparent that, critical to optimal management, there must be awareness that a TMD is rarely an isolated disorder with a single 'cause', but is usually the result of a wide range of interacting adaptations, factors, and influences. Some of these etiological features may be preventable, and/or reversible, while some are historical (injury for example) or inherent. For example, there are unexpected ethnic and racial differences, with a clear discrepancy between the incidence of TMDs amongst, e.g., African Americans (3.8 per cent), mixed-race White/Native Americans (12.7 per cent), and Asians (2 per cent). Other potentially significant influences range from educational, occupational and socioeconomic features, to body weight, physical activities, coexisting conditions, habits such as smoking, as well as biomechanical and psychological factors. Unsurprisingly, these same features are also common risk factors for nonspecific low back pain and chronic neck pain.

The chapters on examining for TMD and orofacial pain clearly describe the need for a comprehensive clinical history, together with a detailed evaluation of the temporomandibular joint itself, the masticatory muscles, and the vital structural and functional connections to the cervicothoracic spine, including possible influences such as posture, neurology, ligamentous stability, arterial dysfunction, segmental ranges of motion and mobility, and the functionality of the deep neck flexor muscles. All, or any, of these topics can potentially be major features in the evolution of TMDs, making their assessment essential for an understanding of the particular influences in any given case.

The chapters covering manual therapy interventions provide evidence-informed details regarding therapeutic exercise, joint manipulation and mobilization, management of referred pain (trigger points), as well as a range of soft tissue methods, postural re-education and training. Among these insightful manual therapy chapters there is also a clear and detailed exposition of the role of fascial anatomy in relation to the cranio-cervico-mandibular region. This chapter includes an extraordinarily detailed and complex outline of fascia in relation to the act of chewing, as a part of the survey of multiple dynamic fascial links, connections and functions in the mouth, throat, head, and neck. Also receiving appropriately detailed coverage in relation to TMD management are dry needling, and – usefully in a separate chapter – acupuncture, as well as current perspectives on pain psychology and treatment of the brain. One of the final chapters – Treating the brain in temporomandibular disorders – includes a fascinating exploration of pain neuroscience education and brain exercises.

As a clinician, this reader now has a far clearer understanding as to the host of influences governing the complex issues around TMDs. This fine textbook has been brilliantly conceived and thoughtfully realized, and all concerned deserve congratulations.

Leon Chaitow ND DO
Honorary Fellow, University of Westminster
London, UK
Editor-in-Chief
Journal of Bodywork and Movement Therapies
Corfu, Greece,
November 2017

FOREWORD by Thomas List

I am very pleased, and honored, to be writing a foreword to this book. The gap between our theoretical knowledge of mechanisms, treatment efficacy, and effectiveness outcomes, and our practical clinical experience in how to apply physical therapy in temporomandibular disorder (TMD) pain patients has long needed such a discussion as this book provides. The wide array of treatment modalities in the domain of physical therapy can be confusing when considering which of the available therapies is best suited to a particular situation. This book focuses on best uses of manual therapy, therapeutic exercises, postural training, dry needling, and acupuncture in the treatment of chronic TMD pain patients.

A large epidemiological study of 46,394 participants in Europe reported that 19 per cent of the population had moderate to severe chronic pain. Two-thirds used non-medication treatments, for example massage (30 per cent), physical therapy (21 per cent) and acupuncture (13 per cent), and 38 per cent reported that it had been extremely helpful. Interestingly, the type of physical therapy and the prevalence of its use ranged widely between countries, indicating large cultural differences. Most physical therapies are designed to treat various musculoskeletal pain disorders in the body. Although many features of the masticatory system are admittedly unique, we have learned that the mechanisms by which nociceptive impulses are initiated, transmitted, and perceived are not, as pain is more or less common throughout the body. This indicates that interventions which have been found to be useful at other sites in the body may also be useful in TMDs. Although evidence is limited, some modalities of physical therapy, such as jaw exercises, have been recommended in Swedish national guidelines in health care and as an integrated part of self-care in several publications. Based upon moderate evidence, the Swedish national guidelines for the treatment of orofacial pain currently recommend

jaw exercises for TMDs, particularly from a health-economic perspective.

Several physical therapy modes are reportedly beneficial because they often activate the endogenous pain inhibitory modulation system; have few side effects; activate the patient by increasing body awareness and providing new pain-relief tools for home use; and facilitate communication with care providers. An additional benefit is that multimodal treatment with other therapies becomes easier and potentially more effective.

Chronic pain is often complex with comorbid pain conditions. An optimum treatment outcome almost always requires multidisciplinary collaboration with other medical disciplines. Although this book provides information on physical therapies useful for TMD patients and targets TMD professionals, such treatment may be delivered by other health professionals who may find the information contained between the covers of this book useful.

The book is divided into four parts, each containing several chapters. The first part deals with the epidemiology and classification of TMDs, nociceptive processing, and the pathophysiology of the masticatory system. These chapters provide the clinician with a deep understanding of the basic science of chronic pain. Part 2 focuses on the clinical case history and the clinical examination of the masticatory system and upper cervical region. The chapters in Part 2 detail the currently tested and accepted methods for assessing and examining the patient. Part 3 reviews various manual therapies for TMDs and neck disorders. This section highlights the available evidence-based literature and provides readers with scientifically sound and effective support for the use of these therapies. Part 4 discusses other interventions, such as acupuncture, and in addition, the final chapter uses a biopsychosocial perspective to set up a framework for integrating physical therapies with other therapies in the management of chronic TMD pain patients.

Although the field of TMDs and orofacial pain has made great strides in the last few decades, clinical situations continue to remind us of the limits to our knowledge. As clinicians, we meet patients seeking help with pain and suffering on a daily basis. We must determine, to the best of our ability – based on the best scientific evidence available, our own clinical experience, and potential value to the patient – the treatment that will best provide an optimal outcome and quality of life for just this patient sitting in our chair. The present book was conceived and written for this purpose.

Treatment needs to be tailored for the individual chronic pain patient; this often implies different approaches or combinations of treatment modes such as behavioral therapies, pharmacologic treatment, occlusal therapy (splints), and physical therapy. One guideline overshadows all else: Select – always –

the most conservative approach, and above all, do no harm. Patients need to feel believed, to know that all attempts to arrive at a correct diagnosis have been made, and to understand that appropriate treatment or referral to other specialists and therapists has been done when necessary.

I congratulate the contributing editors and authors, many of whom are recognized, leading experts in their fields and have contributed significantly to our current knowledge through their research and scientific publications. This book is a gem in its field, providing effective, trustworthy information to clinicians that will help alleviate orofacial pain and the suffering of their patients, and thus to some measure, or substantially, improve the daily experience of chronic pain patients.

Thomas List DDS OdontDr
Professor and Chairman
Department of Orofacial Pain and Jaw Function
Faculty of Odontology, Malmö University,
Malmö, Sweden
November 2017

FOREWORD by Jeffrey P. Okeson

During my professional career, I have had the opportunity to witness some very positive changes for our patients. One of these has been the blending of professional efforts in the area of orofacial pain. As we attempted to better understand pain, we began to appreciate the complexity of this field. Pain is one of the most powerful negative emotions we humans experience, yet we often struggle to help our suffering patients. We have come to learn that pain is far more than a sensation. Instead, pain is actually an experience, far more complex than a simple sensation. We have also learned that common sources of peripheral injury, thought to be the source of most pains, are not the problems we clinicians face. We now understand that when nociception enters the central nervous system it is greatly influenced by excitatory and inhibitory mechanisms. As a result, we have come to appreciate that pain is not exclusive to one medical discipline. Instead, our patients deserve the best that every discipline can offer to reduce their suffering.

This textbook is an example of this progressive thinking as it combines input from three different professions with the idea of providing the best care for our patients. In acute injuries, physical therapy can provide the necessary management that assists in recovery. It is important to recognize that when pain becomes chronic, central factors become a predominant component of maintaining the pain. With these patients, a multiprofessional team adds an important dimension to patient recovery. This textbook offers information from well-known authorities in physical therapy, orofacial pain and clinical psychology, which will help the clinician better understand what each discipline can offer. This multiprofessional effort offers the best possible success for patient management. A text like this is rare and the authors should be commended for their combined work. This professional endeavor is a reflection of the evidence-based science and the state-of-the-art efforts our patients deserve. The information found in this text will help all clinicians better evaluate and manage their patients.

Jeffrey P. Okeson DMD
Provost's Distinguished Service Professor
Professor and Chief, Division of Orofacial Pain
Director, Orofacial Pain Program
College of Dentistry, University of Kentucky
Lexington, Kentucky, USA
October 2017

PREFACE

The term temporomandibular disorder (TMD) encompasses pain in the head and face, a condition which can be highly distressing and disabling for the patient. As clinicians, we should focus our attention on the therapeutic approaches than can help those patients. It is increasingly clear that the value of manual therapy, exercise, and needling therapies can be understood through the emerging concepts of pain neuroscience, and that all these interventions come together in a biopsychosocial model. In fact, manual therapy and exercise is probably the therapeutic combination most commonly used by many health care professionals for treating patients with chronic pain. Today, it is universally accepted that the central nervous system plays a critical role in the personal experience and clinical presentation of pain, and that manual therapy, exercise or needling therapies trigger peripheral and central nervous system responses. It was against this background of a growth in understanding of mechanisms that we were inspired to bring together a wide range of contributors from all over the world to provide a comprehensive and practical account of the diverse approaches to assessing and treating TMDs.

In conceiving and editing this book we have adopted the evidence and clinically informed paradigm. We believe that a combination of evidence and clinical experience should guide all clinicians in the management of individuals with chronic pain. The main feature of the evidence-based paradigm is that diagnosis and management should be guided mainly by the best available scientific evidence; however, the relevance of this doctrine can be limited since there is no good evidence for all intervention or diagnostic procedures that therapists use in daily practice. Although evidence-based practice is in continuous evolution, the evidence-*informed* paradigm is considered more appropriate since the clinician takes the best available scientific evidence and combines it with clinical experience while bearing in mind the patient's expectations and beliefs.

Throughout this textbook, chapter authors have integrated clinical experience and reasoning based on a neurophysiologic rationale with the most up-to-date evidence, thereby in effect combining the best of evidence-based and clinically based paradigms, mimicking what clinicians do in everyday clinical practice. We believe that this approach has created a textbook that truly provides practicing clinicians with what they need to know for real-life screening, diagnosis, and management of patients with TMD pain. This should be especially valuable since the multifactorial etiology and presentation that patients with TMD may exhibit can create a real challenge to the clinician.

The textbook is divided into four parts. In Part 1, several authors review the epidemiology and classification of TMD pain syndromes and the neurophysiological mechanisms underlying craniofacial pain. In Part 2, authors set out the steps for taking a comprehensive history in patients affected by TMD and the basic principles for the physical examination. In this section, authors clearly demonstrate the relevance of regional interdependence by showing why the thoracic and cervical spine should be also assessed in individuals suffering from TMD. The remaining parts cover therapeutic interventions for TMDs. Part 3 describes several manual therapy interventions, including joint, muscle, fascia, and neural interventions, and also therapeutic exercises. Finally, Part 4 covers other therapeutic options, including different needling therapies, by placing the field of these interventions within the context of contemporary pain neurosciences and neuroscience education.

We anticipate that this textbook will become the standard for manual management of individuals with TMDs and we hope that it will bridge apparent differences in opinion. We aim to unite different health care disciplines using manual therapy, exercise, and needling therapies as their therapeutic approach. We hope that the current textbook will ultimately benefit patients worldwide.

Cesar Fernández-de-las-Peñas, Juan Mesa-Jiménez
Madrid, Spain
January 2018

EDITORS

César Fernández-de-las-Peñas PT, DO, MSc, PhD, DrMedSci is Director of the Department of Physical Therapy, Occupational Therapy, Rehabilitation and Physical Medicine at Universidad Rey Juan Carlos, Madrid, Spain. He is the Dean of a pain sciences research group, and has 15 years of clinical experience in private practice in a pain clinic focused on manual approaches to the management of chronic pain. His research activities are on neuroscientific aspects of upper quadrant pain syndromes, particularly head and neck pain conditions. He has published more than 300 scientific publications in peer-reviewed journals and he is first author of approximately 150 of them. He is also editor of several textbooks on headache, migraine, manual therapy and dry needling, and has been invited to present at 50 international conferences.

Juan Mesa-Jiménez PT, MSc, PhD, is Professor in the Faculty of Medicine and Director of the Masters in Cranio-Mandibular Dysfunction and Orofacial Pain at Universidad San Pablo CEU, Madrid, Spain. He has more than 20 years of clinical experience in private practice in a pain clinic focused on the management of patients with orofacial pain. He has published scientific papers in peer-reviewed journals on the topic of orofacial chronic pain and needling intervention for its management, and has been invited to present at conferences around the world.

CONTRIBUTORS

Susan Armijo-Olivo, PT, MSc, PhD
Adjunct Professor, Faculty of Rehabilitation Medicine
and Faculty of Medicine and Dentistry, University of
Alberta, Edmonton; Principal Research Lead,
Institute of Health Economics, Edmonton,
Alberta, Canada

Lars Arendt-Nielsen, PhD, DrMedSci
Center for Sensory-Motor Interaction (SMI®),
Department of Health Sciences and Technology,
Faculty of Medicine, Aalborg University,
Aalborg, Denmark

Brian E. Cairns, PhD, DrMed, ACPR
Professor, Faculty of Pharmaceutical Sciences,
University of British Columbia, Vancouver,
Canada; Professor, Center for Neuroplasticity and
Pain, SMI®, Department of Health Science and
Technology, Faculty of Medicine, Aalborg University,
Aalborg, Denmark

Eduardo Castro-Martín, PT
Professor of Physiotherapy, Department
of Physiotherapy, Universidad de Granada,
Granada, Spain; Physiotherapist, 'VértexCentro,'
Granada, Spain

Joshua A. Cleland, PT, PhD
Professor, Physical Therapy Program,
Franklin Pierce University, Manchester,
New Hampshire, USA

Mike Cummings, MB ChB, DipMedAc
Medical Director, British Medical Acupuncture Society,
United Kingdom

Bill Egan, PT, DPT, OCS, FAAOMPT
Associate Professor of Instruction,
Department of Physical Therapy, Temple University,
Philadelphia, USA

Fernando G. Exposto, DDS, MSc
PhD student, Section of Orofacial Pain and Jaw Function,
Department of Dentistry and Oral Health,
Aarhus University, Denmark; Member,
Scandinavian Center for Orofacial Neurosciences,
Denmark

Blanca Codina García-Andrade, PT, MSc
Lecturer, Masters Program in Orofacial Pain and
Temporomandibular Dysfunction, Universidad San
Pablo CEU, Madrid, Spain

Joe Girard, DPT, DScPT
Assistant Professor, Physical Therapy Program, Franklin
Pierce University, Manchester, New Hampshire, USA

Thomas Graven-Nielsen, DMSc, PhD
Professor, Center for Neuroplasticity and Pain
(CNAP), SMI®, Department of Health Sciences and
Technology, Faculty of Medicine, Aalborg University,
Aalborg, Denmark

Toby Hall, PT, MSc, PhD, FACP
Adjunct Associate Professor, School of Physiotherapy
and Exercise Science, Curtin University, Perth,
Australia; Senior Teaching Fellow, The University of
Western Australia, Perth, Australia

Gary M. Heir, DMD
Clinical and Program Director, Center of
Temporomandibular Disorders and Orofacial Pain,
Rutgers University School of Dental Medicine,
Newark, New Jersey, USA

José L. de-la-Hoz, MD, DMD, MS
Professor and Program Coordinator, Masters
Program in Temporomandibular Disorder and
Orofacial Pain, School of Medicine, Universidad San
Pablo CEU, Madrid, Spain

Abhishek Kumar, BDS, PhD
Postdoctoral Researcher, Department of Dental
Medicine, Karolinska Institutet, Huddinge, Sweden;
Member, Scandinavian Center for Orofacial
Neurosciences, Sweden

Adriaan Louw, PT, PhD
CEO, International Spine and Pain Institute,
Story City, Iowa, USA

Cristina Lozano-López, PT, MSc
PhD student, Department of Physical Therapy,
Occupational Therapy, Physical Medicine and

Rehabilitation, Universidad Rey Juan Carlos, Alcorcón, Madrid, Spain

Megan McPhee, PT
PhD student, Center for Neuroplasticity and Pain (CNAP), SMI®, Department of Health Sciences and Technology, Faculty of Medicine, Aalborg University, Aalborg, Denmark

Ambra Michelotti, DDS Orthod
Associate Professor, Department of Neuroscience, Reproductive Sciences and Oral Sciences, School of Orthodontics, University of Naples Federico II, Naples, Italy

Michael C. O'Hara, PT, DPT, OCS
Senior Physical Therapist,
Good Shepherd Penn Partners, Penn Therapy and Fitness at University City, Philadelphia, USA

Richard Ohrbach, DDS, PhD, Odont Dr(Hons)
Department of Oral Diagnostic Sciences, University at Buffalo School of Dental Medicine, Buffalo, New York, USA

María Palacios-Ceña, PT, CO, PhD
Professor, Department of Physical Therapy, Occupational Therapy, Physical Medicine and Rehabilitation, Universidad Rey Juan Carlos; Clinical Researcher, Cátedra de Docencia e Investigación en Fisioterapia: Terapia Manual y Punción Seca, Universidad Rey Juan Carlos, Alcorcón, Madrid, Spain; Clinical Researcher, Center for Sensory-Motor Interaction (SMI®), Laboratory for Musculoskeletal Pain and Motor Control, Aalborg University, Aalborg, Denmark

Elisa Bizetti Pelai, PT, MSc
PhD student, Movement Science,
Methodist University of Piracicaba (UNIMEP), Piracicaba, São Paulo, Brazil

Harry von Piekartz, PT, BSc, MSc, PhD
Professor, Faculty of Movement and Rehabilitation

Science; Study Director, MSc in Musculoskeletal Therapy, University of Applied Science, Osnabrück, Germany

Andrzej Pilat, PT
Director, Myofascial Therapy School 'Tupimek', Madrid, Spain; Lecturer, Masters Degree Program, ONCE Physiotherapy School,
Universidad Autónoma de Madrid,
Madrid, Spain

Laurent Pitance, PT, PhD
Institute of Experimental and Clinical Research, Neuromusculoskeletal Lab (NMSK),
Catholic University of Louvain, Brussels, Belgium; Oral and Maxillofacial Surgery Department, Saint-Luc University Clinics, Saint-Luc, Brussels, Belgium

Emilio (Louie) Puentedura,
PT, DPT, PhD, OCS, FAAOMPT
Associate Professor and Coordinator for the PhD in Interdisciplinary Health Sciences,
Department of Physical Therapy,
University of Nevada, Las Vegas,
Nevada, USA

Mariano Rocabado, PT, DPT, PhD
Faculty of Dentistry, Universidad de Chile;
Santiago de Chile; Director, Instituto Rocabado, Santiago de Chile

Sonia Sharma, BDS, MS, PhD
Research Assistant Professor, Department of Oral Diagnostic Sciences, University at Buffalo School of Dental Medicine, Buffalo, New York, USA

Peter Svensson, DDS, PhD, Dr Odont
Professor and Head,
Section of Orofacial Pain and Jaw Function, Department of Dentistry and Oral Health, Aarhus University, Aarhus,
Denmark;
Guest Professor,
Department of Dental Medicine,

Karolinska Institute, Huddinge,
Sweden;
Member, Scandinavian Center for Orofacial
Neurosciences, Denmark

Tom Mark Thayer,
BChD, MA(MedEd), FDS RCPS(Glasg), FHEA
Consultant and Honorary Senior Lecturer in Oral Surgery,

Liverpool University Dental Hospital
and School of Dentistry,
University of Liverpool, Liverpool, UK

Hao-Jun You, MD, PhD
Center for Biomedical Research on Pain,
College of Medicine, Xi'An Jiaotong University,
Xi'An, People's Republic of China

ACKNOWLEDGMENTS

After many years working with patients with orofacial pain, and in consultation with Handspring Publishing, we agreed that the time had come to put together a textbook about TMDs. We did not really grasp how many people would eventually become involved in this project, but the result is the current textbook – made possible through the efforts of many individuals.

First, we would like to thank our coauthors, who prepared the chapters, and created a worldwide collaboration. In addition, the authors come from different health care professions, making this book a true multidisciplinary collaboration. Secondly, we would also like to acknowledge our patients who have taught us so much about what it is like to live with acute and chronic persistent TMD pain.

Thirdly, we would like to acknowledge Handspring Publishing for entrusting us with the preparation of this textbook. We have been very impressed with the professionalism and enthusiasm of the folks at Handspring, and much appreciate their guidance and attention to detail.

Lastly, we are grateful to our families, friends, and colleagues. We realize that our professional activities, such as writing book chapters and teaching courses, do take us away from our families and friends. We appreciate their understanding and support for our endeavors.

Cesar Fernández-de-las-Peñas, Juan Mesa-Jiménez
Madrid, Spain
January 2018

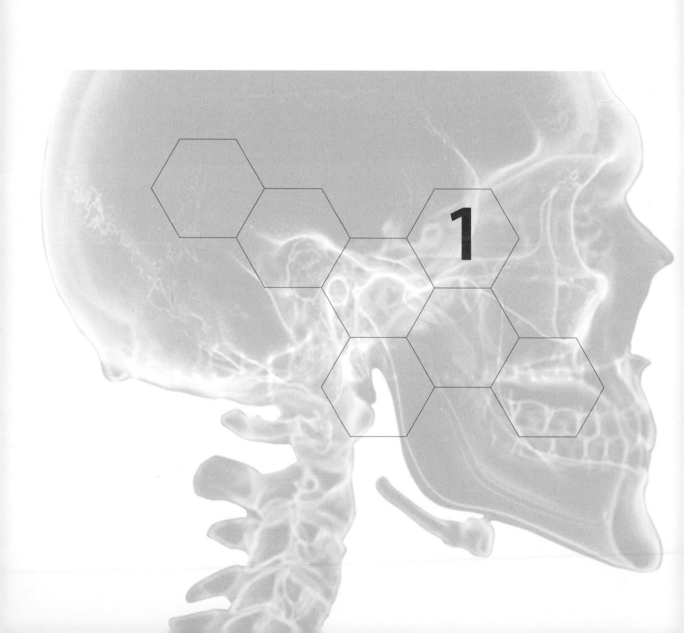

PART 1
Introduction to temporomandibular disorders

Chapter 1

Definition, epidemiology and etiology of painful temporomandibular disorders

Sonia Sharma, Richard Ohrbach

Definition of temporomandibular disorders

Temporomandibular disorders (TMDs) are a group of pain conditions that affect the hard and soft structures of the orofacial region and are characterized principally by pain, limitation in jaw opening, and temporomandibular joint (TMJ) noises (de Leeuw & Klasser, 2013). Based on these principal characteristics, approaches have differed considerably as to how to conceptualize the disorders beyond their basic musculoskeletal character, which has in turn lead to differing diagnostic criteria. In fact, taxonomies and criteria are addressed in Chapter 2 of this textbook; here, we focus on definitions, and how definitions have influenced our understanding of the epidemiology and etiology of TMDs. Furthermore, definitions directly influence taxonomies, criteria, clinical practice, and research, including both the application of clinical research and research focused on classification. In this chapter, we apply the following definitions: 'TMDs' refer to the rubric as a whole, while 'a TMD' is a specific disorder.

According to the most widely accepted diagnostic methods and criteria, TMDs are the second most commonly occurring musculoskeletal condition in the USA after chronic low back pain (Lipton et al., 1993; NIDCR, 2014). In fact, worldwide estimates of their prevalence – approximately 10 per cent of the adult population are affected– appear to mirror those in the USA (Lipton et al., 1993; NIDCR, 2014). How TMDs broadly are defined will substantially influence their prevalence, as discussed in detail in the section on epidemiology later in this chapter; briefly, estimates can be as low as a few per cent if criteria are very restrictive, and as high as 60 per cent if criteria are relaxed. Very restrictive criteria might include requirement of multiple findings of masticatory musculature pain during mobility testing and

palpation, and a high number of days, e.g., 20 in the previous month, with masticatory pain. Very relaxed criteria might be the presence of a single TMD-type symptom, say any TMJ clicking, in the previous six months. Therefore, to address this wide range of possibilities we should consider first the case definition.

Case definition

The purpose of a case definition is to provide an instantiated clarity, even if only temporarily, into a disorder; the clarity of that definition permits separation from other, perhaps more established (though not necessarily valid), diagnostic concepts. The particular case definition is constructed to fit within the context of intended usage in order to maximize reliability (in contrast to clinical diagnosis which is constructed to capture disease as it appears to occur in the natural world), which then permits the meaningful depiction of incidence, prevalence, risk factors, natural history, and clinical course of the disorder, without the burden of restrictions that might be imposed by a conventional diagnosis. An informed case definition is imperative when developing taxonomies and also when revising taxonomies; the instantiated clarity helps avoid circularity when bootstrapping diagnostic concepts from one phase of development to the next phase. In many instances, a given phase of development of a disease taxonomy may represent the current (and best) reference standard for the field; the improvement of a reference standard from one version to the next requires the inclusion of a third perspective.

Prior to the development of the Research Diagnostic Criteria for Temporomandibular Disorders (RDC/TMD) there was no single agreed-upon definition for TMDs as a global term encompassing a variety of subtypes. Several research groups focused on pain in the structures of the temporomandibular region as the defining characteristic of a TMD, and hence the prevalence reported for TMDs has varied widely across studies. Based on the rationale that pain rather than symptoms such as joint sounds or jaw locking had a greater impact on individual suffering, interference with usual activities, increased economic burden due to lost productivity, and seeking health care, Dworkin & LeResche introduced the RDC/TMD (Dworkin et al., 1990; Dworkin & LeResche, 1992). This set of diagnostic criteria revolves around a common case definition for a given type of disorder, standardized examination methods, and standardized methods of gathering self-report information (Dworkin & LeResche, 1992). For further information on this, see the sections below on diagnosing TMDs using the RDC/TMD.

Given the wide differences in the prevalence of TMDs reported, ranging from just a few per cent to up to 60 per cent depending on how the disorders have been variously defined, the determination of the criteria that will correctly identify a 'real' disorder, that is one existing in nature and not just in the mind of the clinician, benefits from the inclusion of a case definition. For research purposes, choosing between a restrictive versus a relaxed approach is generally determined by the research goal for many types of studies. Studies purporting to have clinical generalizability will adhere to standards more suitable for the clinic: tests readily available in the clinic will be given priority. A clinician who believes that even a single episode of a TMJ click is a potential indicator of a subsequent clinical disorder will have a very low threshold for what qualifies as a disorder; a clinician concerned about, for example, the consequences of over-treatment for TMJ clicking that most of the time has very low morbidity will adopt, in contrast, a much higher threshold for severity of symptoms or findings in determining what qualifies as a disorder. Because TMDs, like most chronic pain disorders, have few, if any, pathognomonic markers, there is no clear objective marker of disease to serve as a reference standard by which to determine

pathology versus nonpathology. This is particularly true for the disorders primarily characterized by pain, but even for joint disorders the existing reference standard of imaging only discloses the physical status of the joint structures, and the relationship between imaging-based findings and a disorder with clinical relevance has low diagnostic specificity, with the clinical disorder better explained by behavioral and psychological variables (Dionne et al., 2008; Johansson et al., 2008; Leeuw et al., 2007; Türp et al., 2016; Verkerk et al., 2015; Wasan et al., 2005). Consequently, reasoned decisions for how to construct a case definition, particularly for clinical purposes, revolve around multiple considerations.

Threshold considerations

Based on a simple but widely accepted TMD case definition for epidemiologic purposes, TMDs are associated with pain and disability and affect approximately 5–12 per cent of the population of the USA, and the estimated annual cost is US$4 billion (Lipton et al., 1993; NIDCR, 2014). Here, cost for treatment is determined by the threshold for what constitutes a disorder and, thereby, should be treated. For example, a low threshold for qualifying as a disorder may lead to multiple treatments as trial and error, and thereby increase costs for treatment and consequently lead to over-treating the disorder. A high threshold, in contrast, has the potential to identify the disorder beyond its representation by only simple symptoms and can therefore direct more targeted treatments, thereby reducing costs. Thresholds can be considered from within the disorder or based on the consequences of the disorder.

In order to consider the threshold by which a case definition should identify a clinical disorder, some critical terms require definition. Biomedical vocabulary standards for disease concepts vary widely and consequently for the present purposes we will use a set of definitions developed for ontology (Scheuermann et al., 2009). The selected definitions of primary importance for this chapter are taken verbatim from this source:

- **Disorder.** A causally relatively isolated combination of physical components that is clinically abnormal and not readily reducible to some other entity.

- **Pathological process.** A bodily process that is a manifestation of a disorder.

- **Diseases.** A disposition to undergo a pathological process due to one or more disorders.

- **Sign.** A bodily feature of a patient that is observed in a physical examination and is deemed by the clinician to be of clinical significance.

- **Symptom.** A bodily feature of a patient that is observed by the patient and is hypothesized by the patient to be a realization of a disease.

- **Normal value of a test (or finding).** A value that is based on a statistical treatment of values from a reference population.

- **Preclinical manifestation of a disease.** A disease manifestation that exists prior to its becoming detectable in a clinical history taking or physical examination.

- **Diagnosis.** A conclusion of an interpretative process that has as input a clinical picture of a given patient and as output an assertion to the effect that the patient has a disease of a certain a type.

A case definition needs to be specific to the purpose of what needs to be identified, and within that it can be based on only primary characteristics (for example signs, symptoms or biomarkers), on a combination of primary characteristics, or on the inclusion of secondary characteristics. Table 1.1 gives a summary of pain terminology, representing domains that are widely regarded as primary domains of experienced pain and upon which case definitions are typically based.

One aspect of determining a threshold within the selected characteristics for the purposes of constructing a case definition resides on the normal value of the test or finding, and that in turn depends on a population of values in order to identify normal variability and thereby discriminate abnormality as a possible marker of a pathological process. One example within the diagnosis of masticatory muscle myalgia is whether the evaluation need only disclose one painful masticatory muscle from provocation testing (Diagnostic Criteria for Temporomandibular Disorders [DC/TMD]) or three such muscle sites (RDC/TMD) as a threshold for myalgia within the respective diagnostic systems. This may depend on the presence of a cofactor (for example the provoked pain must replicate the pain of clinical complaint, as in the DC/TMD) in order to protect against false positive diagnoses, given that hyperalgesia is expected in clinically normal individuals due to variations in pain perception, which leads to the ubiquity of simple tenderness from palpation unrelated to any clinical disorder (Dworkin & LeResche, 1992). In this example, the threshold for a disorder is based on the normal value of a test: in the DC/TMD, individuals without pain may have painful muscles due to simply being pain sensitive, but only individuals with a disorder will report familiarity of the provoked pain to some other recent experience (pain recognition); whereas within the RDC/TMD, the threshold of three painful muscle sites was based on the fact that non-cases may report pain from provocation, but statistically no more than two such sites are reported by individuals who did not report a recent history of pain. Normative values help to define an expected prevalence of a disorder versus the prevalence of a finding; for example, if positive findings for anterior disc displacement of the TMJ occur in one-third of the population, then this finding could result in one-third of the population having a disorder if the criteria are based solely on the imaging finding.

The threshold for identifying a disorder can also depend on its consequences, and TMD has three major types of consequences: limitation in function, disability, and chronic pain. Each of these major consequences critically questions what we mean by disorder. As defined above, a disorder is a combination

Table 1.1
Summary of pain terminology (adapted from Blau, 1982).

Pain attributes	Definition	Examples of common terms
Location	Site and spread of pain	Localized Radiating, referred, shooting
Intensity	Magnitude (amount) of pain in a single episode; includes temporal aspects of magnitude	6 out of 10 (on a scale of 0–10) Fluctuating, steady
Duration	Period of time of a single episode, that is, between two pain-free periods	Hours, days, weeks, months
Frequency	Pattern of pain over time	Every morning or evening Continuous (a pain 'episode' that persists for a month or more) Intermittent (two episodes a week)
Quality	Sensory and emotional aspects of an experience	Aching, burning, stabbing Punishing, intolerable
Modifying factors	Factors that initiate, increase, or decrease pain associated with an episode	Touching, washing, coughing, talking, medication, heat, cold
Timecourse	Course of pain over a long period of time	Acute, subacute, chronic, recurrent

of characteristics that are clinically abnormal, but if clinically abnormal characteristics do not disrupt the state of a subject's being, then the characteristics are merely findings. In short, can a constellation of features (symptoms, signs, or both; biomarker-based findings) be a disorder if there is no consequence (Wakefield, 1992)?

TMDs, as musculoskeletal disorders, are assumed to result in functional limitation of the masticatory system, with the extent of functional limitation only somewhat proportional to the severity of the TMD (Ohrbach, 2001; Ohrbach et al., 2008a). Functional limitation includes domains of mastication, jaw mobility, and verbal and emotional expression. If functional limitation is used as a measure of overall severity, individuals with a single positive finding (for example sporadic TMJ clicking) may well report no functional limitation and would correspondingly not be considered to have a painful disorder. An obvious exception would be when isolated clicking has prognostic value for subsequent development of a severe disorder; available data do not support a likely progression from simple clicking to a later disorder that, had the click been 'treated' as a preventive step, the disorder would have been more likely either prevented or minimized. Consequently, both pain and functional limitation represent sensible measures by which a threshold for a disorder may be determined based on available signs, whereas signs alone are poor indicators of a disorder as distinct from either a condition or the range of normal.

Disability is a person-level construct rather than a system-level construct of functional limitation. Disability associated with activities of daily living is a consequence of a TMD. While disability is not likely to occur in the complete absence of any functional limitation, disablement models clearly indicate that disability and functional limitation are not necessarily hierarchically organized (Ohrbach, 2001; Osterweis et al., 1987). The biopsychosocial model of pain indicates that disability due to a disorder is the consequence of not only any biological changes but also necessarily due to contributions from both psychological and social factors (Dworkin, 1991).

A final and relatively common consequence of a TMD is the development of chronic pain associated with that disorder. Three definitions of chronic pain are pertinent: pain that persists beyond the time of usual tissue healing, pain that has not responded to usual treatment for the identified disorder, or, the most commonly used, pain that persists beyond three months or beyond six months (depending on which standard one uses) (Turk & Rudy, 1987). All three of these definitions are useful at different times within both research and clinical practice; all three of these definitions are also more complex than usually regarded. The first definition assumes, based on the IASP pain definition (see below), that some sort of tissue damage (broadly defined) is present prior to the initial perception of pain, and that normal biological factors will result in healing of that tissue damage. Wall's model of injury (Wall, 1979) indicates that if pain persists beyond the normal healing time, then there is the increased probability of developing an acute pain disorder; moreover, Wall also indicates the increased probability of transition from injury to a chronic pain disorder. The possibility during the normal healing stages of transition to either acute or chronic disorder highlights the presence of risk factors occurring early in the normal healing process as well as later in the healing process. The implication of the IASP definition of pain as well as Wall's subsequent insights is that while obvious tissue damage

does heal (and that pain may persist beyond that final healing stage, with the implicit conclusion that with no tissue damage, there should be no remaining source of peripheral nociception), pain may persist, and that pain may be causally related to the initial injury and associated nociception. There are, as Wall's insights suggest, several complications with a simple direct causal pathway. One is that primary nociception (primary and inflammatory; [Woolf, 2004]) may give way to neuropathic pain over time but with the interpretation that the primary tissue injury has healed and a new condition, functional alteration of the nociception-related parts of the nervous system, may emerge. Yet, primary nociception may still remain even after initial tissue healing, and in relation to more complex dysfunctional aspects that appear to now be more clearly defined in the pain research literature. Instead of chronic pain being a disorder of the central nervous system (CNS) in the absence of nociception, given the apparent absence of tissue damage, chronic pain, as a central disorder, may be more likely to co-exist with peripheral disorders that began as some sort of tissue damage (again, broadly defined intentionally here in order to be inclusive) but then progresses to dysfunction of a different sort, associated with nociception, but poorly understood (Moseley, 2003).

The second definition of chronic pain – pain that has not responded to usual treatment – is useful in the clinic for assessing patient factors (for example adherence) and tissue systems treated to date (for example acupuncture but not physical therapy, for a presumed musculoskeletal pain). However, there is a potential but inherent circularity in this definition of chronic pain, as this book points to repeatedly in the various chapters on treatment modalities. That is, this definition assumes that all forms of 'usual treatment' for this patient have already been sufficiently identified and that the usual treatment was provided in a manner consistent with the goal of so-called 'good clinical practices.' Yet, as Moseley indicates, physical forms of treatment to the body can vary enormously in how they focus on the specific tissue system (or part of the tissue system) deemed responsible for presumed ongoing nociception, and a sufficient schema at the treatment level is essential for incorporating all factors (for example psychological, social, or behavioral) into the treatment plan so that a sufficient critical mass of therapies capable of making the kinds of changes necessary to effect change in the individual's chronic pain is included (Moseley, 2003).

The third definition of chronic pain, based on a period of either three or or six months' duration (IASP, 2011), is clearly arbitrary, but in the clinic (or for research purposes) when one has no other milepost to anchor a potential classification of chronic pain for that subject, the time base is at least pragmatic. See Table 1.2 and Figure 1.1 for a summary of pain types according to duration. The classic intervals of three months and six months have emerged largely as a fail-safe approach: the body and

the person have been given the benefit of the doubt for recovery from the initial event that caused the pain, and three months or six months later any persisting pain should therefore be considered evidence of a dysfunctional central pain processing network; treatment should therefore escalate from simply (and often only) focusing on the disorder per se at the bodily level and now incorporate consideration of the many psychological, social, and behavioral factors that can contribute to ongoing pain as well as interfere with response to usual treatments. The primary problem with this approach to defining chronic pain lies in the choice of temporal threshold: emerging data indicate that six months is too long and that three months is probably too long in terms of the factors that can emerge following initial onset, say via injury and which are already active in affecting behavior, interfering with typical treatment response, and perpetuating chronicity. Earlier treatment is superior (Epker et al., 1999).

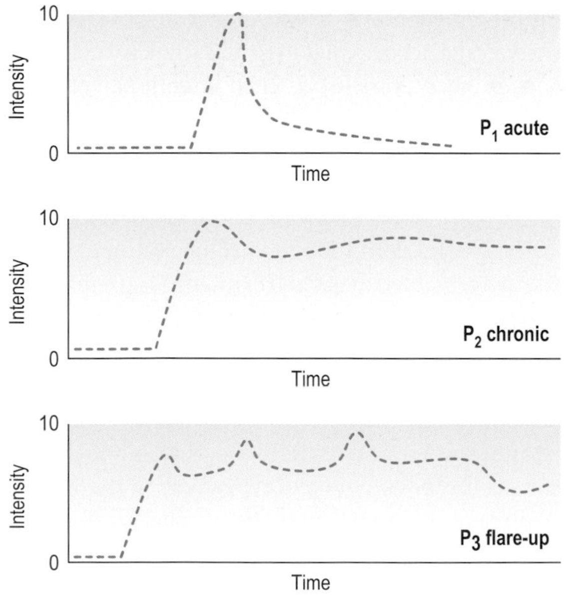

In summary, the threshold for a clinically oriented case definition of a TMD appears to be best based on normative data from the population coupled with functional consequences specific to the identified organ system. The normative data, at this time, should be based on primary symptoms rather than signs, given the absence of prognostic validity for a case definition based solely on signs. Returning to the earlier example, if one-third of the population have anterior disc displacement of the TMJ as disclosed by imaging, but less than 10 per cent of those individuals report symptoms or functional consequences of the disc displacement, then this imaging finding would not constitute a disorder. If, in contrast, the imaging finding has prognostic value for increased risk in the future for developing TMD or for being a factor that contributes to worsening of the TMD after onset, then the imaging finding would constitute a disorder (as per the ontological definition above). Disability associated with a constellation of features is not a useful marker for setting the threshold of whether that constellation of features represents a disorder or

Figure 1.1
Time frame for types of pain.

Table 1.2

Summary of pain types according to duration. Clinical assessment and characterization of an individual's reported pain result in classification within one of these categories. Case definitions also build on these time constructs (adapted from Von Korff, 1994).

Pain type	Definition
Acute	Pain of recent onset that is not recurrent or chronic and that has persisted for less than three months
Subacute	Less recent pain condition, sometimes incorrectly used to depict less severe pain which is in contrast to a severe acute pain
Chronic	Pain that persists for three months or more, or six months or more Pain that persists beyond the time of usual healing Pain that is nonresponsive to usual treatments
Recurrent	New episodes of pain bouts that repeatedly recur after pain-free periods over a longer timescale, for example, menstrual headache Also when pain is present for less than half the days in a specified time period (12 months), occurring in multiple episodes over the year
First-onset	Episode of pain that is the first occurrence of a particular pain disorder in a person's lifetime
Transient	A pain episode of not more than 90 consecutive days that does not recur over a 12-month observation period

not; this is largely due to the inclusion of other factors outside the target disorder contributing to the development of disability. The net effect would probably be a too extreme form of clumping. Similarly, the potential for the emergence of chronic pain may not be a reliable or even valid consideration for how to set the threshold of a disorder for diagnostic purposes.

Disability and chronicity are not integral to the disorder; recognizing this distinction is an important concept regarding the boundary of a disorder, which has, as one of its two core criteria, nonreducibility to another disorder. For example, should a TMD be defined to necessarily also include cervical pain or cervical dysfunction as part of the diagnostic criteria? The DC/TMD has been criticised for not

being sufficiently inclusive because it excludes cervical findings. Certainly, a basis for that criticism could include the well-established neurological and mechanical linkage of symptoms and motor function, respectively, of the masticatory and cervical systems. But because either cervical or masticatory system problems could exist separately from the other system, a case definition based on a combined system would not represent the smallest nonreducible unit of a disorder.

Pain definition

While pain can be informally defined as physical suffering or discomfort caused by illness or injury, the scientific (and far more clinically useful) definition is 'An unpleasant sensory and emotional experience associated with actual or potential tissue damage, or described in terms of such damage' (IASP, 2011). The implications of this definition are that three subtypes of pain exist: pain accompanying actual tissue damage, pain accompanying what is called 'potential tissue damage,' and pain accompanying a description (in some patient reports) involving reference to tissue damage (Smith et al., 2011). In one sense, these three aspects of tissue damage represent the degree of certainty on the part of the patient or provider for whether the initial pain onset was linked to evident nociception from known tissue damage. Note that pain accompanying the least certain form of evident nociception with actual tissue damage, pain described 'in terms of such damage,' has been included in a clinical category termed functional pain (Woolf, 2004) and it is well-known to be the source of much clinical and research speculation as well as confusion. That category probably accounts for the majority of individuals with chronic pain in general and certainly the largest category of individuals with chronic TMD pain. Moreover, it is likely to be the most common type of pain associated with the various disorders identified in this book for targeting via new treatments.

A proposed revised definition of pain is stated as 'pain is a distressing experience associated with actual or potential tissue damage with sensory, emotional, cognitive, and social components' (Williams & Craig, 2016). This definition notably eliminates the complex aspect of the current pain definition, phrased as '…or described in terms of such [tissue] damage'; Williams and Craig acknowledge that this phrase was a part of the current definition to intentionally include individuals who complained of pain in the clear absence of any detectable evidence of tissue damage, suggesting that this was more for political expediency than out of scientific necessity. Nevertheless, the authors further acknowledge that strong evidence of neuroplastic CNS changes in relation to the course of pain supports the wisdom of the decision to previously include that phrase, while further indicating that knowledge advances suggest that such individuals should now

perhaps be classified within a different diagnostic system, reserving 'pain' for only those with actual or potential tissue damage. Yet, clinically more often than not, pain histories associated with, for example a TMD diagnosis, do not identify any particular prior 'actual or potential tissue damage' event strongly associated with known nociception. If such patients are compared to those with a clear history of prior injury, symptom descriptions are typically indistinguishable (aside from specifics related to an injury, if present), and the findings from both types of patients are equivalent in terms of resultant diagnoses (for example, myofascial pain). While the presence or absence of prior tissue damage may suggest differing mechanisms at the time of onset, the mechanisms associated with subsequent stages of transition to an acute pain disorder or further to chronicity may not differ between these types of subjects and consequently, the current definition qualifier of '…or described in terms of such [tissue] damage' appears to remain critically important for an appropriately inclusive domain of pain. Critical analysis of the current IASP definition readily encompasses this broad inclusive framework regarding the marked extremes in examiner certainty about prior injury and associated tissue damage, in that the absence of observable tissue damage does not exclude more subtle levels of tissue damage that we are unable with current methods to assess (Smith et al., 2011). In addition, the relation of a reported injury to nociception known to be determined by tissue damage is not understood; moreover, the range of stimulus, vis-à-vis injury, varies from doubtful tissue injury to certain tissue injury. Consequently, the current pain definition appears to be superior for capturing the relevant clinical phenomena for both diagnosis and treatment, especially in relation to new approaches to treatment using a case definition that builds upon 'pain' as currently defined.

Application of a case definition to development of a diagnostic system

The RDC/TMD system developed in 1992 consists of reliable and validated criteria used to examine, diagnose, and classify most common forms of muscle- and joint-related TMD musculo-skeletal conditions. Based on the biopsychosocial model of pain the RDC/TMD consists of a dual axis approach: Axis I (physical findings) and Axis II (pain-related disability and psychosocial status). The Axis I measures are used to obtain physical diagnosis through a clinical examination which assesses regional pain in the past 30 days as well as current pain from provocation of masticatory musculature and the TMJ via jaw mobility and palpation. The Axis II measures of the RDC/TMD are intended to determine the extent to which cognitive, emotional, or behavioral impairment contribute to the development and maintenance of TMDs. More specifically, these measures assess jaw disability during function, psychological status, and psychosocial level of functioning, and are obtained through reliable and validated behavioral and psychological tests. Based on the RDC/TMD clinical examination protocol, TMDs can include any of the three groups of diagnoses; Group I (muscle disorders), Group II (disc displacements) and Group III (joint disorders) or a combination of any of the subgroups.

In 2010, the RDC/TMD Validation Project was carried out to determine the sensitivity and specificity of the original RDC/TMD. Using a simple case definition of regional pain in the prior 30 days, revised draft diagnostic criteria were developed and two calibrated but independent examiners provided, by consensus, reference standard diagnoses for the pain disorders. According to the Validation Project the following sensitivity and specificity for the Axis I diagnostic algorithms were found for the two main muscle group diagnoses: Group Ia myofascial pain (sensitivity 0.65, specificity 0.92) and Group Ib myofascial pain with limited opening (sensitivity 0.79, specificity 0.92) (Truelove et al., 2010). Realizing that none of the individual diagnostic groups met the target sensitivity of ≥ 0.70 and specificity of ≥ 0.95, and that the targeted sensitivity and specificity were observed only when both Group I diagnoses were combined into any myofascial pain (0.87 and 0.98, respectively), the Validation Project's results strongly suggested a need for developing a revised RDC/TMD (Truelove et al., 2010).

Revising the eight Axis I RDC/TMD diagnostic algorithms subsequently demonstrated the evaluation method to be valid for the most common pain-related TMDs. The criterion measure for this study included a comprehensive history and clinical measures, panoramic radiographs, bilateral TMJ MRIs, and bilateral TMJ computed tomography. A calibrated board-certified radiologist interpreted all images and diagnoses were made by consensus of two TMD experts who independently assessed all participants using the criterion protocol. In case of disagreement final diagnoses were made using the radiologist-interpreted images. The sensitivity and specificity of the revised algorithm for myofascial pain (0.82, 0.99, respectively) and myofascial pain with limited opening (0.93, 0.97, respectively) exceeded the target levels of sensitivity and specificity. On combining diagnoses for any myofascial pain, both sensitivity (0.91) and specificity (1.0) were further increased (Schiffman et al., 2010). Further, the kappa coefficients increased from 0.60 and 0.70 in the original criteria to 0.73 and 0.92 in revised criteria for myofascial pain and myofascial pain with limited opening respectively (Schiffman et al., 2010).

In summary, a broader case definition was more useful than a constricted one for a heterogeneous pain condition such as myofascial pain. For example, the Validation Project recruited individuals with at least one of the three cardinal signs or symptoms of TMD (jaw pain, limited mouth opening, or TMJ noise) as potential cases of TMD; those without TMD signs and symptoms by history and on clinical examination were included as potential controls. This broad inclusion not only helps discriminate between patients with and without TMD pain, but also helps discriminate between patients with TMD pain and patients with orofacial pain complaints of non-TMD origin.

Chapter 1

Epidemiology of temporomandibular disorders

Incidence and prevalence

Epidemiological studies that have used USA nation-wide data such as that from the National Health Interview Survey (NHIS) and the National Health and Nutrition Examination Survey (NHANES) have mostly relied on the self-report of face or jaw pain. In addition to dental oral examinations performed, range of motion and muscle tenderness were also measured in NHANES in the interest of obtaining objective data on TMDs. However, these measures were insufficient to meet the requirements of valid diagnostic criteria of any type of TMD. Due to the use of different case definitions, and due to ambiguity in the use of terminology (such as point prevalence versus period prevalence as boundaries for time) the global prevalence of TMD pain varies considerably across studies. For example, using self-reported information, the prevalence estimates for facial pain have been found to range from 3.7% (Agerberg & Bergenholtz, 1989) and 4.6% (Plesh et al., 2011b) to 12% (Von Korff et al., 1988). Facial pain is often considered to represent TMD pain in large part because TMD pain represents a higher prevalence among orofacial pain compared to other nondental pains.

Attempting to subtype TMD pain based on self-report methods may not be accurate, as the method of capturing potential cases matters greatly in terms of confidence in case ascertainment, and consequently the prevalence of self-reported TMD pain subgroups such as myalgia and arthralgia varies across studies. See Table 1.3 regarding prevalence in adults with ambient TMD pain or functional TMD pain. Using NHIS data, which is based only on self-report, Lipton et al. (1993) reported an overall prevalence of 5%–12% based on subtypes of facial location and pain quality. More specifically with regard to TMD subtypes Lipton et al. (1993) reported a 6.5% prevalence for jaw joint pain and 1.5% prevalence for muscle pain. In contrast, when a validated

clinical examination protocol (for example RDC/TMD) was used, the prevalence of individual diagnostic subgroups of pain-related TMD was found to be higher for a diagnosis of only myalgia at 25% than for TMJ conditions at 4.2%, which included both painful and nonpainful joint diagnoses (Drangsholt & LeResche, 1999). The most likely explanation for this set of contrasting findings is that respondents are unable to reliably distinguish muscle and joint structures when the mode of evaluation is only by self-report. Consequently, examinations are essential for prevalence estimates of subgroups to be accurate, but they may not be feasible in all settings. More general estimates that do not distinguish subtypes are likely reliable via self-report. Furthermore, methodological weakness and limitations of epidemiological studies on TMD pain prevalence do not only lack reporting prevalence estimates by subtypes, but also lack other attributes; see Table 1.4 for further details.

There are a few prospective studies that report TMD incidence. The two studies on adolescents that report incidence of TMD region pain or jaw pain show that the cumulative incidence varies from 1.8% (Heikinheimo et al., 1990) to 2.8% (Kitai et al., 1997) per year for a 3–5 year follow-up interval. The studies on adults aged 18–65 years reported a cumulative incidence of 2.2% (Drangsholt & LeResche, 1999; Von Korff et al., 1993). The above studies highlight that based on self-reported information, estimates of TMD incidence can vary, and again emphasize the importance of valid clinical measure of TMD. More recently the OPPERA study found the incidence rate of lifetime first-onset TMD to be 3.9% per year, based on a median follow-up of 2.8 years following enrollment in participants aged 18–40 years old (Slade et al., 2013). Prospective studies on persistent TMD are scarce, probably because of methodological challenges. One study that assessed for persistent TMD, defined as pain present for ≥ 180 days of the prior 360 days in a group of 1061 Health Maintenance Organization (HMO) enrollees aged 18–65 years, found an incidence rate of 1.2 per 1,000 person-years

Table 1.3

Pain prevalence by type of temporomandibular disorder (TMD).

TMD type	Reference	Disorder definition	Source of sample	Sample size	Age range (years)	Prevalence (%)
Prevalence of ambient TMD pain in adults	Helkimo, 1974	Facial and jaw pain	Finnish Lapps	600	15–65	12
	Molin et al., 1976	Frequent pain in front of ears	Swedish males in the military	253	18–25	5
	Szentpetery et al., 1986	Recent pain in face, neck, or around ears	Hungarians	600	12–85	5.8
Prevalence of functional TMD pain in adults	Agerberg & Carlsson, 1972	Face hurts when yawning	Swedes	1,106	15–74	12
	Osterberg & Carlsson, 1979	Pain when opening the mouth wide to take a large bite	Older Swedes	348	70	3
	Alanen & Kirveskari, 1982	Pain in jaw joint on chewing	Finns	853	18–57	5.2

(Von Korff et al., 1993). Further findings on persistent TMD from the OPPERA study are currently under evaluation and have not yet been published.

Risk factors

In contrast to etiology, risk factors represent a broader domain of factors contributing to a disease, including those that clearly precede disease onset as well as factors that may co-occur at onset or factors that are a consequence of the disease at some stage and which serve to perpetuate the disease. Given the difficulty of research designs in partitioning these various stage-specific roles, we make no distinction here in the timing of the contribution of a particular factor but instead present them as generally identified via cross-sectional designs.

Age and gender

Based on an inclusive definition of TMDs that queries for face or jaw pain in the past three months from the date of interview, the age-specific prevalence patterns for TMDs have been stable over the years. Using the NHIS data, Lipton et al. (1993) reported the following age-specific prevalence for face or jaw pain: 6.5% in those aged 18–34 years, 5.0% in 35–54 year-olds, 4.0% in 55–74 year-olds, and 3.9% among individuals ≥ 75 years old, indicating a slight decrease in TMDs as age increases. According to the

Table 1.4
Methodological weakness and limitations of epidemiological studies on TMD pain prevalence (extracted from Drangsholt & LeResche, 1999).

Methodological weakness or limitation	Studies (n=133) with problem
Inadequate sample size	> 80%
Study is not performed on representative sample of a defined population	> 50%
Case definition does not include pain or depends solely on physical assessment	> 50%
Case definition of pain is not explicit: it does not include severity or duration	> 95%
Age- and gender-specific proportions are not given	> 75%
No mention of spread or dispersion of data; that is, no confidence intervals	> 95%

most recent NHIS, the prevalence of pain in the face or jaw was 4.6% among all persons aged 18 years and older. The age-specific estimates were 5.0% in those aged 18–44 years, 4.6% in 45–64 year-olds, 4.2% in 65–74 year-olds and 2.6% in those ≥ 75 years old, again suggesting a monotonic decrease in prevalent jaw or face pain across the adult life-span (NCHS, 2014). However, it is important to be careful in interpreting estimates from national health surveys of face and jaw pain as necessarily representing TMD pain in that the estimates are based solely on self-report questions focusing on pain location. The only suitable epidemiologic tool that has been developed is a brief set of self-report questions with high sensitivity and specificity for TMDs (Gonzalez et al., 2011).

In contrast, some prospective studies show an increase in incidence of TMD with increase in age. More recently, the OPPERA study enrolled individuals between the ages of 18 and 44 years old who were confirmed to have never had diagnosable TMD, and based on subsequent development of clinically diagnosed TMD, the following age-specific incidence rate of TMD per year emerges: 2.5% for individuals aged 18–24, 3.7% in those aged 25–34, and 4.5% in those aged 35–44. Furthermore, using the age group

of 18–24 years as the reference group, the association (hazard ratio [HR] statistic) between age and TMD showed a 40% increased risk for TMD among individuals aged 25–34 (HR: 1.4, 95% CI 1.0, 1.9) and a 50% increased risk among individuals aged between 35 and 44 years (HR: 1.5, 95% CI 1.0, 2.0) (Slade et al., 2013).

Cross-sectional studies show that prevalence estimates for men (0%–10%) and for women (2%–18%) vary and show that women are 1.5–2 times more likely to be afflicted with TMDs than men (Helkimo, 1974; Plesh et al., 2011a; Von Korff et al., 1988). Recent NHIS data have also shown higher prevalence of face or jaw pain in females (5.8%) than in males (3.4%) (NCHS, 2014). Furthermore, using pooled data from NHIS from the years 2000–2005, Plesh et al. (2011b) reported that females had a significantly higher frequency (odds ratio [OR]: 1.41, P < 0.001) of two or more comorbid pain conditions in comparison to males (Plesh et al., 2011b), indicating that the higher rate of TMD pain in females extends to additional pain disorders. Similar results have been reported in longitudinal studies. For example, Von Korff et al. (1993) also found a higher cumulative incidence of TMDs in women (2.6% per year) compared to men (1.6% per year) in a three-year follow-up. More recently the OPPERA study reported a 3.6 cases of TMD per 100 person-years at-risk incident rate in females compared to males at 2.8 cases of TMD per 100 person-years at risk in a five-year follow-up, but this difference was nonsignificant (HR: 1.3 95% CI0.9, 1.7) (Slade et al., 2013).

Race and ethnicity

As seen with low back pain and neck pain, the prevalence of face or jaw pain is higher in individuals of mixed race. Recent prevalence estimates for jaw or face pain were 4.9% for single-race White adults and 4.0% for American Indian or Alaska Native adults. In contrast, a higher percentage (12.7%) was reported in both mixed-White and American Indian or Alaska Native adults (NCHS, 2014). But among single-race individuals, prevalence rates for Whites were still slightly higher (4.9%) compared to African Americans (3.8%) and Asians (2.1%) (NCHS, 2014). This pattern is the same or nearly the same as observed for back pain. Similarly, the OPPERA study has also shown that the incidence of clinically diagnosed TMD was only slightly higher in African Americans (4.6%) compared to Whites (3.0%). Furthermore, the association between race and TMD was higher for African Americans (HR: 1.4, 95% CI 1.0, 1.9) than for Hispanics (HR: 1.2, 95% CI 0.6, 2.1) (Slade et al., 2013). The prevalence for Whites and African Americans varies across the different studies but stays in the same range and it seems safe to conclude that they are approximately the same. Data indicate that the prevalence in mixed-race people is more limited; this is consistent with their low overall prevalence in the population.

Education and socioeconomic status

Studies on TMD and education or socioeconomic status are scarce. Using a population of health maintenance organization enrollees, education was not associated with any of the five major pain conditions including pain in the face (Von Korff et al., 1988). More recently, the NHIS data regarding education

and jaw pain show that the differences in jaw pain among the different educational groups are minimal. For example, the 2014 NHIS found the following prevalence estimates for face or jaw pain by education level: 5.1% for less than high school diploma, 4.4% for high school diploma, 5.0% for some college education, and 4.4% for bachelor's degree or higher (NCHS, 2014). Furthermore, specifically for TMDs, the OPPERA study did not find significant associations between education and incidence of TMDs. In contrast, association with self-reported rating of satisfaction with material standards of life (a possible surrogate measure of socioeconomic status), showed a decreased association with incidence of TMDs (HR: 0.87, 95% CI 0.76, 0 .98). Similar results were reported when categorizing the variable: greater TMD incidence (HR: 1.71, 95% CI 1.16, 2.51) was found in the individuals with the lowest ratings (0–5) compared to the individuals with highest ratings (9–10) (Slade et al., 2013).

Body weight and physical activity

Literature on body weight and TMDs indicates that body mass index (BMI) is unlikely to be a putative risk factor for TMD pain. A study using participants from the University of Washington Twin Registry assessed the association of excessive weight and obesity with five distinct pain conditions and three pain symptoms, and further examined whether familial influences explained these relationships. After adjustment for age, gender, and depression, overweight twins were more likely to report TMD pain than normal-weight twins (OR: 1.49, 95% CI 1.03, 2.17); however, after further adjustment for familial influences or genetic factors, these associations hardly changed (OR: 1.44, 95% CI 0.99, 2.09) (Wright et al., 2010). Similarly, the OPPERA study found BMI to be a putative risk factor for first-onset TMD in analysis that adjusted for study site and demographic characteristics (HR: 1.13, 95% CI 1.00, 1.26), but its effect was attenuated to statistical nonsignificance after imputation for loss to follow-up (HR: 1.09, 95% CI 0.97, 1.23) (Sanders et al., 2013).

Physical activity has no documented studies regarding its association with TMD, despite emerging models suggesting that increased activity should increase pain resilience (Ambrose & Golightly, 2015; Ahn, 2013).

Comorbidity of pain at other sites

Using pooled data from NHIS from the years 2000–2005, Plesh et al. (2011b) have reported a prevalence of 4.6% for TMD-type pain, and of those who reported TMD-type pain approximately 59% had two or more additional complaints of pain either in the neck, low back, or another joint. Furthermore, with regard to involvement of other body sites across the different races, Plesh et al. (2011b) have also reported that in comparison to Whites, Hispanics (OR: 1.56, P < 0.001) and Blacks (OR: 1.38, P < 0.01) reported significantly higher frequencies of two or more pain complaints in the neck, low back or another joint. Similarly, the OPPERA study also found that incidence of TMD was higher for ≥ 2 comorbidities (HR: 2.70, 95% CI 2.02, 3.59) than that for a single comorbidity (HR: 1.42, 95% CI 1.00, 2.01) compared to no comorbidity. In addition, and compared to no back pain, ≥ 5 back pain episodes strongly predicted TMD risk (HR: 2.20, 95% CI 1.54, 3.14) (Sanders et al., 2013).

Smoking

Studies that have examined the association of smoking with TMDs have found, compared to non-tobacco users, that tobacco users had a higher odds for TMD (OR: 4.56, 95% CI 1.46, 14.24) (Weingarten et al., 2009). Furthermore, a dose-response relationship was noted between smoking and the intensity of TMD pain using a 0–10 numeric rating scale: among light smokers (mean: 5.8 ± 1.8); among moderate smokers (mean: 6.3 ± 2.3) and among heavy smokers (mean: 8.1 ± 1.4) (Melis et al., 2010). Interestingly, among female Caucasians, a stronger association between smoking and TMD occurs in younger women < 30 years (OR: 4.1, 95% CI 1.6, 11.4) than in older women ≥ 30 years (OR: 1.2, 95% CI 0.6, 2.8).

Furthermore, after adjusting for allergy-related conditions, cytokine mediators and psychological variables, the association was reduced by approximately 45% in both younger women (OR: 2.3, 95% CI 0.81, 6.43) and in older women (OR: 0.66, 95% CI 0.26, 1.68). The above findings indicate that the effect of one or more of the explanatory factors was higher among the younger than the older individuals (Sanders et al., 2012).

Occupational factors

The most common occupation potentially related to TMDs appears to be playing musical instruments, which has received widespread consideration albeit mostly based on poor-quality studies (van Selms et al., 2017). Studies on other occupations and their potential relation to TMDs are rare, and therefore for our purposes studies on musicians and TMDs will be further described. A case-control study, notable for its overall methodological quality, found greater prevalence of signs and symptoms of TMDs among a group of violinists than among control subjects who did not play musical instruments (Rodriguez-Lozano et al., 2010). Compared to controls the most commonly and significantly different detected clinical features in the violinists were parafunctional habits such as tongue thrusting, mouth breathing, and biting of nails (26.8%), TMJ sounds (51.2%), and pain on maximum mouth opening (24.4%). Overall, the evidence from association studies of musical instrument playing and TMDs is mixed; associations are more common in studies utilizing clinical examinations for case ascertainment (van Selms et al., 2017). Evidence from experimental trials, however, varies. For example, one study of wind instrument players found that the contractive load on jaw closing muscles measured using EMG activity of jaw muscles was small when playing both medium and high tones on a wind instrument, and playing an instrument for a long time did not induce fatigue of the jaw-closing musculature (Gotouda et al., 2007). An experimental study of 30 musicians that examined the effectiveness of oral splints for TMD found that treatment with oral splints contributed to a significant decrease in dental or TMJ pain in 83% of the participants (Steinmetz et al., 2009). Note: most studies regarding musical instruments and TMDs have focused on TMD symptoms but not TMD diagnosis. A related experimental study found striking evidence among 14 musicians with upper limb pain for increases in same muscle activity in response to pain experience recall and for increases in the opposing trapezius in response to stress imagery (Moulton & Spence, 1992) suggesting that, as stated in our section on etiology, single causes for TMDs (or other musculoskeletal pain) are the exception, and instead the compounding effect of multiple-risk determinants is important.

Psychological factors

An abundance of evidence exists explaining the role that psychological factors play in TMD onset and chronicity. For TMDs specifically, mood disorders and personality disorders are significantly linked to muscle disorders, as opposed to disc or joint disorders (Kight et al., 1999). Studies also show that psychological distress is associated with greater severity and persistence of TMD-related clinical symptoms. More specifically, psychological stress and depression levels are found to be higher in individuals with chronic TMDs (Dworkin et al., 1990; Gatchel et al., 2007; Keefe et al., 2004). Moreover, the OPPERA study found an array of psychological factors that were associated with TMDs, among which the highest hazard ratio was found when using the Pennebaker Inventory of Limbic Languidness – a measure of somatic symptoms, for example aches, soreness, and tightness (HR: 1.44, 95% CI 1.29, 1.60). Among the four identified latent psychological constructs, stress and negative affectivity components (HR: 1.12, 95% CI 0.97, 1.30) and global psychological symptoms (HR: 1.33, 95% CI 1.18, 1.50) were the strongest risk factors, but showed only a modest effect, with a 12% and 33% increase in risk for first-onset TMD respectively (Fillingim et al., 2013). Furthermore,

using repeated measures of stress, the OPPERA study found that stress measured during the same three-monthly period as TMD onset was associated with a 55% increased risk for TMD (HR: 1.55, 95% CI 1.34, 1.79) (Slade et al., 2015). Both of these studies showed that the estimated associations with stress that are measured at enrollment and during the three-monthly follow-up period are likely to be underestimated, because the values measured at both time points do not capture the accumulated effects of stress and global psychological symptoms that are intrinsic to everyday experiences. For example, the increased association with stress reported by Slade et al. (2015) using a measure that is more proximal in time to the outcome still demonstrates a one-time measure of a construct that is transitionally or temporally dynamic and is insufficient to capture its true association.

Etiology of painful temporomandibular disorders

The suspected etiology of TMDs has been as broad as the imagination of both clinician and researcher, but opinions have largely been based on case-series or cross-sectional studies, neither of which represents adequate approaches to the determination of etiology. Here, we address major domains related to the potential etiology of TMDs. Advances in identifying genetic and epigenetic etiological factors associated with pain and TMDs in particular are substantial (Belfer et al., 2013; Diatchenko et al., 2013; Smith et al., 2013); however, this complex area is beyond the scope of the present chapter.

The Bradford Hill criteria for causation and therefore for understanding etiology are appropriate and productive for bacterial diseases, but they are less useful for complex diseases, a category to which TMDs clearly belong (Ohrbach et al., 2015; Rothman & Greenland, 2005). Consequently, in considering the etiology for complex diseases such as TMD, the concept of risk determinants becomes more appropriate. This will perhaps become clearer by the end of this section, as we present the evidence in support of a simple summary:

'TMD is less often a single isolated disorder and rather is more often the result of multiple risk determinants occurring together or in some sequence specific to an individual, such that no single risk determinant is sufficient, on its own, to "cause" TMD.'

— **(Slade et al., 2016)**

Injury

Injuries to the jaw can range from minor laceration of the soft-tissue structures to more severe damage such as fractures of the hard tissues. Moreover, jaw injuries can be brought about by a number of different traumatic events. Among the various traumatic events that have been reported in the literature, assaults are the most frequent at 37% of all facial fractures in emergency department visits, followed by falls at 24.6%, motor vehicle accidents at 12.1%, transport accidents at 2%, and pedal cyclist accidents at 1.6% (Allareddy et al., 2011). In addition to assaults, falls and accidents as sources of injuries to the jaw, other forms of injuries that can affect the jaw include head and neck injuries (Cassidy et al., 2014).

Furthermore, iatrogenic forms of injuries such as oral intubation, laryngoscopies, and dental treatments have also been reported to be sources of dental injuries. However, because dental injuries encompass injuries to structures inclusive of lips, teeth, tongue, etc. it is difficult to parse out from the literature how many injuries affect the jaw bones or muscles specifically. For further details on sources of jaw injuries see the article by Sharma (2017).

Microtrauma

Musculoskeletal microtrauma represents low magnitude forces insufficient to cause sudden disruption in the overt integrity of the involved tissue but which over time lead to physical damage to the body (Fernandez et al., 1995; Hauret et al., 2010). The most common cause of microtrauma appears to be overuse behaviors, with parafunctional habits being a dominant source for the orofacial region and with sports activities being the main source for the remaining body regions. Overuse, in contrast to normal use, is determined based on a combination of extent of load imposed by the behavior, frequency of the behavior, the duration of each particular behavior, the duration of all behaviors per bout, the extent of recovery periods, and the calendar time over which this occurs. In general, no specific measure of overuse behavior exists, and the threshold at which overuse, as opposed to normal use, is identified is generally unknown. Instead, the presence of overuse is often inferred when the threshold for tissue adaptation is exceeded, and either signs or symptoms putatively of microtrauma have appeared. Other potential causes of microtrauma include repeated strain (such as the biological response to repeated external forces on the body, for example from contact sports) and the effects of deconditioning resulting in decreased tissue resilience to load (Nørregaard et al.,1997).

Physical damage may be readily assessable with a disorder such as traumatic arthropathy or tendonitis, often stated to be the result of microtrauma; the clinician may be certain of the diagnosis, and inference leads to the putative etiology of microtrauma based on good evidence in the particular patient of microtrauma-inducing behaviors such as forced marching over long distances, over many days, without rest periods for tissue recovery. In such a context, microtrauma appears to be strongly supported by empirical data (Hauret et al., 2010).

Contrariwise, the presence of physical damage associated with microtrauma as the inferred etiology may not have the same certainty as tendonitis. For example, the clinical presence of findings such as tight bands and myofascial trigger points in the muscle associated with a pain complaint is widely regarded as diagnostic evidence for a myofascial pain disorder. While the clinician may be as certain of the diagnosis here as with, say, tendonitis, despite the softer findings compared to tendonitis, examiner reliability studies indicate that these findings have moderate to poor interexaminer reliability (Gerwin et al., 1997) and the nature of the observed phenomenon is not fully accepted by some authors (Cohen & Quintner, 2008; Quintner et al., 2015). Given, however, the strong role that overuse behaviors have as a stated etiology (Travell & Simons, 1983) as well as the strong role they appear to have empirically in both onset and perpetuation of myofascial pain (Glaros et al., 2016; Ohrbach et al., 2013; Ohrbach et al., 2011), perhaps myofascial pain disorders should be regarded more as a construct comprised of multiple indicators rather than as a simple physical diagnosis. Whether microtrauma is a factor in the formation of the core findings of myofascial pain, taut bands and trigger points, requires more research as well as perhaps more circumspection in the clinic (see Chapter 8 on exploration of the masticatory musculature for discussion of this topic).

Finally, physical damage is sometimes assumed based on presumed microstrain when overuse behaviors are identified, and what might be a behavioral problem with an unknown mechanism for the reported pain (Glaros & Burton 2004; Glaros et al., 2016) is transformed in the clinician's mind to a diagnosed physical disorder with necessary tissue damage as the source of nociception underlying the pain. This inferential pattern of using any sort of abnormal finding to support the belief that physical damage has occurred (and therefore must be the focus of physical intervention) follows that which has been endemic in the TMD field for decades, and it stems from inadequate assessment as well as not considering levels of diagnosis (Ohrbach & Dworkin, 2016). It is worth noting, however, that microtrauma as a source of pain 'described in terms of such damage' remains a critically important possibility for the TMD pain problems that have onset without known cause (Slade et al., 2016).

With these preliminaries, microtrauma has been an often-stated initial cause of TMDs, particularly for disorders affecting the TMJ, but this appears to

be largely based on speculation rather than evidence. Some compelling evidence from one lab points to one pathway for microtrauma to emerge and affect the TMJ. Healthy females (compared to males) have higher energy densities within the TMJ disc during normal closing movement of the jaw (Iwasaki et al., 2017b); women with disc displacements (compared to those without displacements) have higher TMJ energy density (Iwasaki et al., 2017a); and women with disc displacement and pain (compared to those without either) exhibit longer periods of muscle contraction and a higher duty factor during an episode of sleep bruxism (Wei et al., 2017). Collectively, these findings would suggest that TMJ disc displacements and regional pain influence joint biomechanics, such that women may be more susceptible to the repeated forces of sleep bruxism, which would appear to fall into the microtrauma range. These findings may have implications for the potential microtrauma effects of other types of overuse behaviors on TMDs.

Psychological and behavioral factors

It is not hyperbole to state that probably every cross-sectional study examining a set of psychological variables in relation to TMDs has found at least one of the target variables to have a significant association with any of the TMDs, and with the painful TMDs dominating this picture. A comprehensive evaluation of nearly all known TMD-relevant psychological variables confirmed prior associations with chronic painful TMDs, with standardized odds ratios (SOR) ranging from 1.3–2.4 (Fillingim et al., 2011); such a cross-sectional design does not provide any insight into etiology, however. The same variables when examined for predicting who would subsequently develop painful TMDs exhibited significant albeit weak associations, with standardized hazard ratios ranging from 1.1–1.4 with TMD onset (Fillingim et al., 2013). In the chronic cohort, the strongest predictors were physical body symptoms, with SOR: 2.4 distinct from all others; yet, none of the predictors of incident TMDs were notable in comparison to the others. These findings, taken together, highlight that a psychological etiology of painful TMDs exists primarily as a rubric representing general distress or psychosocial dysfunction, whereas once pain begins, the burden of pain serves to substantially aggravate all psychological processes, some more than others, among subjects with painful TMDs. Consistent with the application of the biopsychosocial model to pain conditions and with special reference to orofacial pain broadly, these findings also indicate that comprehensive multiaxial assessment is essential for both clinical and research subjects in order to better understand the many aspects involved in pain processing (Durham et al., 2015; Ohrbach & Durham, 2017).

A frequently regarded behavioral variable for the etiology of TMDs is parafunctional habits, described previously under the microtrauma section as overuse behaviors. A substantial cross-sectional literature attests to the potential importance of these behaviors in association with TMDs. Experimental studies demonstrate that maintaining a behavioral pattern at a sufficient magnitude, duration, and frequency reliably leads to pain symptoms consistent with a myalgia diagnosis (Glaros, 2007; 2008). Ambulatory studies demonstrate that stress reactivity includes parafunctional behaviors, which lead to pain (Glaros et al., 2016; Glaros et al., 2005). In terms of actual prediction of painful TMDs, individuals with oral parafunctional behaviors with scores above 25 (representing 30% of the total possible score), according to the Oral Behaviors Checklist (Kaplan & Ohrbach 2016; Markiewicz et al., 2006; Ohrbach et al., 2008b) are 75% more likely to develop first-onset painful TMDs, compared to individuals with a score below 17. These findings also indicate that only when a sufficient density of behaviors, based on the number of behaviors and their respective frequency, exists do these behaviors reliably matter; this is consistent with the prior discussion regarding microtrauma.

Alterations in the pain processing system

Considerable evidence across multiple pain disorders exists regarding changes in the pain processing system emerging with pain chronicity. These changes can be measured in multiple domains: pressure pain thresholds, thermal pain thresholds and tolerance, thermal windup and after-sensations, cutaneous pinprick threshold, and cutaneous windup and after-sensations (see Chapter 6 of the current text). These changes in each of these domains are measurable in individuals with chronic painful TMDs (Greenspan et al., 2011). In contrast, alterations in pain processing are less notable prior to painful TMD onset, with smaller changes across fewer measurement domains (Greenspan et al., 2013). In particular, for both chronic and incident TMDs, alterations in pain processing measured by the modality of pressure are most notable, but interestingly changes in pressure pain sensitivity fluctuate with painful TMD onset and do not predict onset (Slade et al., 2014).

Pain comorbidity

Distinguishing a pain condition local to one system (e.g., TMD within the masticatory system with an otherwise negative medical history for relevant factors) versus a pain condition existing within a set of general health factors or other pain disorders is critical and necessary based on substantial empirical data. General health factors exhibit strong association with chronic TMDs and also strongly predict new TMD onset (Aggarwal et al., 2010; Ohrbach et al., 2011; Sanders et al., 2013). These factors include other pain disorders, neurosensory disorders, respiratory disorders, and tobacco use for both new onset and chronic TMD (Ohrbach et al., 2011; Sanders et al., 2013). In addition, increasingly poor sleep over time is a substantial predictor of new onset TMDs (Sanders et al., 2016). Among these general health factors, other pain disorders (such as low back pain, irritable bowel syndrome, headache, and genital pain) are perhaps the most investigated and substantiated risk factors for painful TMDs. Early insights into the compounding effects of two or more co-occurring pain disorders informed the subsequent gate control theory and, later, neuromatrix theory of pain (Livingston, 1998; Melzack, 1989; Melzack & Wall, 1965), with the implication that multiple-pain disorders do not have an additive effect but have a multiplicative effect on the consequences of pain, including the intensity of pain experienced, psychological variables such as mood and catastrophizing, pain-related disability, and risk for subsequent onset of yet another pain disorder (Aggarwal et al., 2006; Creed et al., 2012; Macfarlane et al., 2003; McBeth et al., 2002; Raphael et al., 2000). These findings also suggest that TMD as a local disorder, existing in isolation from other comorbid pain disorders, and TMD as a disorder mixed with other pain disorders would respond differently to condition-specific treatment. And, indeed, strong evidence points to oral appliances, for example, as treatment for sleep bruxism having notably lower efficacy when widespread pain is also present (Raphael & Marbach, 2001).

TMD, as a musculoskeletal pain condition, occurs in the facial region situated between two other major structures, each with its own complex pain disorders: the head and headache, and the cervical spine and neck pain. In addition to the link with other pain disorders via more general CNS mechanisms associated with the pain processing system broadly, TMDs share specific mechanism-overlap with both headache and cervical problems (Ballegaard et al., 2008; Häggman-Henrikson et al., 2016; Häggman-Henrikson et al., 2002; Wiesinger et al., 2013). The mechanism overlap includes peripheral nerve convergence in the trigeminal nucleus caudalis, mechanical activity-based motor control strategies subserving basic functions such as mastication, and gross structure overlap such as the temporal region that is home to the temporalis muscle of jaw function and is the site of a large proportion of headaches.

Conclusion

In summary, musculoskeletal conditions as a group are exemplified by nonspecific back pain, neck pain, and TMD pain, and the conditions have in common two main risk factors, psychological factors and injury, and one probable risk factor of smoking, conclusions nicely summarized elsewhere (McLean et al., 2010; Taylor et al., 2014; Sharma, 2017). Herewith, we take a broader perspective on painful TMD and regard it as only one among other musculoskeletal conditions. Of the two main risk factors, it appears that psychological characteristics have played the most robust role in not only initiating the development of such conditions, but also in the persistence of pain symptoms and the development of chronic pain. This stronger role for psychological characteristics may also be a function of more and better research examining those characteristics in contrast to the more limited research focusing on injury. Smoking is a common risk factor for back pain and TMDs; while it is often regarded as a potential proxy for poorer social or health conditions, the evidence also suggests direct effects on pain. Occupational factors play a major role in back pain, whereas occupational factors have a much weaker or nonexistent role in TMDs and an unclear role at present in neck pain. Similarly, education, socioeconomic status, and physical activity have shown stronger associations with back pain than with neck pain or TMDs.

The role of case definitions and its impact on research has differed not only for TMDs, but across these other two musculoskeletal pain types, and with the same effect. In contrast to the recent extremely well-operationalized and reliable definitions for TMDs, the varying level of validity in the case definitions for back pain and for neck pain may have impeded the respective research programs. It is notable that the well-standardized definitions for TMDs that have now been developed have allowed research into TMD pain to move forward at a relatively rapid pace (Ohrbach & Dworkin, 2016).

Furthermore, taken together the available information suggests that risk factors for musculoskeletal pain conditions may have a more complex dynamic relationship over time, which also includes reciprocal causation. Musculoskeletal pain conditions are now considered complex diseases, and a collective picture of complex causation emerges. Only recently has one aspect of the complexity become clearer through the OPPERA studies, and that is that one single risk factor alone is not sufficient to cause a pain disorder. While that understanding about musculoskeletal pain has so far been restricted to TMDs, there is no evidence to suggest that TMDs are unique among musculoskeletal pain problems. However, to date, mechanisms underlying the transition from risk factors to pain disorders remain poorly understood. Lung cancer provides a good example of what is missing in the pain literature. For lung cancer, risk factors such as smoking and asbestos are sufficient and readily explainable in biological terms, for which a tissue-level correspondence can be found and which makes for clearer public health implications. Although the characteristics of individual risk factors have been presented based on the existing studies on TMDs, there are major neurobiological processes underlying the multivariable predictors at play in the development of musculoskeletal pain conditions in general, and the nature of the causal processes are complex indicating a higher level interaction across these factors. We close this chapter with the emphasis on the importance of multiple-risk determinants, acting together and over time, in the development of painful TMDs and their persistence into chronicity.

References

Agerberg G, Bergenholtz A. Craniomandibular disorders in adult populations of West Bothnia, Sweden. Acta Odontol Scand 1989; 47: 129–140.

Agerberg G, Carlsson GE. Functional disorder of the masticatory system: I. Distribution of symptoms according to age and sex as judged from investigation by questionnaire. Acta Odontol Scand 1972; 30: 597–613.

Aggarwal VR, McBeth J, Zakrzewska JM, Lunt M, Macfarlane GJ. The epidemiology of chronic syndromes that are frequently unexplained: do they have common associated factors? Int J Epidemiol 2006; 35: 468–476.

Aggarwal VR, Macfarlane GJ, Farragher TM, McBeth, J. Risk factors for onset of chronic oro-facial pain: results of the North Cheshire oro-facial pain prospective population study. Pain 2010; 149: 354–359.

Ahn AH. Why does increased exercise decrease migraine? Current Pain and Headache Reports 2013; 17: 379.

Alanen P, Kirveskari P. Stomatognathic dysfunction in a male Finnish working population. Proc Finnish Dental Society 1982; 78: 184–188.

Allareddy V, Allareddy V, Nalliah RP. Epidemiology of facial fracture injuries. J Oral Maxillofac Surg 2011; 69: 2613–2618.

Ambrose KR, Golightly YM. Physical exercise as non-pharmacological treatment of chronic pain: Why and when. Best Practice & Research. Clinical Rheumatology 2015; 29: 120–130.

Ballegaard V, Thede-Schmidt-Hansen P, Svensson P, Jensen R. Are headache and temporomandibular disorders related? A blinded study. Cephalalgia 2008; 28; 832–841.

Belfer I, Segall SK, Lariviere W et al. Pain modality- and sex-specific effects of COMT genetic functional variants. Pain 2013; 154: 1368–1376.

Blau JN. How to take a history of head or facial pain. Br Med J 1982; 285: 1249–1251.

Cassidy JD, Boyle E, Carroll L. Population-based, inception cohort study of the incidence, course, and prognosis of mild traumatic brain injury after motor vehicle collisions. Arch Phys Med Rehabil 2014; 95: S278–285.

Cohen M, Quintner J. The horse is dead: let myofascial pain syndrome rest in peace. Pain Med 2008; 9: 464–465.

Creed FH, Davies I, Jackson J et al. The epidemiology of multiple somatic symptoms. J Psychosom Res 2012; 72: 311–317.

de Leeuw R, Klasser GD. Orofacial Pain: Guidelines for Assessment, Diagnosis, and Management. 5th ed. Hanover Park, IL: Quintessence Publishing; 2013.

Diatchenko L, Fillingim RB, Smith SB Maixner W. The phenotypic and genetic signatures of common musculoskeletal pain conditions. Nature Rev Rheumatol 2013; 9: 340–350.

Dionne CE, Dunn KM, Croft PR et al. A consensus approach toward the standardization of back pain definitions for use in prevalence studies. Spine 2008; 33: 95–103.

Drangsholt M, LeResche L. Temporomandibular disorder pain. In Crombie IK, Croft PR, Linton SJ, LeResche L, Von Korff M (eds). Epidemiology of Pain. Seattle, WA: International Association for the Study of Pain; 1999.

Durham J, Raphael KG, Benoliel R, Ceusters W, Michelotti A, Ohrbach R. Perspectives on next steps in classification of oro-facial pain – part 2: role of psychosocial factors. J Oral Rehabilitation 2015; 42: 942–955.

Dworkin SF. Illness behavior and dysfunction: review of concepts and application to chronic pain. Can J Physiol Pharmacol 1991; 69: 662–671.

Dworkin SF, Huggins KH, LeResche L et al. Epidemiology of signs and symptoms in temporomandibular disorders: clinical signs in cases and controls. J Am Dent Assoc 1990; 120: 273–281.

Dworkin SF, LeResche L. Research diagnostic criteria for temporomandibular disorders: review, criteria, examinations and specifications, critique. J Craniomandib Disord 1992; 6: 301–355.

Epker J, Gatchel RJ, Ellis E. A model for predicting chronic TMD: practical application in clinical settings. JADA 1999; 130: 1470–1475.

Fernandez JE, Fredericks TK, Marley RJ. The psychophysical approach in upper extremities work. In Robertson SA (ed.) Contemporary Ergonomics. London: Taylor & Francis; 1995, pp. 456–461.

Fillingim RB, Ohrbach R, Greenspan JD et al. Potential psychosocial risk factors for chronic TMD: descriptive data and empirically identified domains from the OPPERA case-control study. J Pain 2011; 2: T46-T60.

Fillingim RB, Ohrbach R, Greenspan JD et al. Psychological factors associated with development of TMD: the OPPERA prospective cohort study. J Pain 2013; 14: T75-T90.

Gatchel RJ, Peng YB, Peters ML, Fuchs PN, Turk DC. The biopsychosocial approach to chronic pain: scientific advances and future directions. Psychol Bull 2007; 133: 581–624.

Gerwin RD, Shannon S, Hong CZ, Hubbard D, Gevirtz R. Interrater reliability in myofascial trigger point examination. Pain 1997; 69: 65–73.

Glaros AG. EMG biofeedback as an experimental tool for studying pain. Biofeedback 2007; 35: 50–53.

Glaros AG. Temporomandibular disorders and facial pain: a psychophysiological perspective. Appl Psychophysiol Biofeedback 2008; 33: 161–171.

Glaros AG, Burton E. Parafunctional clenching, pain, and effort in temporomandibular disorders. J Behav Med 2004; 27: 91–100.

Glaros AG, Williams K, Lausten L. The role of parafunctions, emotions and stress in predicting facial pain. JADA 2005; 136: 451–458.

Glaros AG, Marszalek JM, Williams KB. Longitudinal multilevel modeling of facial pain, muscle tension, and stress. J Dent Res 2016; 95: 416–422.

Gonzalez YM, Schiffman E, Gordon SM et al. Development of a brief and effective temporomandibular disorder pain screening questionnaire: reliability and validity. J Am Dent Assoc 2011; 142: 1183–1191.

Gotouda A, Yamaguchi T, Okada K, Matsuki T, Gotouda S, Inoue N. Influence of playing wind instruments on activity of masticatory muscles. J Oral Rehabil 2007; 34: 645–651.

Greenspan JD, Slade GD, Bair E et al. Pain sensitivity risk factors for chronic TMD: descriptive data and empirically identified domains from the OPPERA case-control study. J Pain 2011; 12: T61-T74.

Greenspan JD, Slade GD, Bair E et al. Pain sensitivity and autonomic factors associated wtih development of TMD: the OPPERA prospective cohort study. J Pain 2013; 14: T63-T74.

Häggman-Henrikson B, Zafar H, Eriksson PO. Disturbed jaw behavior in whiplash-associated disorders during rhythmic jaw movements. J Dent Res 2002; 81: 747–751.

Häggman-Henrikson B, Lampa E, Marklund S, Wänman A. Pain and disability in the jaw and neck region following whiplash trauma. J Dental Res 2016; 95: 1155–1160.

Hauret KG, Jones BH, Bullock SH, Canham-Chervak M, Canada S. Musculoskeletal injuries: description of an under-recognized injury problem among military personnel. Am J Prev Med 2010; 38 S61-S70.

Heikinheimo K, Salmi K, Myllarniemi S, Kirveskari P. A longitudinal study of occlusal interferences and signs of craniomandibular disorder at the ages of 12 and 15 years. Eur J Orthod 1990; 12: 190–197.

Helkimo M. Studies on function and dysfunction of the masticatory system. IV. Age and sex distribution of symptoms of dysfunction of the masticatory system in Lapps in the north of Finland. Acta Odontol Scand 1974; 32: 255–267.

IASP. IASP Taxonomy, 2011. [Online] Available: https://www.iasp-pain.org/Education/Content. aspx?ItemNumber=1698&navItemNumber=576 [Oct 22, 2017].

Iwasaki L, Gonzalez Y, Liu Y et al. Mechanobehavioral scores in women with and without TMJ disc displacement. J Dent Res 2017a; 96: 895–901.

Iwasaki L, Gonzalez Y, Liu Y et al. TMJ energy densities in healthy men and women. Osteoarthritis and Cartilage 2017b; 25: 846–849.

Johansson AC, Gunnarsson LG, Linton SJ et al. Pain, disability and coping reflected in the diurnal cortisol variability in patients scheduled for lumbar disc surgery. Eur J Pain 2008; 12: 633–640.

Kaplan SEF, Ohrbach R. Self-report of waking-state oral parafunctional behaviors in the natural environment. J Oral Facial Pain Headache 2016; 30: 107–119.

Keefe FJ, Rumble ME, Scipio CD, Giordano LA, Perri LM. Psychological aspects of persistent pain: current state of the science. J Pain 2004; 5: 195–211.

Kight M, Gatchel RJ, Wesley L. Temporomandibular disorders: evidence for significant overlap with psychopathology. Health Psychol 1999; 18: 177–182.

Kitai N, Takada K, Yasuda Y, Verdonck A, Carels C. Pain and other cardinal TMJ dysfunction symptoms: a longitudinal survey of Japanese female adolescents. J Oral Rehabil 1997; 24: 741–748.

Leeuw M, Goossens ME, Linton SJ, Crombez G, Boersma K, Vlaeyen JW. The fear-avoidance model of musculoskeletal pain: current state of scientific evidence. J Behav Med 2007; 30: 77–94.

Lipton JA, Ship JA, Larach-Robinson D. Estimated prevalence and distribution of reported orofacial pain in the United States. J Am Dent Assoc 1993; 124: 115–121.

Livingston WK. Pain and Suffering. Seattle: IASP Press; 1998.

Macfarlane TV, Blinkhorn AS, Davies R, Kincey J, Worthington H. Factors associated with health care seeking behaviour for orofacial pain in the general population. Community Dent Health 2003; 20: 20–26.

Markiewicz MR, Ohrbach R, Mccall WD Jr. Oral behaviors checklist: reliability of performance in targeted waking-state behaviors. J Orofac Pain 2006; 20: 306–316.

McBeth J, Macfarlane GJ, Silman AJ. Does chronic pain predict future psychological distress? Pain 2002; 96: 239–245.

McLean SM, May S, Klaber-Moffett J, Sharp DM, Gardiner E. Risk factors for the onset of non-specific neck pain: a systematic review. J Epidemiol Community Health 2010; 64; 565–572.

Melis M, Lobo SL, Ceneviz C et al. Effect of cigarette smoking on pain intensity of TMD patients: a pilot study. Cranio 2010; 28:187–192.

Melzack R. Phantom limbs, the self and the brain. Can Psychol 1989; 30: 1–16.

Melzack R, Wall PD. Pain mechanisms: a new theory. Science 1965; 150: 971–979.

Molin C, Carlsson GE, Friling B, Hedegard B. Frequency of symptoms of mandibular dysfunction in young in young Swedish men. J Oral Rehabil 1976; 3: 9–18.

Moseley GL. A pain neuromatrix approach to patients with chronic pain. Man Ther 2003; 8: 130–140.

Moulton B, Spence SH. Site-specific muscle hyper-reactivity in musicians with occupational upper limb pain. Behav Res Ther 1992; 30: 375–386.

NCHS. Summary Health Statistics Tables for the U.S. Population: National Health Interview Survey, 2014 (12/2015) [Online]. CDC/ National Center for Health and Statistics. Available: http://www.cdc.gov/nchs/nhis/SHS/ tables.htm [Oct 22, 2017].

NIDCR. Facial Pain. [Online] National Institutes of Health, 2014. Available: http://www.nidcr.nih.gov/DataStatistics/ FindDataByTopic/FacialPain/ [Oct 22, 2017].

Nørregaard J, Lykkegaard JJ, Mehlsen J, Danneskiold-Samsøe B. Exercise training in treatment of fibromyalgia. J Musculoskeletal Pain 1997; 5: 71–79.

Ohrbach R. Disability assessment in temporomandibular disorders and masticatory system rehabilitation. J Oral Rehabil 2001; 37: 452–480.

Ohrbach R, Durham J. Biopsychosocial aspects of orofacial pain. In Farah CS, Balasubramaniam R, Mccullough MJ (eds). Contemporary oral medicine. Heidelberg, Germany: Springer Meteor; 2017.

Ohrbach R, Dworkin SF. The evolution of TMD diagnosis: past, present, future. J Dental Res 2016; 95: 1093–1101.

Ohrbach R, Larsson P, List T. The jaw functional limitation scale: development, reliability, and validity of 8-item and 20-item versions. J Orofac Pain 2008a; 22: 219–230.

Ohrbach R, Markiewicz MR, Mccall WD. Waking-state oral parafunctional behaviors: specificity and validity as assessed by electromyography. Eur J Oral Sciences 2008b; 116: 438–444.

Ohrbach R, Fillingim RB, Mulkey F et al. Clinical findings and pain symptoms as potential risk factors for chronic TMD: descriptive data and empirically identified domains from the OPPERA case-control study. J Pain 2011; 12: T27-T45.

Ohrbach R, Bair E, Fillingim RB et al. Clinical orofacial characteristics associated with risk of first-onset TMD: the OPPERA prospective cohort study. J Pain 2013; 14: T33-T50.

Ohrbach R, Blasberg B, Greenberg MS. Temporomandibular disorders. In Glick M (ed.) Burket's Oral Medicine. 12th ed. Shelton, CT: PMPH-USA; 2015.

Osterberg T, Carlsson GE. Symptoms and signs of mandibular dysfunction in 70-year old men and women in Gothenburg, Sweden. Community Dent Oral Epidemiol 1979; 7: 315–321.

Osterweis M, Kleinman A, Mechanic D (eds). Pain and disability: clinical, behavioral, and public policy perspectives. Institute of Medicine (US) Committee on Pain, Disability, and Chronic Illness Behavior. Washington DC: National Academies Press; 1987.

Plesh O, Adams SH, Gansky SA. Racial/ethnic and gender prevalences in reported common pains in a national sample. J Orofac Pain 2011a; 25: 25–31.

Plesh O, Adams SH, Gansky SA. Temporomandibular joint and muscle disorder-type pain and comorbid pains in a national US sample. J Orofac Pain 2011b; 25: 190–198.

Quintner JL, Bove GM, Cohen ML. A critical evaluation of the trigger point phenomenon. Rheumatology 2015; 54; 392–399.

Raphael KG, Marbach JJ. Widespread pain and the effectiveness of oral splints in myofascial face pain. J Am Dental Assoc 2001; 132: 305–316.

Raphael KG, Marbach JJ, Klausner J. Myofascial face pain: Clinical characteristics of those with regional vs widespread pain. JADA 2000; 131: 161–171.

Rodriguez-Lozano FJ, Saez-Yuguero MR, Bermejo-Fenoll A. Prevalence of temporomandibular disorder-related findings in violinists compared with control subjects. Oral Surg Oral Med Oral Pathol Oral Radiol Endod 2010; 109: e15–19.

Rothman KJ, Greenland S. Causation and causal inference in epidemiology. Am J Public Health 2005; 95: S144-S150.

Sanders AE, Maixner W, Nackley AG et al. Excess risk of temporomandibular disorder associated with cigarette smoking in young adults. J Pain 2012; 13: 21–31.

Sanders AE, Slade GD, Bair E et al. General health status and incidence of first-onset temporomandibular disorder: the OPPERA prospective cohort study. J Pain 2013; 14: T51-T62.

Sanders AE, Akinkugbe AA, Bair E et al. Subjective sleep quality deteriorates before development of painful temporomandibular disorder. J Pain 2016; 17: 669–677.

Scheuermann RH, Ceusters W, Smith B. Toward an ontological treatment of disease and diagnosis. Proceedings of the 2009 AMIA summit on translational bioinformatics, 2009; 116–120.

Schiffman EL, Ohrbach R, Truelove EL et al. The Research Diagnostic Criteria for Temporomandibular Disorders. V: methods used to establish and validate revised Axis I diagnostic algorithms. J Orofac Pain 2010; 24: 63–78.

Sharma S. The associations of injury and stress with temporomandibular disorders. University at Buffalo; 2017 [Online]. Available: https://www.researchgate.net/profile/Sonia_Sharma6 [Oct 22, 2017].

Slade GD, Bair E, Greenspan JD, et al. Signs and symptoms of first-onset TMD and sociodemographic predictors of its development: the OPPERA prospective cohort study. J Pain 2013; 14: T20-T32.

Slade GD, Sanders AE, Ohrbach R et al. Pressure pain thresholds fluctuate with, but do not usefully predict, the clinical course of painful temporomandibular disorder. Pain 2014; 155: 2134–2143.

Slade GD, Sanders AE, Ohrbach R et al. COMT Diplotype amplifies effect of stress on risk of temporomandibular pain. J Dent Res 2015; 94: 1187–95.

Slade GD, Ohrbach R, Greenspan JD et al. Painful temporomandibular disorder: decade of discovery from OPPERA Studies. J Dental Res 2016; 95: 1084–1092.

Smith B, Ceusters W, Goldberg LJ, Ohrbach, R. Towards an ontology of pain. In Okada M (ed). Proceedings of the Conference on Logic and Ontology. Tokyo: Keio University Press; 2011.

Smith SB, Mir E, Bair E et al. Genetic variants associated with development of TMD and its intermediate phenotypes: the genetic architecture of TMD in the OPPERA prospective cohort study. J Pain 2013; 14: T91-T101.

Steinmetz A, Ridder PH, Methfessel G, Muche B. Professional musicians with craniomandibular dysfunctions treated with oral splints. Cranio 2009; 27: 221–230.

Szentpetery A, Huhn E, Fazekas A. Prevalence of mandibular dysfunction in an urban population in Hungary. Community Dent Oral Epidemiol 1986; 14:177–180.

Taylor JB, Goode AP, George SZ, Cook CE. Incidence and risk factors for first-time incident low back pain: a systematic review and meta-analysis. Spine J 2014; 14: 2299–2319.

Travell JG, Simons DG. Myofascial Pain and Dysfunction: The Trigger Point Manual. Baltimore: Williams and Wilkins; 1983.

Truelove E, Pan W, Look JO et al. The Research Diagnostic Criteria for Temporomandibular Disorders. III: validity of Axis I diagnoses. J Orofac Pain 2010; 24: 35–47.

Turk DC, Rudy TE. Towards a comprehensive assessment of chronic pain patients. Behav Res Ther 1987; 25: 237–249.

Türp JC, Schlenker A, Schröder J, Essig M, Schmitter M. Disk displacement, eccentric condylar position, osteoarthrosis – misnomers for variations of normality? Results and interpretations from an MRI study in two age cohorts. BMC Oral Health 2016; 16: 124.

van Selms M, Ahlberg J, Lobbezoo F, Visscher C. Evidence-based review on temporomandibular disorders among musicians. Occup Med (Lond) 2017; 67: 336–343.

Verkerk K, Luijsterburg PaJ, Heymans MW et al. Prognosis and course of pain in patients with chronic non-specific low back pain: A 1-year follow-up cohort study. Eur J Pain 2015; 19: 1101–1110.

Von Korff M. Studying the natural history of back pain. Spine (Phila Pa 1976) 1994; 19 (18 Suppl): 2041s–2046s.

Von Korff M, Dworkin SF, Le Resche L, Kruger A. An epidemiologic comparison of pain complaints. Pain 1988; 32: 173–183.

Von Korff M, Le Resche L, Dworkin SF. First onset of common pain symptoms: a prospective study of depression as a risk factor. Pain 1993; 55: 251–258.

Wakefield J. The concept of mental disorder: on the boundary between biological facts and social values. Am Psychologist 1992; 47: 373.

Wall PD. On the relation of injury to pain. Pain 1979; 6: 253–264.

Wasan AD, Davar G, Jamison R. The association between negative affect and opioid analgesia in patients with discogenic low back pain. Pain 2005; 117: 450–461.

Wei F, Van Horn MH, Coombs MC et al. A pilot study of nocturnal temporalis muscle activity in TMD diagnostic groups of women. J Oral Rehabil 2017; 44: 517–525.

Weingarten TN, Iverson BC, Shi Y, Schroeder DR, Warner DO, Reid KI. Impact of tobacco use on the symptoms of painful temporomandibular joint disorders. Pain 2009; 147: 67–71.

Wiesinger B, Häggman-Henrikson B, Hellström F, Wänman A. Experimental masseter muscle pain alters jaw–neck motor strategy. Eur J Pain 2013; 17: 995–1004.

Williams AC de C, Craig KD. Updating the definition of pain. Pain 2016; 157: 2420–2423.

Woolf CJ. Pain: moving from symptom control toward mechanism-specific pharmacologic management. Annals Intern Med 2004; 140: 441–451.

Wright LJ, Schur E, Noonan C, Ahumada S, Buchwald D, Afari N. Chronic pain, overweight, and obesity: findings from a community-based twin registry. J Pain 2010; 11: 628–635.

Chapter 2
Classification of temporomandibular disorders

Ambra Michelotti, Peter Svensson

Introduction

Definition

Temporomandibular disorders (TMDs) encompass a group of musculoskeletal and neuromuscular conditions that involve the temporomandibular joints (TMJs), the masticatory musculature and all associated tissues. They are characterized by regional acute or persistent pain in the facial and preauricular areas, or by limitation or interference of orofacial neuromuscular functions such as eating, yawning, talking, etc. Signs and symptoms may include pain in the masticatory muscles or TMJs, reproduced during the clinical examination, and noises or sounds in the TMJs. The most common TMD subtypes include pain-related disorders (myalgia and arthralgia), and disorders associated with the TMJ (internal derangements and degenerative joint disease). The patient often suffers from other painful disorders (comorbidities), for example headaches, neck and shoulder pain, widespread pain, and fibromyalgia. TMDs are no longer considered a solely local disorder but rather are the outcome of multiple-risk determinants (Svensson & Kumar 2016; Slade et al., 2013). Among risk factors it is important to evaluate the biopsychosocial domain, since the chronic forms of TMD pain may lead to absence from or impairment of work or social interactions, resulting in an overall reduction in the quality of life, susceptibility to medication overuse or even abuse, and increased frequency of treatment seeking (Ohrbach & Dworkin, 2016; Verkerk et al., 2015; AADR, 2015).

Purpose of classification

From a clinical perspective, it is widely accepted that an appropriate treatment of any disease or disorder requires an accurate diagnosis (Ceusters et al., 2015a). From a research point of view accurate diagnosis and classification are prerequisites for collecting reliable information to expand existing knowledge bases. Anatomically, TMD conditions are included under the wider umbrella of orofacial pain. The International Headache Society (IHS), the American Academy of Orofacial Pain (AAOP) and the International RDC/TMD Consortium Network are all constantly monitoring and revising their respective classifications due to the evolving understanding and scientific knowledge of the disorders (Renton et al., 2012). The most commonly used research classification system for TMD has been the Research Diagnostic Criteria for Temporomandibular Disorders (RDC/TMD) (Dworkin & LeResche, 1992). These criteria came from the need for a diagnostic system that could not only distinguish, for epidemiologic and clinical research purposes, cases from controls but also differentially define and diagnose common subtypes of chronic pain-related TMDs. The main principles underlying this diagnostic approach included the biopsychosocial model with a dual-axis system. This is composed of physical diagnoses based on TMD clinical signs and symptoms (Axis I) and psychosocial profiles (Axis II) describing aspects of the person who had the disorder to classify disease and illness. The diagnoses are based on strict operational definitions of terms, including precise specifications for the clinical examination.

Moving from Research Diagnostic Criteria (RDC) to Diagnostic Criteria (DC)

The RDC/TMD is a milestone contribution in the field of TMD clinics and research and has been used and cited extensively. The evolution of the RDC/TMD came approximately 20 years later as the result of a longitudinal process of research and data analyses. The resulting publications included the Diagnostic Criteria for Temporomandibular Disorders (DC/TMD) (Schiffman et al., 2014), which provided reliable and valid criteria for common TMDs for clinical and research settings, and the expanded DC/TMD

(Peck et al., 2014), which provided criteria for the less common TMDs. In summary, when compared with the RDC/TMD, the DC/TMD has advanced to an evidence-based system with greater validity for clinical use. In particular, the DC/TMD was built on evidence including the reliability and validity of the diagnosed disorders. However, while diagnostic tests for pain-related common TMDs exhibit sensitivity and specificity of > 0.90 (Schiffman & Ohrbach, 2016), the link between the test and underlying pathophysiology of the disorder remains poorly understood. Nevertheless, the DC/TMD provides a common language for clinicians and researchers. The definition of classification and diagnostic criteria is important for a better understanding of TMD prevalence, incidence, and other characteristics in populations around the world. In clinical practice, the classification is needed especially when the diagnosis is uncertain and when a patient receives more than one diagnosis; for research, the classification is indispensable in order to allow comparisons between different studies.

Description of Diagnostic Criteria: Axis I and Axis II

The following new evidence-based DC/TMD Axis I encompasses the most common TMD diagnoses with an acceptable estimate of sensitivity and specificity (ideal values: sensitivity of ≥ 70% and specificity of ≥ 95%). Namely, pain-related TMDs – arthralgia, myalgia, myofascial pain with referral, and headache attributed to TMD; and intra-articular TMDs – disc displacement (DD) with reduction, DD with reduction with intermittent locking, DD without reduction with limited opening, DD without reduction without limited opening, degenerative joint disease, and subluxation or luxation. In addition, two other diagnoses, namely local myalgia and myofascial pain, are also considered in the muscle pain related diagnoses, accepting a content validity; however, in contrast to all other diagnoses in the DC/TMD, they do not have established measures of validity, that is, at present the sensitivity and specificity are not known.

The new DC/TMD Axis II protocol has also been expanded. New instruments have been added to evaluate pain behavior, psychological status, and psychosocial functioning, and include assessments ranging from screening to comprehensive expert evaluation.

Axis I temporomandibular diagnoses

Axis I screening questionnaire

The Axis I TMD Pain Screener (Gonzalez et al., 2011) is a simple, reliable, and valid self-report six-item questionnaire used to assess the presence of pain-related TMDs, with sensitivity and specificity of ≥ 0.95 (see Table 7.1 in Chapter 7). This questionnaire assesses the reporting of pain and factors that may affect the pain, including jaw function and oral parafunction. The routine use of this self-report questionnaire is recommended in dental practice to intercept pre-existing TMD, to prevent chronicity, and to facilitate informed consent regarding potential complications from dental treatment. It identifies patients who have a pain-related TMD or who are at risk of exacerbating their pre-existing pain during dental treatments and may be in need of treatment. It is useful for informing the patient about any TMD-related symptoms that may occur during treatment, and for informing the dentist so that he or she can take appropriate precautions to protect the patient's jaw.

Axis I physical diagnoses

The DC/TMD diagnoses can be considered the 'core' diagnoses in the evaluation of patients with orofacial pain complaints because they are very prevalent and because they are the best described. Figure 2.1 attempts to capture the relation of DC/TMD diagnoses to other types of TMD diagnoses, orofacial pain, and headache. A more detailed description of the specific painful and nonpainful DC/TMD diagnoses is provided below.

Myalgia

Myalgia is muscle pain that is localized in the jaw, temple, in the ear, or in front of ear, and that is

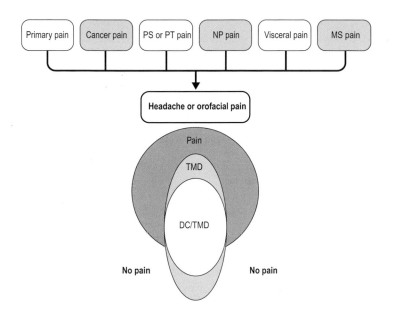

Figure 2.1
The DC/TMD diagnosis is a well-described subset of all types of TMDs. Only a subset of TMD diagnoses is painful which fit into the category of headaches and orofacial pain according to the IASP classification. Six other types of chronic pain categories can co-exist or overlap with chronic orofacial pain. DC, Diagnostic Criteria; MS, musculoskeletal pain; NP, neuropathic; PS, postsurgical; PT, post-traumatic; TMD, temporomandibular disorder.

affected by jaw movement, function, or parafunction. Replication of this pain (familiar pain) occurs with provocation testing of the masticatory musculature (muscle palpation and/or mouth opening). The sensitivity is 0.90, and specificity is 0.99. Myalgia is differentiated into three subtypes according to the provocation testing based on standardized muscle palpation:

- **Local myalgia** is a myalgia with report of pain localized to the site of palpation. For this diagnosis sensitivity and specificity have not been established.

- **Myofascial pain** is a myalgia with report of pain spreading beyond the site of palpation but within the boundary of the muscle. For this diagnosis sensitivity and specificity have not been established.

- **Myofascial pain with referral** is a myalgia, with report of pain at a site beyond the boundary of the muscle being palpated. The sensitivity is 0.86, and specificity is 0.98.

Arthralgia

Arthralgia is pain of TMJ origin that is affected by jaw movement, function, or parafunction. Replication of this pain (familiar pain) occurs with

provocation testing of the TMJ (joint palpation and/or mouth opening). The sensitivity is 0.89, and specificity is 0.98.

Headache attributed to temporomandibular disorder

This is headache in the temple area secondary to pain-related TMD that is affected by jaw movement, function, or parafunction. Replication of this headache (familiar headache) occurs with provocation testing of the masticatory system (palpation of the temporalis muscle and/or mouth opening). The sensitivity is 0.89, and specificity is 0.87. In fact, 'Headache attributed to TMD' is included as a new disorder type to replace 'Headache or facial pain attributed to TMJ disorder' as described in the International Classification of Headache Disorders II (ICHD-II, 2004) and has been incorporated into the beta version of the ICHD-III (2013).

Temporomandibular joint disc displacement and degenerative joint disease

Disc displacement with reduction is an intracapsular biomechanical disorder involving the disc–condyle complex. In the closed-mouth position, the disc is in an anterior, medial or lateral position relative to the condylar head and the disc reduces upon opening of the mouth. Clicking, popping, or snapping noises may occur with disc reduction. Without imaging the sensitivity is 0.34, and specificity is 0.92. TMJ magnetic resonance imaging is the reference standard for this diagnosis.

Disc displacement with reduction with intermittent locking is an intracapsular biomechanical disorder involving the disc–condyle complex. In the closed-mouth position, the disc is in an anterior, medial or lateral position relative to the condylar head, and the disc intermittently reduces with opening of the mouth. When the disc does not reduce with opening of the mouth, intermittent limited mandibular opening occurs. When limited opening occurs, a maneuver may be needed to unlock the TMJ. When this disorder is present clinically, examination is positive for inability to open the mouth to a normal range, even momentarily, without the clinician or patient performing a maneuver to reduce the lock. Clicking, popping, or snapping noises may occur with disc reduction. Without imaging the sensitivity is 0.38, and specificity is 0.98. Imaging is the reference standard for this diagnosis.

Disc displacement without reduction with limited opening is an intracapsular biomechanical disorder involving the disc–condyle complex. In the closed-mouth position, the disc is in an anterior, medial or lateral position relative to the condylar head, and the disc does not reduce with opening of the mouth. This disorder is associated with persistent limited mandibular opening that does not reduce when the clinician or patient performs a manipulative maneuver. This is also referred to as 'closed lock.' This disorder is associated with limited mandibular opening severe enough to interfere with the ability to eat. The maximum assisted opening (passive stretch) movement, including vertical incisal overlap, is <40 mm. Without imaging the sensitivity is 0.80, and specificity is 0.97. Imaging is the reference standard for this diagnosis.

Disc displacement without reduction without limited opening is an intracapsular biomechanical disorder involving the disc–condyle complex. In the closed-mouth position, the disc is in an anterior, medial or lateral position relative to the condylar head and the disc does not reduce with opening of the mouth. This disorder is NOT associated with current limited opening with maximum assisted opening (passive stretch) movement including vertical incisal overlap of ≥40 mm. Without imaging the sensitivity is 0.54, and specificity is 0.79. Imaging is the reference standard for this diagnosis.

Degenerative joint disease is a degenerative disorder involving the joint characterized by deterioration of articular tissue with concomitant osseous changes in the condyle and/or articular eminence. During clinical examination crepitus is detected with palpation during at least one of the following movements: opening, closing, right or left lateral, or protrusive. Without imaging the sensitivity is 0.55, and specificity is 0.61. TMJ computed tomography imaging is the reference standard for this diagnosis.

Subluxation is a hypermobility disorder involving the disc–condyle complex and the articular eminence. In the open-mouth position, the disc–condyle complex is positioned anterior to the articular eminence and is unable to return to a normal closed-mouth position without a manipulative maneuver. The duration of dislocation may be momentary or prolonged. When the patient can reduce the dislocation by himself or herself, this is referred to as subluxation.

Luxation or complete dislocation is a condition in which the condyle is positioned anterior to the articular eminence and is unable to return to a closed position without a specific maneuver by the clinician. Pain may occur at the time of dislocation with residual pain following the episode. This disorder is also referred to as 'open lock.' The sensitivity and specificity have been established for only subluxation. Without imaging and based only on history the sensitivity is 0.98, and specificity is 1.00.

Axis II evaluation

According to the International Association for the Study of Pain (IASP), pain is defined as 'An unpleasant sensory and emotional experience associated with actual or potential tissue damage, or described in terms of such damage' and 'Chronic pain in one or more anatomical regions is characterized by significant emotional distress (anxiety, anger, frustration or depressed mood) and functional disability (interference in daily life activities and reduced participation in social roles).' Since biological, psychological and social factors all contribute to the pain condition, responses to pain are quite independent of the source of their pain. Axis I addresses the nociceptive inputs from peripheral tissues. However, pain as an experience is modulated by activity in multiple areas of the central nervous system; consequently, the whole person needs to be assessed. The Axis II protocol is based on the biopsychosocial model that characterizes pain and assesses effects including cognitive, psychosocial, and behavioral factors that also can complicate treatment outcome and contribute to chronicity. It is therefore important to assess the psychosocial factors, especially when the patient presents with chronic diseases. The DC/TMD recommends screening instruments to assess the psychosocial functioning associated with any pain condition and jaw dysfunction. The criteria used to select these instruments were reliability, validity, interpretability, patient and clinician acceptability, patient burden, and feasibility, as well as availability of translated versions for different languages and cultures (Durham et al., 2015).

Axis II screeners

Five simple self-report screening instruments are available for detection of pain that is related to psychosocial and behavioral functioning.

Patient Health Questionnaire-4

PHQ-4 is a short, reliable, and valid screening instrument for detecting 'psychological distress' due to anxiety and/or depression in patients in any clinical setting. A cut-off value of >6, suggesting moderate psychological stress, should be interpreted as warranting observation, while a cut-off value of >9, suggesting severe psychological distress, should be interpreted as warranting either further assessment or referral.

Graded Chronic Pain Scale

GCPS is a short, reliable, and valid instrument that assesses pain intensity and pain-related disability. The two GCPS subscales are: 1) Characteristic Pain Intensity (CPI), which reliably measures pain intensity, with ≥ 50/100 considered as 'high intensity,' and 2) the pain-disability rating, which is based on the number of days that pain interferes with activity and the extent to which it interferes with social, work, or normal daily activities. High pain and high interference, or moderate to severe disability (classified as Grades 3 or 4), should be interpreted as disability due to pain, warranting further investigation, and suggests that TMD is having a significant impact on the individual's life.

Pain drawing

This consists of drawing all the symptoms experienced in the head, jaw, and body and allows the patient to report the location of the main pain complaint. Widespread pain suggests the need for comprehensive assessment of the patient.

Jaw Functional Limitation Scale

The JFLS is a reliable and valid short form (consisting of eight items) using the Jaw Functional Limitation Scale. It assesses global limitations across mastication, jaw mobility, and verbal and emotional expression.

Oral Behaviors Checklist

The OBC is an instrument for assessing the frequency of oral parafunctional behaviors.

Chapter 2

Comprehensive Axis II instruments

The Axis II instruments are to be used when indicated by clinical specialists or researchers in order to obtain a more comprehensive evaluation of psychosocial functioning. They are based on the Initiative on Methods, Measurement, and Pain Assessment in Clinical Trials (IMMPACT) recommendations. Pain drawing and the OBC (see above) are also components of the comprehensive assessment.

Graded Chronic Pain Scale

The GCPS is used to measure pain intensity and pain disability.

Jaw Functional Limitation Scale

The JFLS is a 20-item scale used to measure disease-specific physical functioning.

Patient Health Questionnaire-9

PHQ-9 is used for assessing depression. Cut-offs of 5, 10, 15, and 20 represent, respectively, mild, moderate, moderately severe, and severe levels of depression.

Generalized Anxiety Disorder-7

GAD-7 is used for evaluating anxiety. Cut-offs of 10 and 15 represent, respectively, moderate and severe levels of anxiety.

Patient Health Questionnaire-15

PHQ-15 is used for determining physical symptoms. Cut-offs of 5, 10, and 15 represent low, medium, and high somatic symptom severity respectively.

From RDC/TMD to DC/TMD: What's new?

Several topics have evolved from the original RDC/TMD (Dworkin & LeResche, 1992) to the new DC/TMD (Schiffman et al., 2014; Peck et al., 2014) as outlined below:

1. A valid and reliable Axis I screening questionnaire for identifying pain-related TMDs is now included in the criteria.

2. Valid and reliable Axis I diagnostic algorithms for the most common pain-related TMDs and for the most common intra-articular disorders have been introduced. All TMD-pain-related diagnoses present an excellent sensitivity and specificity. Diagnostic criteria for all but one intra-articular disorder lack adequate validity for clinical diagnoses but can be used for screening purposes.

3. Axis II core assessment instruments assessing pain intensity, pain-related disability, jaw functioning, psychosocial distress, parafunctional behavior, and widespread pain have also been introduced.

4. A patient report of pain modified, that is, made better or worse, by jaw function, movement, or parafunction is now a requirement for all pain-related TMD diagnoses. Pain modification is especially important in differential diagnosis when comorbid conditions may be present, especially other pain conditions of the trigeminal system. A patient report of familiar pain is required with pain provoked by jaw movement or palpation to diagnose all pain-related TMDs, including arthralgia, myalgia, the three types of myalgia, and headache attributed to TMD. The intent is to replicate the patient's chief complaint of pain in order to minimize false positive findings from pain-provoking tests in asymptomatic subjects and incidental findings in symptomatic patients. It must be stressed that the presence of familiar pain is not associated exclusively with the diagnoses of arthralgia, myalgia, and the three types of myalgia, as other conditions may cause familiar pain (such as infection and rheumatoid disease affecting the TMJ).

5. For myalgia and the three types of myalgia diagnoses, palpation of only the temporalis and masseter muscles is now required, and

mandatory palpation of the temporalis tendon, lateral pterygoid area, submandibular region, and posterior mandibular region has been eliminated because of its poor reliability.

6. For the same reason, palpation of the posterior aspect of the TMJ through the external auditory meatus has also been eliminated, but can be used when indicated.

7. TMJ noises can be difficult to detect, even with auscultation using a stethoscope, and may be sporadically present. It has been concluded that patient differentiation of noise such as clicking, crunching, grinding, or grating noises (crepitus) is an inconsistent source of clinical information.

8. The distinction between coarse and fine crepitus has been omitted because these sounds cannot be reliably distinguished and the distinction does not contribute to the diagnostic accuracy of degenerative joint disease.

Expanding the taxonomy of Diagnostic Criteria for TMDs

The DC/TMD described in the previous section provides a standardized assessment for a limited set of TMDs with validated criteria useful both for researchers and for clinicians. However, there is a need to expand the classifications to include less common but clinically important disorders. In fact, most of the latter are described in the classifications determined by the American Academy of Orofacial Pain (AAOP, 2008) without the same standardized approach. In order to develop a consensus-based classification system and associated diagnostic criteria that have clinical and research utility for less common TMDs a working group (members of the International RDC/TMD Consortium Network of the International Association for Dental Research (IADR), the Orofacial Pain Special Interest Group (SIG) of the International Association for the Study of Pain (IASP), and other professional societies) reviewed disorders for inclusion based on clinical significance and the availability of plausible

diagnostic criteria. Other disorders with sensitivity and specificity not yet established were added to the DC/TMD, included in the expanded taxonomy, and placed in the following categories: TMJ disorders, masticatory muscle disorders, headache disorders, and disorder affecting associated structures (Peck et al., 2014).

Temporomandibular joint disorders

Arthritis

Arthritis is pain of joint origin with clinical characteristics of inflammation or infection over the affected joint: edema, erythema, and/or increased temperature. Associated symptoms can include dental occlusal changes. There is no history of systemic inflammatory disease.

Hypomobility disorders other than disc disorders: adhesions and ankylosis

Intra-articular fibrous adhesions (or adherence) and ankylosis are mainly characterized by restricted mandibular movements with deflection to the affected side on opening. In the case of bilateral involvement, asymmetries in mandibular movements during clinical examination will be less pronounced or absent. The condition is not usually associated with pain. Adhesions may occur secondary to joint inflammation that results from direct trauma, excessive loading or systemic conditions, such as a polyarthritic disease, and are typically associated with disc disorders. The most frequent cause of TMJ ankylosis is macrotrauma; less frequent causes are infection of the mastoid or middle ear, systemic disease and inadequate surgical treatment of the condylar area.

Systemic arthritides

These are generalized systemic inflammatory diseases, which cause joint inflammation resulting in pain or structural changes, e.g., rheumatoid arthritis, juvenile idiopathic arthritis, spondyloarthropathies (ankylosing spondylitis, psoriatic arthritis, infectious arthritis, Reiter's syndrome), and crystal-induced arthritis (gout, chondrocalcinosis). Other rheumatologically related diseases that may affect the TMJ include autoimmune disorders and other mixed connective tissue diseases (scleroderma, Sjögren's syndrome, lupus erythematosus). Therefore, this group of arthritides includes multiple diagnostic categories that are best diagnosed and managed by rheumatologists using general or systemic therapy. Clinical signs and symptoms of ongoing chronic (TMJ) inflammation are variable among patients and often vary over time for a single patient. They can vary from no signs or symptoms to only pain, or swelling/exudate, or tissue degradation, or growth disturbance. Resorption of condylar structures may be associated with malocclusion such as a progressive anterior open bite or mandibular asymmetry. Imaging in the early stages of the disease may not show any osseous findings.

Condylysis or idiopathic condylar resorption

Condylysis is resorption of the condyles, which leads to the idiopathic loss of condylar height, and a progressive anterior open bite. The condition is almost always bilateral and predominantly occurs in adolescent and young adult females. The presence of pain or articular sounds is variable. In the early stages, dental occlusal changes may not be evident but imaging findings would be positive. The cause is unknown, although it has been suggested that estrogen may be implicated.

Osteochondritis dissecans

This is a joint condition in which there are loose osteochondral fragments within the joint. The pathophysiology is unclear. It occurs usually in the knee and elbow and is often related to sports. The clinical presentation may be a combination of pain, swelling, joint noises, and limitation of jaw movements.

Osteonecrosis

Osteonecrosis is a painful condition that is found in the mandibular condyle and manifests on MRI as decreased signal in T1-weighted or proton density images and in T2-weighted images (sclerosis pattern) and can be combined with increased signal in T2 images (edema). This condition has also been referred to in the literature as avascular necrosis (AVN).

Neoplasms

Neoplasms result from tissue proliferation with histological characteristics and may be benign (chondroma or osteochondroma) or malignant (primary or metastatic). They may present with swelling, pain during function, limited mouth opening, crepitus, occlusal changes, and/or sensory and motor changes. Facial asymmetry with a midline shift may occur as the lesion expands. Diagnostic imaging, typically using computed tomography (CT) or cone beam computed tomography (CBCT) and/or MRI, and biopsy are essential when a neoplasm is suspected.

Synovial chondromatosis

Synovial chondromatosis is a cartilaginous metaplasia of the mesenchymal remnants of the synovial tissue of the joint. Its main characteristic is the formation of cartilaginous nodules that may be pedunculated and/or detached from the synovial membrane becoming loose bodies within the joint space. The disease may be associated with malocclusion, such as a progressive ipsilateral posterior open bite. Imaging is needed to establish the diagnosis.

Fracture

A fracture is a nondisplaced or displaced break in bone involving the joint (for example, the temporal bone and/or mandible). The fracture may include the cartilage. The most common is the subcondylar fracture. The condition may result in a malocclusion (contralateral posterior open bite) and impaired function (uncorrected ipsilateral deviation with opening or restricted contralateral jaw movement), and typically results from a traumatic injury.

Congenital or developmental disorders

Aplasia is typically a unilateral absence of condyle and incomplete development of the articular fossa and eminence, resulting in facial asymmetry. It is commonly associated with other congenital anomalies (Goldenhar syndrome, hemifacial microsomia and Treacher Collins syndrome). It is occasionally bilateral and in such cases, asymmetry is not present but micrognathia is the dominant clinical manifestation. The condition may be associated with malocclusion, which may include open bite.

Hypoplasia is an incomplete development or underdevelopment of the mandibular condyle. It can be secondary to facial trauma, and also to the same congenital anomalies associated with aplasia. Facial asymmetry or micrognathia occur and the condition may be associated with malocclusion (for example nonhorizontal occlusal plane and contralateral posterior open bite in unilateral cases or anterior open bite in bilateral cases).

Hyperplasia is an overdevelopment of the cranial bones or mandible. There is a nonneoplastic increase in the number of normal cells. Hyperplasia is typically unilateral with localized enlargement such as condylar hyperplasia, or overdevelopment of the entire mandible or side of the face.

Masticatory muscle disorders

Tendonitis

Tendonitis is pain of tendon origin affected by jaw movement, function, or parafunction, and replication of this pain with provocation testing of the masticatory tendon. Limitation of mandibular movement secondary to pain may be present. The temporalis tendon may be a common site of tendonitis and refer pain to the teeth and other nearby structures. Tendonitis could also apply to other masticatory muscle tendons.

Myositis

Myositis is pain of muscle origin with clinical characteristics of inflammation or infection such as edema, erythema, and/or increased temperature. It generally arises acutely following direct trauma of the muscle or from infection, or chronically with autoimmune disease. Limitation of unassisted mandibular movements secondary to pain is often present. Calcification of the muscle can occur (myositis ossificans).

Spasm

Spasm is a sudden, involuntary, reversible tonic contraction of a muscle. It may affect any of the masticatory muscles. Acute malocclusion may be present.

Contracture

Contracture is the shortening of a muscle due to fibrosis of tendons, ligaments, or muscle fibers. It is usually not painful unless the muscle is overextended. A history of radiation therapy, trauma, or infection is often present. It is more commonly seen in the masseter or medial pterygoid muscle.

Hypertrophy

Hypertrophy is an enlargement of one or more masticatory muscles, and is usually not associated with pain. It can be secondary to overuse and/or chronic tensing of the muscle(s). Some cases are familial or genetic in origin. Diagnosis is based on clinician assessment of muscle size and needs consideration of craniofacial morphology and ethnicity.

Neoplasms

Neoplasms result from tissue proliferation with histologic characteristics, and may be benign (myoma) or malignant (rhabdomyosarcoma, or metastatic). They are uncommon. They may present with swelling, spasm, pain during function, limited mouth opening, and/or sensory or motor changes (paresthesia, weakness). Diagnostic imaging, typically using CT/ CBCT and/or MRI, and biopsy are essential when a neoplasm is suspected.

Movement disorders

Orofacial dyskinesia is involuntary, mainly choreatic (dance-like) movements that may involve the face, lips, tongue, and/or jaw.

Oromandibular dystonia is an excessive, involuntary and sustained muscle contraction that may involve the face, lips, tongue, and/or jaw.

Movement disorders have been included in the expanded DC/TMD taxonomy because, in some cases, they may present primarily as masticatory muscle disorders.

Masticatory muscle pain attributed to systemic or central pain disorders

Fibromyalgia is a widespread pain condition with concurrent masticatory muscle pain.

Disorders affecting associated structures

Coronoid hyperplasia is a progressive enlargement of the coronoid process that impedes mandibular opening when it is obstructed by the zygomatic process of the maxilla.

General comments and future direction

General comments on temporomandibular disorder pain

The diagnostic algorithms in the new DC/TMD for arthralgia and myalgia now include criteria for *modification of pain by function, movement, or parafunction*. Indeed it has been shown that subjects reporting multiple parafunctional behaviors in the Oral Behaviors Checklist questionnaire had 16 times the odds of chronic TMD as subjects who reported only

a few (Slade et al., 2016). Care needs to be taken to distinguish between self-reported parafunctional activity, for example, bruxism with teeth clenching or grinding, and electrophysiologically documented jaw muscle activity (in polysomnographic recordings, audio and video monitoring, etc.) because there is a poor correlation between what the patient may report and what the patient actually does (for a review see Svensson et al., 2008; Lobbezoo et al., 2013; Castrillon et al., 2016). The clinical examination includes *provocation tests of pain* with any jaw movement, muscle and/or TMJ palpation. Pain from these provocation tests must replicate the patient's pain complaint. *Familiar pain* is pain that is like or similar to the pain complaint the patient has experienced in the last 30 days. *Familiar headache* is pain that is like or similar to the patient's headache complaint. The time frame for assessing pain-related TMD diagnoses including headache is 'in the last 30 days' since the validity was established using this time frame.

Muscle pain

The palpation pressure for myalgia is 1 kg for two seconds, but to differentiate the three types of myalgia the duration of the 1 kg of palpation pressure is increased to five seconds to allow more time to elicit spreading or referred pain if present. Assessing for myofascial pain with referral is useful in cases of nonodontogenic 'tooth' pain because jaw muscles can refer pain to the teeth. When using the Axis I diagnoses, the clinician must first rule out odontogenic disease and other pain disorders that can occur in the masticatory system. Numbness, swelling, and redness typically are not present with the common TMDs, and when they are present, the clinician must rule out clinically significant disease, including infections, neoplasms, and systemic conditions. In addition, the clinician also must consider the uncommon TMDs.

The subdivision of myalgia into three subclasses (local myalgia, myofascial pain, and myofascial pain with referral) was proposed to assess a possible temporal progression of muscle pain from a localized myalgia to more widespread pain. However, it is not yet known whether myofascial pain can be considered a singular disorder, or whether clinically important subtypes exist, and, if they do, what the mechanisms and clinical implications of defining these pain subtypes are (Svensson et al., 2015). The biologically plausible argument is that these three disorders could respond differently to treatment and have a different prognostic value. Although this is a valid reasoning, it is important to elaborate on the fact that the distinction between the four muscle pain-related diagnoses may not be clear from a mechanistic point of view or from a management point of view. While it may be plausible that local myalgia could evolve into myofascial pain with spreading and on to myofascial pain with referral, there is currently no evidence to support such a hypothesis. Spreading of muscle pain could be related to the observation in animal studies of increases in receptive fields of second-order neurons in the trigeminal brainstem sensory nuclear complex, and referral of pain could be related to central convergence of nociceptive afferent inputs onto second-order neurons (Sessle, 2000), and also to central sensitization and ultimately changes in descending inhibitory pathways (Svensson & Graven-Nielsen, 2001; Graven-Nielsen, 2006). However, it is known from human experimental studies that some subjects exposed to painful injections into the masseter muscle may experience a spread of the pain within the boundaries of the injected muscle, but also that other subjects with the exact same type of painful stimulation of the masseter muscle may experience referred pain in the teeth, TMJ, or temple. This simple observation with acute muscle pain calls for caution because both types of responses (spreading or referrals) could simply be epiphenomena of deep noxious inputs (Svensson & Kumar, 2016). Criterion validity for myalgia is established and excellent, as it is for the clinical subtype 'myofascial pain with referral.' It seems that thorough palpation of the muscles

is likely to uncover the presence of painful points when applying pressure for at least five seconds. If pain referral is no longer a required criterion for the identification of such particular points, 'myofascial pain' and 'myofascial pain with referral' are then potentially the same disorder and similar to the 'myofascial pain syndrome' known to occur in other parts of the body. It should be noted that the term 'trigger points' was avoided in this context because the precise definition, diagnostic validity and underlying pathophysiology are still unclear. Finally, although centrally mediated myalgia has been a distinct clinical entity in the AAOP classification system, it was not included in the expanded taxonomy because it overlaps with the 'myofascial pain with referral' and fibromyalgia. Centrally mediated myalgia may represent less a disorder and perhaps more a mechanism, such as in the widespread pain disorder. The distinctive myalgia subtypes should be assessed through well-designed research protocols based on the multidimensional, integrated approach recently proposed in the ACTTION-American Pain Society Pain Taxonomy (AAPT) (Fillingim et al., 2014). Hence for each myalgia subtype, distinguishing features must be delineated according to five major dimensions:

1. core diagnostic criteria

2. common features

3. potential common medical comorbidities

4. neurobiological, psychosocial, and functional consequences, and

5. putative neurobiological and psychosocial mechanisms, risk factors and protective factors.

This approach may be the key for clearly substantiating whether both types of myofascial pain as per the DC/TMD are a single disorder representing a distinctive clinical entity of local myalgia due to significant differences in pathophysiological and psychosocial mechanisms, response to treatment and prognosis (Michelotti et al., 2016).

Chapter 2

Arthritis

Arthritis presents an unspecific pathophysiology and it is not possible to determine whether it belongs to the joint pain diagnostic group or the joint disease group (Michelotti et al., 2016). A definition of TMJ arthritis should include the cardinal signs of inflammation (edema, erythema, increased temperature over the joint and articular pain); however, swelling, edema, and increased temperature are only seldom seen. Indeed, chronic TMJ inflammation may not show any of the cardinal signs even if the disease progresses, but it can present as loss of function and tissue degradation or growth disturbance. On the one hand, TMJ arthritis might cause arthralgia, but arthralgia could also be due to other factors which trigger articular nociceptors. An important goal to be achieved is an early diagnosis of ongoing TMJ arthritis. According to the American College of Rheumatology, clinical symptoms and signs that should be considered for an early and more specific diagnosis could be pain from the TMJ on jaw movement, pain from the TMJ on loading, and recent progressive occlusal changes. TMJ resting pain, TMJ pain on palpation or TMJ movement pain has high sensitivity for inflammatory activity in the TMJ; no TMJ resting pain, TMJ pain on palpation or TMJ movement pain has a high specificity for inflammatory activity; and TMJ movement pain is strongly related to the degree of inflammatory activity in the TMJ. In the future, biomarkers may provide a more objective identification of these disorders, and radiographic imaging could be required to detect TMJ cartilage or bone tissue destruction (Ceusters et al., 2015b). However, today it is not possible to make a radiological differential diagnosis to distinguish inflammatory TMJ conditions.

Headache attributed to temporomandibular disorders

The current DC/TMD 'Headache attributed to TMD' (HA-TMD) has excellent criterion validity (sensitivity of 89% and specificity of 87%). With the same reference standard, the criterion validity of the ICHD-II has a sensitivity of 84% and a specificity of 33%. The low specificity of the ICHD-II was due, in part, to the need for a positive imaging finding of intra-articular TMJ disorders, reduced or irregular opening and TMJ noise – all of which can be present in headache patients without other TMD signs or symptoms, including head pain. The DC/TMD for HA-TMD does not require imaging findings to demonstrate the presence of a TMJ disorder. The criteria require instead that the patient has a pain-related TMD diagnosis. This approach seems more logical because it directly links TMD-related headache to pain-related TMD rather than imaging findings, which can be present in asymptomatic individuals (Michelotti et al., 2016). Caution may still be needed when using the term 'attributed' because recent findings also suggest that painful TMDs can be attributed to headaches and the cause–effect relationship between TMDs and headaches may require more research to better understand the underlying pain mechanisms (Conti et al., 2016).

General comments on joint disease

The clinical procedures for assessing 'disc displacement (DD) with reduction,' 'DD without reduction without limited opening,' and 'degenerative joint disease (DJD)' lead to clinical diagnoses based on procedures that exhibit low sensitivity but good to excellent specificity (Schiffman et al., 2014). Therefore, the tests can be used only for screening purposes to render preliminary diagnoses of DD or DJD. Consequently, for treatment decision–making in selective cases, confirmation of a provisional clinical diagnosis requires imaging: definitive diagnoses require TMJ MRI for DD and TMJ CT for DJD. Taking as an example the diagnosis of DD with reduction, the clinical criteria for this diagnosis have low sensitivity but high specificity relative to findings from TMJ MRI. Many patients with MRI-depicted DD with reduction do not have any clinically detectable joint noise or have only sporadic occurrence of these noises, which is why the diagnostic criteria for this disorder have low sensitivity. In contrast, the clinical procedures for assessing DD without reduction with limited opening have acceptable sensitivity and specificity, and the clinical evaluation may be sufficient for the initial working diagnosis. However, certainty for this diagnosis requires MRI because these diagnostic criteria have not been assessed for criterion validity in patients with other disorders that result in limited opening. In the past, the criteria for DD without reduction with limited opening included other findings, such as deviation with opening to the affected side, but these findings are not consistently present and thus were not included. As for DJD, crepitus can occur without frank osseous changes, and crepitus is not always present with DJD. MRI is an excellent imaging technique for DD and joint effusions, but the sensitivity for detecting DJD is only 59% when CT is used as the reference standard. Thus, CT is needed to assess for DJD accurately to address the false negative results that occur when using MRI. Finally, panoramic radiographs are typically available in dental offices. However, these radiographs have a sensitivity of 26% for detection of DJD compared with that of CT and thus have a clinically significant number of false negative results.

TMJ noise by history is a recommended criterion for assessing the intra-articular disorders of DD with reduction and DJD. This history criterion may be met by the patient's report of any joint noise (click or crepitus) during the 30 days prior to the examination, or by the patient's detection of any joint noise with jaw movements during the clinical examination. In addition, a diagnosis of DD with reduction requires examiner detection of clicking, popping, or snapping noises during the clinical examination. Establishing a diagnosis of DJD is dependent on the detection of crepitus (crunching, grinding, or grating noises) during the examination. For DJD, no distinction between fine versus coarse crepitus is made. Finally, for DD without reduction, an assisted opening measurement (including the amount of vertical incisal overlap) of < 40 mm yields the subtype of 'with limited opening,' while the measurement ≥ 40 mm yields the subtype of 'without limited opening.' DD with reduction with intermittent locking and TMJ subluxation are included as new disorders. The diagnostic algorithms for these disorders include specific criteria from the patient history, including current intermittent locking with limited opening for DD with reduction with intermittent locking and jaw locking in the wide-open position for TMJ subluxation. The terms osteoarthritis and osteoarthrosis are considered to denote subclasses of DJD.

Disc–condyle complex disorders

Disc–condyle complex disorders typically result in changes in jaw mobility, including hypomobility and hypermobility (Michelotti et al., 2016). Some joint disorders are relatively common (for example disc displacements are at 18%–35% in a nonclinical population); however, epidemiological data that may be important in evaluating the etiology and progression of these disorders are not available. A recent study demonstrated no association between an individual's intra-articular status and reported pain, function and disability (Chantaracherd et al., 2015). While a limited subset of disc displacements with reduction progress to a nonreducing state (Schiffman et al., 2017), the progression of other disorders such as dislocations is unknown. Neither is it known whether the disorders represent unique entities that require specific interventions, or if they can be grouped and then managed in the same manner. While the etiologies and pathophysiologies of these disorders are not clearly and fully understood, it is assumed that the anatomical (structural) and the biomechanical (functional) environments contribute to these disorders. Cross-sectional studies suggest that those anatomical variables contributing to the etiology include a steep anterior wall of the condylar fossa, a high articular eminence, incongruence between condyle–disc and fossa, ligament laxity, muscle angulation and lateral pterygoid attachment to the TMJ disc. Putative biomechanical etiological contributors include high compressive, tensile and/or shear forces resulting from, for example oral parafunction, trauma or impaired joint lubrication.

Diagnostic criteria for disc–condyle complex disorders have been proposed; however, four of them have not been assessed for criterion validity and as for the others the diagnostic criteria do not have acceptable sensitivity and specificity for a definitive diagnosis (that is, sensitivity of > 70% and specificity of > 95%). Diagnostic schemes that produce relatively high false negatives (those with low sensitivity) are not necessarily a priority research area if the disorder has little clinical consequence, such as disc displacements with reduction. Research should focus on whether the disc–condyle complex disorders are distinct entities and on the management strategies that are effective in reducing impact or preventing the disorder's progression.

General comments on the biopsychosocial domain

For screening purposes, selected contributing factors were targeted in Axis II questionnaires (Schiffman et al., 2014; Durham et al., 2015; Michelotti et al., 2016). If these potential contributing factors are present, then the clinician needs to assess these further or refer the patient to a mental health care professional for a comprehensive assessment that should be included in the treatment plan. Conversely, the clinician can use these screening questionnaires to triage the patient and, when clinically significant findings are present, refer the patient to clinicians with more expertise rather than initiate treatment that may have a high risk of failure. If referral is not an option, then the clinician can explain the challenges that exist and that complete resolution of pain may not be possible. In this way, the patient receives comprehensive information and can provide informed consent regarding the potential contributing factors

to their pain complaints before treatment is initiated. The reference standard for diagnosing psychological distress is an assessment by a mental health care professional – ideally a health psychologist – when pain is an issue. The GCPS assesses both pain intensity and pain-related disability with regard to the degree the pain interferes with the patient's life. High levels of pain suggest the need to rule out clinically significant disease first but may indicate that the patient has amplification of symptoms because of emotional distress or central sensitization. The JFLS, as a specific measure of the masticatory system, assesses functional limitation and complements the findings from the GCPS. The JFLS has a short form for global assessment of patient-reported ability to use the jaw for mastication, mobility, and other functions and a long form that can group the findings into three constructs: mastication, mobility, and emotional and verbal expression.

Pain drawing assesses for local, regional, or widespread pain. Local pain is limited to the masticatory area, and regional pain often is present because many patients with TMD also have concurrent cervical conditions. When cervical pain is present, then medical assessment, including evaluation by a physician or physical therapist, can be considered. Widespread pain throughout the body is suggestive of systemic pain disorders such as rheumatic diseases, including rheumatoid arthritis and fibromyalgia. When widespread pain is present, assessment of the systemic condition may be needed to have a clinically significant effect on the 'local' TMD. However, widespread and multiple bodily complaints may indicate that the patient has amplification of pain from central sensitization and emotional dysregulation, and these patients need multidisciplinary treatment teams. Finally, comprehensive assessment of parafunctional behaviors (for example, oral habits) is important because they can overload the masticatory structures. The available evidence supports a clinical suspicion that such behaviors can cause or perpetuate the patient's pain.

Further development of orofacial and temporomandibular disorder pain classification

Currently the IASP Task Force is working on a simple and pragmatic classification model of chronic pain with seven proposed main categories (Treede et al., 2015) (Figure 2.1):

1. primary pain

2. cancer pain

3. postsurgical and post-traumatic pain

4. neuropathic pain

5. headache and orofacial pain

6. visceral pain, and

7. musculoskeletal pain.

The significance of this new pain classification is that TMD pain could have multiple 'parents,' that is, TMD pain could be considered to be a primary type of pain (idiopathic pain), but it could also be a musculoskeletal (muscle, joint, ligaments, tendons) type of pain, in addition to obviously also being an orofacial (anatomical) type of pain. Moreover, TMD pain may be comorbid with many other chronic pain conditions. It should be noted that 'chronic' in accordance with the new definition means longer than three months' duration instead of the old IASP definition of six months' duration. The subgroup of headaches and orofacial pain will follow the ICHD-III and the DC/TMD classification and will allow for more emphasis on the remaining types of chronic orofacial pain. A final note is that this new IASP classification system is a compromise between a mechanistic classification (neuropathic pain), a topographical classification (headache and orofacial pain), and tissue classification (visceral and musculoskeletal pain). Nevertheless, this classification is sufficiently pragmatic and clinically applicable and, importantly, will be adopted by the International Classification of Diseases.

Given that this endeavor is inherently multidisciplinary, debates are welcome and compromises required. Hopefully the current progress in classification of not only the TMDs but also chronic pain will lead to improved research studies focusing on risk factors and underlying pain mechanisms in addition to better management of patients with TMD pain.

References

AADR – American Association for Dental Research. Temporomandibular disorders (TMD). Science Policy, 2015. Available: http://www.iadr.org/AADR/About-Us/Policy-Statements/Science-Policy#TMD [Oct 23, 2017].

AAOP – American Academy of Orofacial Pain. de Leeuw R (ed.) Orofacial Pain: Guidelines for Assessment, Diagnosis and Management. 4th ed. Chicago, IL: Quintessence Publishing Co., Inc.; 2008.

Castrillon EE, Ou KL, Wang K et al. Sleep bruxism: an updated review of an old problem. Acta Odontol Scand 2016; 74: 328–334.

Ceusters W, Michelotti A, Raphael KG, Durham J, Ohrbach R. Perspectives on next steps in classification of orofacial pain – Part 1: role of ontology. J Oral Rehabil 2015a; 42: 926–941.

Ceusters W, Nasri-Heir C, Alnaas D et al. Perspectives on next steps in classification of orofacial pain – Part 3: biomarkers of chronic orofacial pain – from research to clinic. J Oral Rehabil 2015b; 42: 956–966.

Chantaracherd P, John MT, Hodges JS, Schiffman EL. Temporomandibular joint disorders' impact on pain, function, and disability. J Dent Res 2015; 94: 79S-86S.

Conti PC, Costa YM, Gonçalves DA, Svensson P. Headaches and myofascial temporomandibular disorders: overlapping entities, separate managements? J Oral Rehabil 2016; 43: 702–715.

Durham J, Raphael KG, Benoliel R et al. Perspectives on next steps in classification of orofacial pain – Part 2: role of psychosocial factors. J Oral Rehabil 2015; 42: 942–955.

Dworkin SF, LeResche L. Research diagnostic criteria for temporomandibular disorders: review, criteria, examinations and specifications, critique. J Craniomandib Disord 1992; 6: 301–355.

Fillingim RB, Bruehl S, Dworkin RH et al. The ACTTION-American Pain Society Pain Taxonomy (AAPT): an evidence based and multidimensional approach to classifying chronic pain conditions. J Pain 2014; 15: 241–249.

Gonzalez YM, Schiffman EL, Gordon SM et al. Development of a brief and effective TMD-pain screening questionnaire: Reliability and validity. J Am Dent Assoc 2011; 24: 1183–1191.

Graven-Nielsen T. Fundamentals of muscle pain, referred pain, and deep tissue hyperalgesia. Scand J Rheumatol 2006; 122: S1-S43.

ICHD-II. Headache Classification Subcommittee of the International Headache Society (IHS). The International Classification of Headache Disorders, 2nd ed. Cephalalgia 2004; 24: S9-S160.

ICHD-III. Headache Classification Committee of the International Headache Society (IHS). The International Classification of Headache Disorders, 3rd ed. Cephalalgia 2013; 33: 629–808.

Lobbezoo F, Ahlberg J, Glaros AG et al. Bruxism defined and graded: an international consensus. J Oral Rehabil 2013; 40: 2–4.

Michelotti A, Alstergren P, Goulet JP et al. Next steps in development of the diagnostic criteria for temporomandibular disorders (DC/TMD): Recommendations from the International RDC/TMD Consortium Network workshop. J Oral Rehabil 2016; 43: 453–467.

Ohrbach R, Dworkin SF. The evolution of TMD diagnosis: past, present, future. J Dental Res 2016; 95: 1093–1101.

Peck CC, Goulet J-P, Lobbezoo F, et al. Expanding the taxonomy of the diagnostic criteria for temporomandibular disorders. J Oral Rehab 2014; 41: 2–23.

Renton T, Durham J, Aggarwal VR. The classification and differential diagnosis of orofacial pain. Expert Rev Neurother 2012; 12: 569–576.

Schiffman E, Ohrbach R, Truelove E et al. Diagnostic criteria for temporomandibular disorders (DC/TMD) for clinical and research applications: recommendations of the International RDC/TMD Consortium Network and Orofacial Pain Special Interest Group. J Oral Facial Pain Headache 2014; 28: 6–27.

Schiffman E, Ohrbach R. Executive summary of the diagnostic criteria for temporomandibular disorders for clinical and research applications. J Am Dent Assoc 2016; 147: 438–445.

Schiffman EL, Ahmad M, Hollender L et al. Longitudinal stability of common TMJ structural disorders. J Dent Res 2017; 9: 270–276.

Sessle BJ. Acute and chronic craniofacial pain: brainstem mechanisms of nociceptive transmission and neuroplasticity, and their clinical correlates. Crit Rev Oral Biol Med 2000; 11: 57–91.

Slade GD, Fillingim RB, Sanders AE et al. Summary of findings from the OPPERA prospective cohort study of incidence of first-onset temporomandibular disorder: implications and future directions. J Pain 2013; 14: S116–S124.

Slade GD, Ohrbach R, Greenspan JD, et al. Painful temporomandibular disorder: decade of discovery from OPPERA Studies. J Dent Res 2016; 95: 1084–1092.

Svensson P, Graven-Nielsen T. Craniofacial muscle pain: review of mechanisms and clinical manifestations. J Orofac Pain 2001; 15: 117–145.

Svensson P, Jadidi F, Arima T, Baad-Hansen L, Sessle BJ. Relationships between craniofacial pain and bruxism. J Oral Rehabil 2008; 35: 524–547.

Svensson P, Michelotti A, Lobbezoo F, List T. The many faces of persistent orofacial muscle pain. J Oral Facial Pain Headache 2015; 29: 207–208.

Svensson P, Kumar A. Assessment of risk factors for oro-facial pain and recent developments in classification: implications for management. J Oral Rehabil 2016; 43: 977–989.

Treede RD, Rief W, Barke A, et al. A classification of chronic pain for ICD-11. Pain 2015; 156: 1003–1007.

Verkerk K, Luijsterburg PA, Heymans MW et al. Prognosis and course of pain in patients with chronic non-specific low back pain: a 1-year follow-up cohort study. Eur J Pain 2015; 19: 1101–1110.

Chapter 3
Trigeminal nociceptive processing
Brian E. Cairns

Pathway of trigeminal nociception

Pain reported by patients with temporomandibular disorders (TMDs) is often localized in the temporomandibular joint (TMJ), masseter and temporalis muscles, although involvement of other masticatory musculature (for example medial pterygoid, digastric, and mylohyoid) and spread to other craniofacial tissues may be reported. The masticatory muscles and TMJ are supplied by branches of the mandibular nerve (V3). Small diameter unmyelinated (C fibers) and myelinated (Aδ fibers) fibers with free nerve endings are thought to be the principal transducers of nociceptive stimuli from these tissues. In fact, these tissues are also innervated by Aβ fibers that play an important role in sensing non-noxious mechanical stimulation of the muscle and joint, and likely contribute to the localization of pain in these tissues. In addition, the jaw closer muscles are innervated by spindle afferent fibers, which play an important role in reflex modulation of jaw muscle activity as well as in proprioception. The jaw opener muscles generally lack spindle afferent fibers and thus the jaw does not have the same opposing reflex drives as other joints (for example the knee) (Capra et al., 2007). Although not directly involved in the transduction of nociceptive stimulation, pain in the masticatory muscles modifies the output of spindle afferent fibers, which leads to altered jaw muscle reflex activity such as an enhancement of masseteric stretch reflex (Capra et al., 2007).

The small diameter afferent fibers from the masticatory muscles and TMJ project by way of the trigeminal ganglion to the ipsilateral brainstem where second and higher order trigeminal sensory neurons are located. The trigeminal ganglion contains the cell bodies (soma) of nerve fibers that innervate the craniofacial region. These trigeminal ganglion neurons are round and lack synapses (Figure 3.1). They are completely encircled by a number of small accessory cells called satellite glial cells (SGCs), which are thought to play a role similar to astrocytes, a type of glial cell, in the central nervous system (Ohara et al., 2009; Takeda et al., 2009). Trigeminal ganglion neurons that innervate the jaw closer muscles have been studied and have been found to express a large number of receptors including N-methyl-D-aspartate (NMDA) and purinoceptor 3 (P_2X_3) receptors, commonly associated with nociceptive neurons in the central nervous system (Kondo et al., 1995; Sahara et al., 1997; Quartu et al., 2002; Dong et al., 2007; Wang et al., 2012; Cairns et al., 2014). The SGCs function in a similar way to astrocytes in the central nervous system in that they remove ions and neurotransmitters from the extracellular space around the ganglion neurons, and supply neurotrophic and other factors to maintain the health and functioning of the trigeminal nerve fibers (Takeda et al., 2009). This is consistent with the concept that SGCs control the microenvironment surrounding the ganglion neuron (Takeda et al., 2009; Ohara et al., 2009; Goto et al., 2016). Interestingly, SGCs contain neurotransmitters, such as glutamate and adenosine triphosphate (ATP) that activate NMDA and P_2X_3 receptors, which may mean that there is communication between ganglion neurons and their surrounding SGCs in the trigeminal ganglion that may modify nociceptive input before it enters the central nervous system.

The brainstem trigeminal sensory nuclear complex (TSNC) has a tubular shape and is composed of neurons which take input from the craniofacial region. The TSNC is composed of several subnuclei, which appear to have different functions in orofacial pain processing. The three rostral subnuclei are called principalis (main sensory), oralis, and

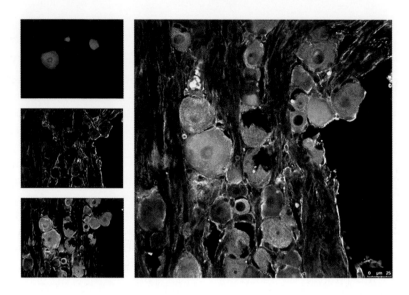

Figure 3.1

The images show trigeminal ganglion neurons that project to the temporalis muscle and their associated satellite glial cells (SGCs) (main image). The ganglion neurons were identified by injection of the fluorescent dye fast blue into the temporalis muscle (top left image). SGCs are identified by their expression of glutamine synthetase (middle left image) and it can be seen that these cells surround the soma of the ganglion neuron. The expression of the receptor for fractalkine, a chemotactic cytokine (chemokine), is shown in the lower left image. Fractalkine is proposed to contribute to crosstalk between trigeminal ganglion neurons and SGCs (Cairns et al., 2017).

interpolaris, and play an important role in motor reflex coordination and innocuous thermal and mechanical sensory input from the face, underlying muscles and joints, as well as receiving innocuous and noxious input from the oral cavity (Figure 3.2). In contrast, trigeminal neurons that respond to nociceptive input from the orofacial region outside of the oral cavity are generally found in the posterior third of the interpolaris, and in the most caudal subnucleus of the TSNC, the caudalis (Sessle, 2005). The structure of the caudalis becomes organized into lamina as it nears the cervical spinal cord, and thus resembles the structure of the spinal dorsal horn. As a result, the caudalis is often referred to as the medullary dorsal horn (Sessle, 2005). Small-diameter afferent fibers from the masticatory muscles and the

TMJ have been shown to project principally to this region of the TSNC as well as to the rostral part of the cervical dorsal horn (Nishimori et al., 1986; Capra & Dessem, 1992).

A subgroup of neurons found in the interpolaris and caudalis respond to noxious stimulation of the orofacial region, including the masticatory muscles and TMJ. Nociceptive information then ascends, via the trigeminothalamic tract, to the ventrobasal complex, the posterior group of nuclei and the medial part of the thalamus, where thalamic neurons that respond to noxious orofacial stimulation are found (Sessle, 2005). There are also important projections from the caudal TSNC to the motor nuclei, the parabrachial nucleus and the reticular formation,

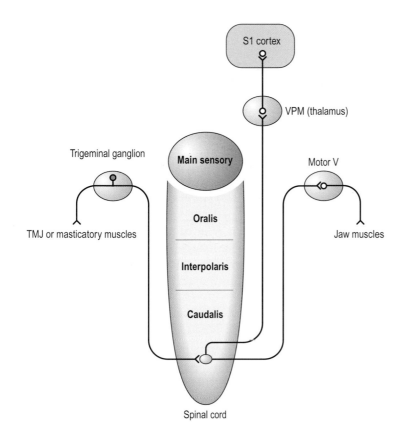

S1 cortex

VPM (thalamus)

Trigeminal ganglion

Main sensory

Motor V

TMJ or masticatory muscles

Oralis

Jaw muscles

Interpolaris

Caudalis

Spinal cord

Figure 3.2
Trigeminal afferent fibers that innervate the craniofacial region project by way of the trigeminal ganglion to the TSNC, where second order neurons that integrate sensory information are located. The subnucleus caudalis receives the majority of nociceptive input from the masticatory muscles and TMJ. The major output from the TSNC is to the ventral posteromedial nucleus of the thalamus, which itself projects to various regions of the cortex.

which are involved in motor and autonomic control respectively (Sessle, 2005). From the thalamus, the main projection of nociceptive responsive thalamic neurons is to the primary somatosensory cortex, where pain perception is thought to occur.

Functional characteristics of masticatory muscle and temporomandibular nociceptors and the role of peripheral sensitization

Aδ and C fibers that innervate the TMJ and masticatory musculature respond to noxious mechanical and chemical stimuli with action potential discharges consistent with the role of these fibers in nociception. These deep-tissue nociceptors are activated by mechanical stimulation at or above the intensity required to produce withdrawal reflexes in rats or pain reports in humans (Cairns, 2007). Mechanical nociceptors of the TMJ are also activated by excessive protrusion, lateral movement or jaw rotation of the joint, and begin to discharge as these motions exceed the normal range of jaw movement (Cairns, 2007). Sustained noxious mechanical stimulation of the muscle or joint results in prolonged action potential discharges in these afferent fibers that, in some cases, continue after the cessation of the stimulus (after discharges). Tissue injury also results in the release of a number of substances, which include prostaglandins, neurotransmitters and cytokines that activate the endings of nociceptors resulting in action potential discharge (Sessle, 2005). Many of these same fibers also exhibit robust responses to injection of one or more algogenic substances into the muscle or joint tissue, which suggests that they function as polymodal nociceptors. For example, masticatory muscle injection of glutamate, which is acutely painful in humans, causes prolonged action potential discharges which can be attenuated by NMDA receptor antagonists, such as ketamine (Cairns et al., 2002a; Cairns et al., 2003; Castrillon et al., 2007). In addition to producing action potential discharges, glutamate injection also decreases the mechanical threshold for activation of the nerve ending; an effect termed peripheral sensitization. In the case of injection of glutamate, this peripheral sensitization can last for many hours after a single injection.

Research has demonstrated that a number of other putative pain-causing substances, which include serotonin, ATP, prostaglandin E2, nerve growth factor, tumor necrosis factor alpha, and potassium, when injected into the masticatory muscle or TMJ, produce peripheral sensitization (Gerdle et al., 2014). At least two of these substances, glutamate and serotonin, have been shown to be elevated in the masticatory muscles of patients with TMD, and there is some evidence that antagonists for the NMDA and 5-HT3 receptor, selectively, can attenuate pain in certain TMD sufferers (Castrillon et al., 2008; Chrisditis et al., 2015). Further, NSAIDs, which block the synthesis of prostanglandins, appear to be effective analgesics for some TMD-related pain. Elevation of nerve growth factor, which is important for maintaining the health of the nerves, in the masticatory muscles has been demonstrated to produce a particularly prolonged peripheral sensitization, which can last days to weeks in both animals and humans (Svensson et al., 2003; Wong et al., 2014). The mechanism of nerve growth factor appears to involve a 'phenotypic' switch, whereby previously non-nociceptive afferent fibers begin behaving more like nociceptors (Wong et al., 2014). The extent to which peripheral sensitization contributes to ongoing pain in TMD remains a subject of debate; however, it is likely that this mechanism is important not only for initiating jaw muscle and joint pain but also for maintaining it.

The endings of nociceptors have vesicles that can, upon excitation of the ending, fuse with the cell membrane and release neuromodulatory substances into a particular tissue. These substances include neuropeptides, for example substance P or calcitonin gene-related peptide (CGRP), as well as neurotransmitters such as glutamate (Ichikawa et al., 1990; Kido et al., 1995; Lundeberg et al., 1996; Loughner et al., 1997). The neuropeptides produce vasodilation and plasma protein extravasation, while neurogenic release of glutamate results in excitation and sensitization of the afferent ending (Gazerani et al., 2010). This effect is referred to as neurogenic inflammation, and while it has been proposed to contribute to migraine headache, it is unknown if it also contributes significantly to pathogenesis of TMDs.

The trigeminal ganglia were once thought to be a passive conduit of action potentials to the central nervous system. However, activation of ganglion neurons results in alterations in the expression of ion channel proteins and neuropeptides, which suggests that these cells may not be as passive as once thought (Goto et al., 2016). Further, it has been proposed that SGCs modulate the activity of ganglion neurons by releasing neuroactive substances into a gap of about 20 nm between the neuronal and SGC cell membranes (Ohara et al., 2009; Takeda et al., 2009). Glutamate receptors have been found in trigeminal ganglion neurons (Kondo et al., 1995; Sahara et al., 1997; Quartu et al., 2002; Dong et al., 2007; Wang et al., 2012; Cairns et al., 2014) and it has been suggested that glutamate may serve as a 'neuro-glial' transmitter in the trigeminal ganglion (Kung et al., 2013) (Figure 3.3). Trigeminal ganglion neurons as well as SGCs release glutamate when activated (Puil & Spigelman, 1988; Kung et al., 2013; Laursen et al., 2014). Ganglion neurons that innervate the jaw muscles fire action potentials when the concentration of glutamate in the trigeminal ganglion is increased (Laursen et al., 2014). Increased action potential discharge in afferent fibers that innervate the masticatory muscles and TMJ could then lead to increased glutamate concentrations in the trigeminal ganglion resulting in ectopic firing of

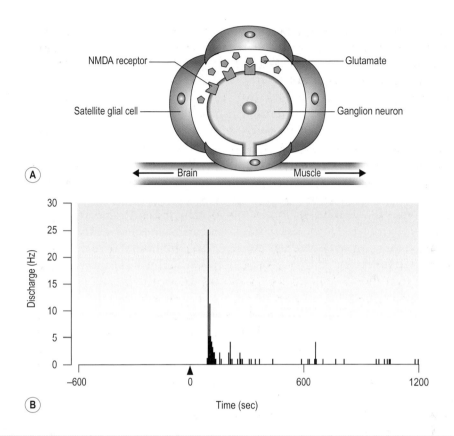

Figure 3.3

(A) The image illustrates how elevation of glutamate in the trigeminal ganglion could induce ectopic action potential discharge in a trigeminal ganglion neuron that innervated the temporalis muscle. (B) Injection of glutamate into the ganglion at time 0 (arrow head) produced a short, but robust action potential discharge followed by a prolonged period of sporadic action potential discharge from this ganglion neuron.

trigeminal ganglion neurons. This may serve to further amplify the pain signal. This suggests the possibility of neuroplastic changes in the sensory ganglia that may alter transmission of sensory information from tissues to the brain to affect sensation.

Elevation of intraganglionic glutamate concentration also decreases the mechanical threshold of the afferent endings in the masticatory muscles (Laursen et al., 2014). This mechanical sensitization was subsequently found to last for more than three hours after

a single injection of glutamate, and was mediated through activation of NMDA receptors. The underlying mechanism for this effect has not been determined; however, it does not appear to involve central nervous system activation as it occurs even when input from the trigeminal ganglion to the caudal brainstem is blocked with a local anesthetic (Laursen et al., 2014). It also does not appear to require action potentials to be generated in the ganglion neuron under study, as intraganglionic injection of a nitric oxide donor or fractalkine (a molecule proposed to mediate ganglion neuron-SGC communication in sensory ganglia) both induced prolonged mechanical sensitization of masticatory muscle afferent fibers without evoking action potential discharge (Cairns et al., 2014; Cairns et al., 2017). Nitric oxide-induced changes appeared to be mediated through prostaglandin E2 release by SGCs (Laursen et al., 2013; Cairns et al., 2014). One explanation for how activity in the trigeminal ganglion can affect the afferent endings so far away from it is that neurons or SGCs are able to release neuromodulatory substances into the systemic circulation. If true, this would mean that sensory ganglia have an endocrine-organ-like role that influences sensory transmission and perhaps other physiological functions.

It has also been suggested that ganglion neurons can communicate with each other through SGCs (Takeda et al., 2009; Goto et al., 2016). Some trigeminal ganglion neurons and their associated SGCs release ATP (Villa et al., 2010; Goto et al., 2016). It has been proposed that the released ATP acts on ATP receptors expressed by SGCs, causing SGCs to release more ATP that can affect neighboring SGCs, which then release this neurotransmitter to act on the ganglion neuron they surround, to pass the signal from one ganglion neuron to the next (Goto et al., 2016). Elevation of ATP levels in the trigeminal ganglion also leads to peripheral sensitization. The spread of an excitatory neurotransmitter, such as ATP or glutamate, through the trigeminal ganglion could lead to activation of adjacent ganglion neurons that innervate different tissues and lead to pain expansion and referral. Taken together, these recent studies are suggesting that some features of TMD pain such as secondary hyperalgesia and pain referral may be partly generated in the peripheral nervous system as well as in the central nervous system.

Trigeminal nociceptive neurons

As in the spinal cord, the response properties of neurons in the TSNC fall into three functional categories: low-threshold mechanoreceptive neurons, wide dynamic range neurons, and nociceptive-specific neurons (Sessle, 2005). Low-threshold mechanoreceptive (LTM) neurons are activated by innocuous mechanical stimulation applied to the face or head, and respond maximally to stimulation that is below the nociceptive threshold. Wide dynamic range (WDR) neurons are characterized by their ability to code the intensity of mechanical stimulation through increased action potential discharge from innocuous through noxious mechanical cutaneous stimulation. Nociceptive-specific (NS) neurons, as their name implies, are only activated by noxious cutaneous stimulation. Although some NS and WDR neurons that respond to noxious stimulation of the oral cavity (for example the teeth) are found in the rostral TSNC, the vast majority of NS and WDR neurons that respond to noxious activation of the masticatory muscles and TMJ are found the interpolaris and caudalis (Sessle, 2005). These nociceptive trigeminal neurons are commonly activated by innocuous and/or noxious stimulation of both the skin and deep craniofacial tissues. This convergence of input from different craniofacial tissues on a single neuron may, in part, explain not only pain referral, whereby intense noxious stimulation of the masticatory muscles or TMJ results in pain being felt in other regions of the face, but also the generally poor localization of pain from deeper structures in the craniofacial region (Sessle, 2005).

Most trigeminal nociceptive neurons can be activated by stimulation of discrete areas of the face and specific deep tissues. The area of a tissue that can be stimulated to activate trigeminal nociceptive neurons is called its receptive field. Tissue injury induces a sustained noxious input that has been shown to lower the stimulus intensity within the receptive field required to activate trigeminal nociceptive neurons as well as expand the size of their receptive fields and occasionally result in the emergence of novel receptive fields (regions of the face that did not result in neuronal action potential discharge prior to injury). These injury-induced changes in neuronal response properties are referred to as 'central sensitization,' and are manifested in patients with TMD as hyperalgesia and referral. Importantly, central sensitization can be produced in trigeminal nociceptive neurons by noxious stimulation of the craniofacial region outside of the receptive field of the neuron. Damage to deep tissues, specifically masticatory muscle or the TMJ, is substantially more effective in producing central sensitization than noxious stimulation of the skin (Sessle, 2005). This effect is thought to underlie the generalized increased sensitivity to painful stimulation of the craniofacial region and other regions of the body reported by some TMD patients.

It is now being recognized that there is considerable crosstalk between neurons and glial cells, which contributes to the long-term changes in central nervous system excitability that occur due to sustained noxious input from craniofacial tissues (Ren & Dubner, 2016). Glial cells (that is, astrocytes and microglia) exhibit increased activity after injury to TMJ or masticatory muscles and are thought to contribute to the mechanisms that initiate and maintain central sensitization (Ren & Dubner, 2016). It has been proposed that intense input to sensory neurons results in the release of fractalkine, which activates microglia through the fractalkine receptor (CX3CR1) (Ren & Dubner, 2016). This increase in glial activity is accompanied by elevated levels of inflammatory cytokines (for example interleukins (IL) 1b and 6) as well as glutamate and ATP in the TSNC that increase neuronal excitability. Inhibitors of glial activation, such as methionine sulfoximine and minocycline, can greatly attenuate the sensitization of TSNC neurons that occurs after tissue injury, which indicates a significant role for glial cell mechanisms in this phenomenon.

It is also possible to modulate the activity of nociceptive neurons in the TSNC. A number of brain centers are involved in the descending modulation of TSNC neuronal activity, for example periaqueductal gray, rostral ventromedial medulla, and the sensorimotor cortex. Activation of these centers can either facilitate or inhibit the activity of nociceptive WDR and NS neurons as a result of increased levels of neurochemicals, such as serotonin, enkephalins and g-aminobutyric acid (GABA), in the TSNC. Further, it is also possible to decrease the excitability of trigeminal nociceptive neurons by applying noxious stimulation outside of the orofacial region – a phenomenon termed diffuse noxious inhibitory controls (DNIC). It has been speculated that part of the enhanced pain sensitivity in TMD patients is due to decreased endogenous pain control mechanisms (King et al., 2009).

Thalamic processing of nociceptive input from the orofacial region

A subset of neurons in the nucleus ventralis posteromedialis (VPM), posterior group and medial thalamus respond to noxious stimulation of the craniofacial region (Sessle, 2005). These neurons can also be subdivided into WDR and NS categories, similar to neurons in the TSNC (Sessle, 2005). However, unlike nociceptive neurons in the subnucleus caudalis, these thalamic nociceptive neurons are much more likely to exhibit spontaneous action potential discharge. VPM nociceptive neurons have connections with the somatosensory cerebral cortex compatible with a function of localization and discrimination of painful stimuli. VPM neurons can also undergo a process of central sensitization after tissue injury, but this only occurs when the subnucleus caudalis is intact (Park et al., 2006), suggesting that it may be driven by changes to caudalis neurons described previously. Nociceptive neurons in the intralaminar and medial thalamic nuclei are connected to areas such as the hypothalamus and anterior cingulate cortex, which suggests that they may be more involved in mediating the affective or motivation dimensions of craniofacial pain (Sessle, 2005; Sugiyo et al., 2006).

Cortical regions associated with the processing of orofacial nociceptive information

The principal projection of thalamic neurons that respond to noxious stimulation of the face is to the primary somatosensory area (SI) of the cerebral cortex.

As in the brainstem and thalamus, cortical neurons in this region can be excited by noxious orofacial stimulation and exhibit WDR and NS-like response properties (Sessle, 2005; Takeda et al., 2010). These cortical neurons are thought to code the sensory-discriminative dimension of pain. Other regions of the cortex, such as the anterior cingulate cortex and insula also contain nociceptive neurons. Neurons in these regions of the cortex are limited in their ability to indicate stimulus location and intensity and thus are thought to contribute to affective, attentional and motivational components of chronic orofacial pain.

Trigeminal pain processing and temporomandibular disorder pain

Most of what is known about neural processing of pain from the masticatory musculature and TMJ has been derived from animal models where acute, often inflammatory injury has been made. In this respect, pain mechanisms derived from these models may not be applicable to chronic TMD pain. Some attempts have been made to create longer lasting models of masticatory muscle and TMDs. For example, unilateral ligation of the tendon on the anterior-superior part of the masseter muscle causes over eight weeks of mechanical sensitization in this region of the muscle (Guo et al., 2010). This model produces central sensitization that includes a robust activation of astrocytes and microglia in the subnucleus caudalis. Another model uses discrete injection of nerve growth factor (NGF), which is released upon tissue injury, into the masseter muscle. This model is of interest because it produces a punctate region of muscle mechanical sensitization that is confined to the injection site in the absence of gross tissue inflammation. Injection of NGF produces rapid sensitization of muscle nociceptors to mechanical stimulation that is mediated through activation of the tropomysin receptor kinase A (TrkA) receptor, a neurotrophin receptor that selectively binds NGF. NGF appears to induce a phenotypic change in non-nociceptive afferent fibers that innervate the

muscles so that they begin to exhibit properties of nociceptors (Wong et al., 2014). It has also been possible to assess the effect of intramuscular injections on healthy human subjects. Subjects injected with NGF report a discrete area of muscle tenderness at the site of injection that does not spread, and is only painful upon palpation or occasionally when opening the jaw (for example when yawning or chewing). This sensitization lasts several weeks after a single injection and is greater in women than in men. This model is, therefore, valuable for studying localized tender areas in the masticatory muscles, which are a consistent feature of myofascial TMD.

A majority of TMD sufferers attending pain clinics are women. It has been suggested for many years that sex hormones, and in particular estrogens, may be responsible for sex-related differences in the prevalence of TMDs (LeResche et al., 1997; LeResche et al., 2003). Both peripheral and central neural sites of action for estrogen modulation of nociception have been identified. Estrogen receptors are expressed by trigeminal ganglion neurons that innervate masticatory muscle (Wang et al., 2012), as well as in nociceptive neurons in the subnucleus caudalis (Amandusson & Blomqvist, 2010). Noxious stimulation of the TMJ or the masticatory muscles evokes greater afferent fiber discharges and reflex jaw muscle activity in females than in males (Cairns et al., 2002b; Dong et al., 2007). This effect appears to be mediated in part by estrogens, since female ovariectomy eliminates, while estrogen-replacement therapy restores, these sex-related differences. Taken together, these findings support the view that there is an enhanced responsiveness to injury of the masticatory muscles and TMJ in females as compared with males.

Current pharmacological treatment of TMD-related pain remains largely empirical due to a paucity of well-designed clinical trials. Systemically, locally or topically administered nonsteroidal anti-inflammatory drugs (NSAIDs), such as naproxen, ibuprofen and diclofenac, may be useful for the treatment of TMD pain. Evidence also indicates that in addition to inhibiting prostaglandin production, local administration of diclofenac and ketorolac may competitively inhibit the NMDA subtype of the glutamate receptor, which is found on masticatory muscle and TMJ nociceptors (Cairns et al., 2002b; Dong et al., 2007). This mechanism may contribute to the effectiveness of diclofenac-containing topical preparations for TMD-related pain.

Conclusion

The pathogenesis of TMD pain remains uncertain (Cairns, 2010). There continues to be considerable debate about the relative importance of peripheral versus central mechanisms in the development and maintenance of muscle and joint pain in TMD patients. It is clear that central sensitization plays a critical role in the underlying mechanisms of some characteristics of TMD-related pain and, in particular, explains why

some of these patients have lowered thresholds for pain at sites outside of the craniofacial region. Central sensitization may also underlie the unusual pattern of pain referral found in some TMD patients. For example, pain in the deep masseter muscle may be referred to the posterior maxillary teeth, while pain from the anterior temporalis or middle masseter muscles can be referred to the anterior maxillary teeth. However, symptoms of localized muscle or joint pain and tenderness may be more reflective of peripheral sensitization. Recent work makes it conceivable that even some of the unusual referral patterns of TMD pain could also be produced by a peripheral mechanism, for example through neuronal-SGC interactions in the trigeminal ganglion. Determining the relative contributions of peripheral and central pain mechanisms to pain in individual TMD patients can help determine which treatments are likely to be most beneficial.

References

Amandusson A, Blomqvist A. Estrogen receptor-alpha expression in nociceptive-responsive neurons in the medullary dorsal horn of the female rat. Eur J Pain 2010; 14: 245–258.

Cairns BE. Nociceptors in the orofacial region (temporomandibular joint & masseter muscle). In Schmidt RF, Willis WD (eds). Encyclopedia of Pain. Heidelberg, Germany: Springer-Verlag; 2007.

Cairns BE. Pathophysiology of TMD pain: basic mechanisms and their implications for pharmacotherapy. J Oral Rehabil 2010; 37: 391–410.

Cairns BE, Gambarota G, Svensson P, Arendt-Nielsen L, Berde CB. Glutamate-induced sensitization of rat masseter muscle fibers. Neuroscience 2002a; 109: 389–399.

Cairns BE, Sim Y, Bereiter DA, Sessle BJ, Hu J. Influence of sex on reflex jaw muscle activity evoked from the rat temporomandibular joint. Brain Res 2002b; 957: 338–344.

Cairns BE, Svensson P, Wang K et al. Activation of peripheral NMDA receptors contributes to human pain and rat afferent discharges evoked

by injection of glutamate into the masseter muscle. J Neurophysiol 2003; 90: 2098–2105.

Cairns BE, Laursen JC, Dong XD, Gazerani P. Intraganglionic injection of a nitric oxide donor induces afferent mechanical sensitization that is attenuated by palmitoylethanolamide. Cephalalgia 2014; 34: 686–694.

Cairns BE, O'Brien M, Dong XD, Gazerani P. Elevated fractalkine (CX3CL1) levels in the trigeminal ganglion mechanically sensitize temporalis muscle nociceptors. Mol Neurobiol 2017; 54: 3695–3706.

Capra NF, Dessem D. Central connections of trigeminal primary afferent neurons: topographical and functional considerations. Crit Rev Oral Biol Med 1992; 4: 1–52.

Capra NF, Hisley CK, Masri RM. The influence of pain on masseter spindle afferent discharge. Arch Oral Biol 2007; 52: 387–390.

Castrillon EE, Cairns BE, Ernberg M et al. Effect of a peripheral NMDA receptor antagonist on glutamate-evoked masseter muscle pain and mechanical sensitization in women. J Orofac Pain 2007; 21: 216–224.

Castrillon EE, Cairns BE, Ernberg M et al. Effect of peripheral NMDA receptor blockade with ketamine on chronic myofascial pain in temporomandibular disorder patients: a randomized, double-blinded, placebo-controlled trial. J Orofac Pain 2008; 22: 122–130.

Christidis N, Omrani S, Fredriksson L et al. Repeated tender point injections of granisetron alleviate chronic myofascial pain – a randomized, controlled, double-blinded trial. J Headache Pain 2015; 16: 104.

Dong XD, Mann MK, Kumar U et al. Sex-related differences in NMDA-evoked rat masseter muscle afferent discharge result from estrogen-mediated modulation of peripheral NMDA receptor activity. Neuroscience 2007; 146: 822–832.

Gazerani P, Au S, Dong X et al. Botulinum neurotoxin type A (BoNTA) decreases the mechanical sensitivity of nociceptors and inhibits neurogenic vasodilation in a craniofacial muscle targeted for migraine prophylaxis. Pain 2010; 151: 606–616.

Gerdle B, Ghafouri B, Ernberg M, Larsson B. Chronic musculoskeletal pain: review of mechanisms and biochemical biomarkers as assessed by the microdialysis technique. J Pain Res 2014; 7: 313–326.

Goto T, Oh SB, Takeda M et al. Recent advances in basic research on the trigeminal ganglion. J Physiol Sci 2016; 66: 381–386.

Guo W, Wang H, Zou S et al. Long lasting pain hypersensitivity following ligation of the tendon of the masseter muscle in rats: a model of myogenic orofacial pain. Mol Pain 2010; 6: 40.

Ichikawa H, Matsuo S, Wakisaka S, Akai M. Fine structure of calcitonin gene-related peptide-immunoreactive nerve fibres in the rat temporomandibular joint. Arch Oral Biol 1990; 35: 727–730.

Kido MA, Kiyoshima T, Ibuki T et al. A topographical and ultrastructural study of sensory trigeminal nerve endings in the rat temporomandibular joint as demonstrated by anterograde transport of wheat germ agglutinin-horseradish peroxidase (WGA-HRP). J Dent Res 1995; 74: 1353–1359.

King CD, Wong F, Currie T et al. Deficiency in endogenous modulation of prolonged heat pain in patients with irritable bowel syndrome and temporomandibular disorder. Pain 2009; 143: 172–178.

Kondo E, Kiyama H, Yamano M, Shida T, Ueda Y, Tohyama M. Expression of glutamate (AMPA type) and gamma-aminobutyric acid (GABA)A receptors in the rat caudal trigeminal spinal nucleus. Neurosci Lett 1995; 186: 169–172.

Kung LH, Gong K, Adedoyin M et al. Evidence for glutamate as a neuroglial transmitter within sensory ganglia. PLOS One 2013; 8: e68312.

Laursen JC, Cairns BE, Kumar U et al. Nitric oxide release from trigeminal satellite glial cells is attenuated by glial modulators and glutamate. Int J Physiol Pathophysiol Pharmacol 2013; 5: 228–238.

Laursen JC, Cairns BE, Dong XD et al. Glutamate dysregulation in the trigeminal ganglion: a novel mechanism for peripheral

sensitization of the craniofacial region. Neuroscience 2014; 256: 23–35.

LeResche L, Saunders K, Von Korff MR, Barlow W, Dworkin SF. Use of exogenous hormones and risk of temporomandibular disorder pain. Pain 1997; 69: 153–160.

LeResche L, Mancl L, Sherman JJ, Gandara B, Dworkin S. Changes in temporomandibular pain and other symptoms across the menstrual cycle. Pain 2003; 106: 253–261.

Loughner B, Miller J, Broumand V, Cooper B. The development of strains, forces and nociceptor activity in retrodiscal tissues of the temporomandibular joint of male and female goats. Exp Brain Res 1997; 113: 311–326.

Lundeberg T, Alstergren P, Appelgren A et al. A model for experimentally induced temporomandibular joint arthritis in rats: effects of carrageenan on neuropeptide-like immunoreactivity. Neuropeptides 1996; 30: 37–41.

Nishimori T, Sera M, Suemune S et al. The distribution of muscle primary afferents from the masseter nerve to the trigeminal sensory nuclei. Brain Res 1986; 372: 375–381.

Ohara PT, Vit JP, Bhargava A et al. Gliopathic pain: when satellite glial cells go bad. Neuroscientist 2009; 15: 450–463.

Park SJ, Zhang S, Chiang CY et al. Central sensitization induced in thalamic nociceptive neurons by tooth pulp stimulation is dependent on the functional integrity of trigeminal brainstem subnucleus caudalis but not subnucleus oralis. Brain Res 2006; 1112: 134–145.

Puil E, Spigelman I. Electrophysiological responses of trigeminal root ganglion neurons in vitro. Neuroscience 1988; 24: 635–646.

Quartu M, Serra MP, Ambu R, Lai ML, Del Fiacco M. AMPA-type glutamate receptor subunits 2/3 in the human trigeminal sensory ganglion and subnucleus caudalis from prenatal ages to adulthood. Mech Ageing Dev 2002; 123: 463–471.

Ren K, Dubner R. Activity-triggered tetrapartite neuron-glial interactions

following peripheral injury. Curr Opin Pharmacol 2016; 26: 16–25.

Sahara Y, Noro N, Iida Y, Soma K, Nakamura Y. Glutamate receptor subunits GluR5 and KA-2 are coexpressed in rat trigeminal ganglion neurons. J Neurosci 1997; 17: 6611–6620.

Sessle BJ. Peripheral and central mechanisms of orofacial pain and their clinical correlates. Minerva Anestesiol 2005; 71: 117–136.

Sugiyo S, Takemura M, Dubner R, Ren K. Demonstration of a trigeminothalamic pathway to the oval paracentral intralaminar thalamic nucleus and its involvement in the processing of noxious orofacial deep inputs. Brain Res 2006; 1097: 116–122.

Svensson P, Cairns BE, Wang K, Arendt-Nielsen L. Injection of nerve growth factor into human masseter muscle evokes long-lasting mechanical allodynia and hyperalgesia. Pain 2003; 104: 241–247.

Takeda M, Takahashi M, Matsumoto S. Contribution of the activation of satellite glia in sensory ganglia to pathological pain. Neurosci Biobehav Rev 2009; 33: 784–792.

Takeda M, Takahashi M, Nasu M, Matsumoto S. In vivo patch-clamp analysis of response properties of rat primary somatosensory cortical neurons responding to noxious stimulation of the facial skin. Mol Pain 2010; 6: 30.

Villa G, Fumagalli M, Verderio C, Abbracchio MP, Ceruti S. Expression and contribution of satellite glial cells purinoceptors to pain transmission in sensory ganglia: an update. Neuron Glia Biol 2010; 6: 31–42.

Wang MW, Kumar U, Dong XD, Cairns BE. Expression of NMDA and oestrogen receptors by trigeminal ganglion neurons that innervate the rat temporalis muscle. Chin J Dent Res 2012; 15: 89–97.

Wong H, Kang I, Dong XD et al. NGF-induced mechanical sensitization of the masseter muscle is mediated through peripheral NMDA receptors. Neuroscience 2014; 269: 232–344.

Chapter 4
Pathophysiology of temporomandibular pain

Abhishek Kumar, Fernando G. Exposto, Hao-Jun You, Peter Svensson

Basic pain research related to temporomandibular disorders

Pioneers in the field of basic pain research into temporomandibular disorders (TMDs) over the last four decades have carefully and systematically dissected the trigeminal nociceptive system. Research in this field has judiciously characterized the peripheral nociceptors, afferent fiber properties, trigeminal brainstem sensory nuclei, thalamic nuclei and cortical networks (Sessle, 2000; Woda, 2003; Stohler & Zubieta, 2010; Ren & Dubner, 2011). The susceptibility of the nociceptive system together with the inherent property of neuroplasticity leading to peripheral and central sensitization has been convincingly demonstrated and is certainly a key element in much of this research (Hucho & Levine, 2007; Woolf, 2011; Denk et al., 2014). Neuroplasticity in the present context refers to the change in the input–output relation between external stimuli and the neuronal and behavioral output. The term 'plasticity' essentially means that the (nociceptive) system remains changed (that is, is irreversible); however, several animal and human studies have shown that 'neuroplastic' changes may be temporary and can revert to baseline conditions (that is, they are reversible). The question therefore is: do current animal and human experimental pain models adequately represent (reversible) 'neuro-elasticity' as opposed to (irreversible) 'neuroplasticity'?

In TMD pain, peripheral sensitization can occur both at the level of muscle and joint nociceptors (Cairns, 2010; Sessle, 2011). For the joint, peripheral sensitization can occur due to increased loading and remodeling which leads to the release of inflammatory substances such as substance P, calcitonin gene-related peptide (CGRP), tumor necrosis factor alpha (TNFα), and interleukins (Alstergren et al., 1998). This mix of substances is usually referred to as neurogenic inflammation, and is in turn responsible for the major signs and symptoms of inflammation such as redness, edema, temperature increase and pain (Takahashi et al., 1998; Sato et al., 2004; Takeuchi et al., 2004; Sato et al., 2007). Regarding the muscle, it is thought that adenosine triphosphate (ATP) and protons can cause the activation of muscle nociceptors and in turn release similar substances as when joint nociceptors are activated, for example substance P, CGRP, bradykinin, TNFα and nerve growth factor (NGF). Because of the release of these substances in both the joint and the muscle, nociceptors become sensitized and as such a lower threshold for nociceptor depolarization is present leading to hyperalgesia (increased sensitivity to stimuli that usually cause pain) (Cairns, 2010; Sessle, 2011). As a consequence, a higher susceptibility to stimuli, for example evoked by normal jaw function, can occur, causing pain with chewing, yawning, and talking.

If this peripheral sensitization state persists with a sufficient intensity, it can lead to sensitization of both nociceptive-specific and wide-dynamic range neurons of the subnucleus caudalis within the central nervous system which is termed central sensitization. Indeed central sensitization could be responsible for the phenomenon of allodynia (pain triggered by non-noxious stimuli) (Woolf, 2011; Chichorro et al., 2017). If this sensitization is contained within the trigeminal system, the hyperalgesia and allodynia will be limited to the areas innervated by the trigeminal nerve. If it spreads to third-order neurons in the thalamus, then this could lead to hypersensitivity in more widespread areas that are not innervated by the trigeminal nerve (Burstein et al., 2000; Woolf, 2011).

Clinically, it is has been shown that TMD patients (both myogenous and arthralgic) have lowered pain thresholds in the painful area compared to healthy controls (Svensson et al., 2001; Vierck et al., 2014). This can be explained through peripheral sensitization caused by the release of the algogenic substances discussed above. On the other hand, studies looking at psychophysical correlates of central sensitization such as temporal summation in patients with TMD have shown mixed results. There have been studies that have shown increased temporal summation of pain (Sarlani et al., 2004a; Sarlani et al., 2004b) and decreased pain thresholds in extracranial body sites in TMD patients when compared to healthy controls (Ayesh et al., 2007; Fernández-de-las-Peñas et al., 2009). On the other hand, there have also been studies failing to show increased temporal summation in TMD patients when compared to controls (Pfau et al., 2009; Garrett et al., 2013). This could mean that there are different subtypes of TMD patients with some patients showing only peripheral involvement while others show both peripheral and central involvement. Pfau et al. (2009) seem to confirm this as they found that TMD patients with tender points throughout the body have lowered pressure and thermal pain thresholds when compared to TMD patients without tender points or with fewer tender points throughout the body.

In addition, the endogenous pain modulatory systems, both inhibitory and facilitatory, have been shown to have a profound impact on the responsiveness of nociceptive cells and nocifensive behaviors in animals (Millan, 2002; Ren & Dubner, 2002) and humans (Bushnell et al., 2013; Yarnitsky et al., 2014). In terms of the complex endogenous modulatory mechanisms in pain and nociception, a novel hypothesis has been proposed; the so-called supraspinal nociceptive discriminator located within the thalamic mediodorsal and ventromedial nuclei (You et al., 2010). From anatomical and physiological perspectives, this concept for the first time suggests that peripheral nociception evoked by mechanical and heat stimuli can be monitored and distinguished by the thalamic mediodorsal and ventromedial nuclei respectively. However, the generation and control of endogenous

pain modulation – both inhibitory and facilitatory effects organized by these thalamic nociceptive discriminators – are physiologically inactive or 'silent.' Triggering the process of endogenous descending modulation requires sufficient afferents mediated by C fibers, in particular capsaicin-sensitive fibers, associated with gain effects from both central temporal and spatial summation. Most importantly, noxious mechanically mediated activities could be controlled by descending facilitation, whereas heat elicited responses could be governed by descending inhibition. The significance of such a thalamic nociceptive discriminator is that it helps to explain the clinical finding that secondary heat hyperalgesia, unlike secondary mechanical hyperalgesia, is rarely reported in the literature. In addition, this concept helps to explain the complexity of responses observed in, for example TMD pain patients both in terms of psychophysical (quantitative sensory testing) outcomes and conditioned pain modulation studies (Lei et al., 2017).

Furthermore, experimental evidence has shown that the nociceptive system interacts with both glial cells (Chiang et al., 2011) and the immune system (Marchand et al., 2005). In actual fact, there are robust indications of interactions between the nociceptive system and several other biological systems including, motor function (Graven-Nielsen & Arendt-Nielsen, 2008; Hodges & Smeets, 2015), autonomic function (Drummond, 2013), sleep (Lavigne et al., 2011), emotions (Tracey & Mantyh, 2007), and cognitive function (Moriarty et al., 2011).

Woolf et al. (1998) published a landmark paper on the concept of classification of pain mechanisms suggestively categorizing pain into transient, inflammatory, neuropathic, and functional pain, although these classifications can be considered an oversimplification of complex and possibly overlapping mechanisms, and more than one mechanism could be at play at the same time. Nevertheless, classification provides a clinically relevant framework for understanding the different types of orofacial pain. More importantly, the article pointed towards a mechanism-based management of the different types of pain. For example, if an orofacial pain complaint emanates from an inflammatory mechanism it would be logical and rational to manage the inflammation irrespective of whether the pain was localized in the tooth pulp (pulpitis) or synovial tissue (synovitis) of the temporomandibular joint (TMJ). In this example, the approach and the tools used would obviously differ for both conditions but eliminating the inflammatory component would be the ultimate goal for both of them. Figure 4.1 schematically illustrates the proposed classification of pain mechanisms modified for the orofacial region.

In 1992, Dworkin and LeResche proposed a landmark paper on the dual axes system for the clinical classification of TMDs. Accordingly, Axis I was the physical presentation of the problem and Axis II the psychosocial distress part of the problem for the patient (Dworkin & LeResche, 1992). The importance of this classification was that for the first time TMD pain was recognized as a biopsychosocial problem, or perhaps even more correctly a 'psycho-bio-social' problem, thus also recognizing that psychological

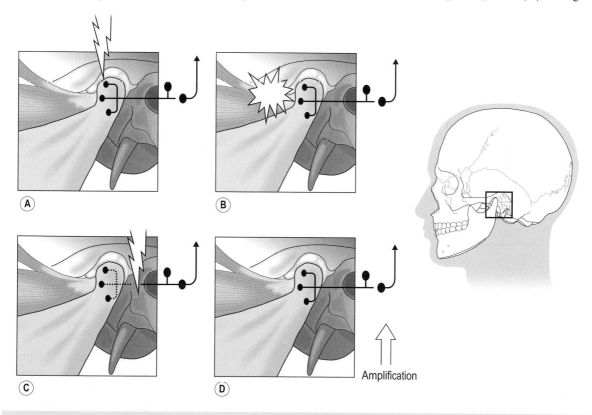

Figure 4.1

Simplified overview of the putative mechanism of pain with implications for classification (Modified from Woolf et al. 1998 with permission). (A) Nociceptive pain. (B) Inflammatory pain. (C) Neuropathic pain. (D) Functional pain.

issues such as depression and anxiety may contribute significantly to the clinical picture. In addition to this, the emergence of new information relating to TMD pain, for example on genetic markers, indicates a possible third axis, which will be discussed later in this chapter.

In an urge to translate the basic research findings in the orofacial region into clinical concepts, scientists and researchers have attempted to identify biomarkers and risk factors for a number of clinical orofacial pain conditions including both specific and nonspecific TMDs. Some of these studies have been summarized in the following paragraphs and Table 4.1.

Biomarkers and risk factors for temporomandibular disorders

The term biomarker is generally used to refer to a measurable indicator of some biological state or condition. According to the Institute of Medicine, biomarker is defined as: '…characteristics that are objectively measured and evaluated as indicators of normal biological processes, pathogenic processes or response to an intervention.' A combined effort from the International Research Diagnostic Criteria for TMD (RDC/TMD) Consortium Network and the Special Interest Group for Orofacial Pain under the International Association for the Study of Pain (IASP) outlined several putative biomarkers for orofacial pain in a symposium in 2011. Primarily based on available techniques, the following seven domains were suggested:

1. Tissue-based assays (blood, saliva, muscle dialysate, tissue, etc.);

2. Brain imaging (electroencephalography, positron emission tomography, magnetoencephalography, functional magnetic resonance imaging);

3. Non-brain imaging (computerized tomography scans, ultrasound, magnetic resonance imaging);

4. Neurophysiological measures (trigeminal reflexes, microneurography, electromyography);

5. Psychophysical measures (conditioned pain modulation, quantitative sensory testing);

6. Psychophysiological measures (heart rate variability, blood pressure); and,

7. Jaw function measures (bite force, jaw tracking).

These biomarkers were assessed according to invasiveness, costs, availability and potential for large-scale studies. Subsequently, and with the reservation that many putative biomarkers are emerging, it was considered that at present biological samples, structural imaging of tissues, functional brain imaging, quantitative sensory testing (Chapter 6) and conditioned pain modulation would sufficiently qualify as potential biomarkers (Ceusters et al., 2015). Nevertheless, these biomarkers are not ideal because issues such as complexity, cost, time consumption, and also reproducibility hinder their research and consistency in clinical use.

Risk factors can be defined as variables that are associated with an increased risk of developing a disease, for example orofacial pain, and can be expressed as odds ratios (OR), as explained by Szumilas: 'The OR represents the odds that an outcome will occur given a particular exposure, compared to the odds of the outcome occurring in the absence of that exposure. Odds ratios are most commonly used in case-control studies, however they can also be used in cross-sectional and cohort study designs as well (with some modifications and/or assumptions)' (Szumilas, 2010). Even though the presence of biomarkers and/or risk factors do not necessarily imply causation, it is still important to understand the multiple variables associated with orofacial pain and keep them in mind when doing research or assessing patients.

A search for the terms 'risk factor,' 'odds ratio,' 'temporomandibular disorders,' and 'orofacial pain' provides a lengthy list of published original research studies. Table 4.1 shows the preliminary overview of

Table 4.1
Risk factors for specific and nonspecific TMDs.

	Risk factor	Author and year	TMD
1.	Trauma	Huang et al. (2002) Choi et al. (2002)* Ohrbach et al. (2011)*	
2.	Malocclusion	Pullinger et al. (1993) Marklund & Wanman (2010) Miamoto et al. (2011)*	Osteoarthrosis, myalgia, disc displacement Signs and symptoms of TMD
3.	Gender	Michelotti et al. (2010) Marklund & Wanman (2010) Huang et al. (2002) Chang et al. (2015)* Pereira et al. (2010)*	Myofascial pain Myofascial pain Myofascial pain with arthralgia
4.	Bruxism	Marklund & Wanman (2010) Fernandes et al. (2012) Choi et al. (2002)*	Signs and symptoms of TMD Myofascial pain and arthralgia
5.	Headache and migraine	Akhter et al. (2013) Stuginski-Barbosa et al. (2010) Gonçalves et al. (2013)* Choi et al. (2002)* Slade et al. (2013b)*	Clicking, TMJ pain, difficulty in mouth opening Tenderness in the masticatory muscles and joints
6.	Clenching or grinding	Marklund & Wanman (2010) Michelotti et al. (2010) Miyake et al. (2004) Huang et al. (2002)	Signs and symptoms of TMD Myofascial pain and disc displacement TMJ noise and pain, impaired mouth opening Myofascial pain with arthralgia
7.	Catastrophizing and depression	Velly et al. (2011)	Progression of temporomandibular muscle and joint pain
8.	Genetic factors	Smith et al. (2011)*	
9.	Smoking	Sanders et al. (2012)* Sanders et al. (2013)*	
10.	Obesity	Jordani et al. (2017)	
* nonspecific TMD			

such common findings. Even though the included studies used different definitions of TMD and pain, it can be seen that many different risk factors (trauma, malocclusion, gender, bruxism, headache, catastrophizing, depression, genetics, etc.) are pertinent and they exist with different degrees of strength, as shown by the varying OR. In fact, the Orofacial Pain Prospective Evaluation and Risk Assessment (OPPERA) study is a unique attempt to identify risk factors amongst several different domains – clinical, autonomic, genetic, somatosensory and psychological (Fillingim et al., 2011a; Maixner et al., 2011; Slade et al., 2013a). The term 'risk factor' in the OPPERA studies reflects both the events and experiences that can lead to the onset of TMD and also those that can lead to the persistence and exacerbation of TMD (Maixner et al., 2011), and in this sense is a blend of risk factors and biomarkers. The initial sample of participants in this study was of approximately 3,300 healthy individuals. These individuals were extensively characterized with somatosensory, autonomic and genetic tests, questionnaires and clinical examination. Following these tests, the participants were followed up at regular intervals to ascertain the

number of TMD cases that had developed. From analyses of baseline variables, estimates of risk factors expressed as odds ratios were determined. The OPERRA study has so far shown a wide range of risk factors for the development of TMDs, such as clinical risk factors where a total of 59 out of 71 variables demonstrated significant associations between baseline characteristics and new onset TMD pain patients, for example:

- History of trauma, parafunctional behaviors, and higher frequency of other pain conditions including headache (Ohrbach et al., 2011);

- Genetic risk factors such as COMT, serotonin receptor HTR2A, and more than 20 other SNPs (out of 3,295 SNPs);

- Autonomic risk factors (e.g., heart rate);

- Somatosensory risk factors (e.g., pressure pain and heat pain) – a total of 14 out of 39 variables; and ultimately

- Psychological risk factors (e.g., psychological distress, stress and catastrophizing, and somatic awareness) (Fillingim et al., 2011b).

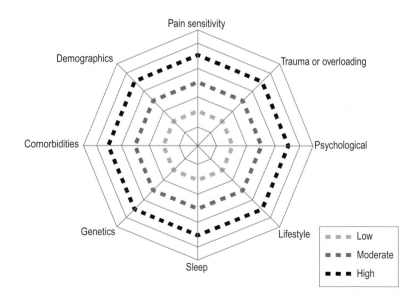

Figure 4.2

Risk assessment diagram of orofacial pain (RADOP) (Svensson & Kumar 2016). Eight overall dimensions of orofacial/TMD pain are aligned in a radar or spider chart where each dimension can be categorized into low, moderate or high risk. Personalized versions of the diagram will allow an immediate overview of the current condition of the patient.

As it is difficult to make sense of all this research information either from OPPERA studies or other studies in a clinical setting, we are proposing a new risk assessment diagram for orofacial pain (RADOP). The original idea came from periodontology where a six-spoke spider chart of risk factors for periodontitis was developed. Applying this idea in periodontology has been shown to have a positive impact on patient management. In order to encompass the different domains of orofacial pain risk factors, an eight-spoke spider chart is proposed (Figure 4.2). Currently the labeling of the different spokes is arbitrary but it can be modified according to needs and new research information. For example, in terms of 'pain sensitivity' the suggested biomarkers quantitative sensory testing (QST) and conditioned pain modulation (CPM) could be used. In this spoke, it could be defined that if one out of three tests is positive, the patient has a low risk in terms of pain sensitivity. If, on the other hand, all three tests are positive the patient would be at higher risk and this would indicate increased pain sensitivity. The proposal is open for formalized studies to address the clinical usefulness of this approach.

While the RADOP diagram attempts to capture in a simple and easy fashion the complexity of orofacial pain patients, it does not provide a conceptual model that explains how these different risk factors interact with each other and how these interactions may change over time. Therefore, to explain this, a new model based on stochastic variation is presented below (Svensson & Kumar, 2015; Svensson & Kumar, 2016).

Stochastic variation as a model for temporomandibular disorders

The inspiration for this approach to explain complex systems comes from microbiology where bacteria with host-protective or host-damaging capacities would randomly interact to determine if gingivitis, periodontitis or caries would be the consequence (Manji & Nagelkerke 1989). Accordingly,

let us assume that there would be 100 meaningful factors for a given individual to determine if he or she would become an orofacial pain patient. These factors could be categorized as both *risk factors* that facilitate the development or maintenance of TMD pain or *protective factors* that inhibit or counteract the development of TMD pain. Furthermore, each of these factors could have different potency ranging from 0 (neutral) to 100 being enormously potent. If these factors occur in a random way, and the protective and risk factors balance each other out, then they would basically be representing 'noise' in the system. Furthermore, if the risk factors had an additive effect, but the protective mechanisms counterbalanced these effects, then due to stochastic process these factors would just oscillate in a nonpainful state, never crossing an arbitrary threshold for symptom development and clinical manifestations of pain (Figure 4.3A–C). It is thus easy to see that different patterns may emerge and, due to random variation, a pattern in which the risk factors are additive and the protective factors do not compensate for this may occur. If this occurs, the pain condition could become 'persistent' whereas in other cases (patients) the random interaction would generate only brief and transient types of pain such as that experienced in headache disorders. Figure 4.3 illustrates some of the theoretical outcomes of a simple stochastic process created by adding randomly generated integers.

The practical challenge of the stochastic variation model for orofacial pain is first of all to determine the most important or significant risk factors; secondly, to describe their relative potency; and, lastly, to establish biological models supported by bioinformatics to determine the timecourse of the interactions. Obviously this is a daunting task but future research may be encouraged to take this approach. The principle of stochastic variation is also currently being discussed in connection with various neurodegenerative diseases such as Alzheimer's disease. The proposed model is intended to start a discussion on different ways to think about orofacial pain

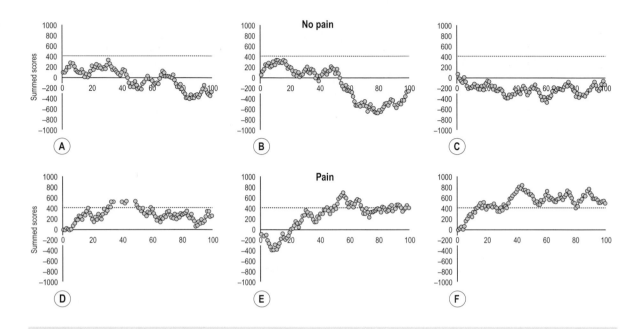

Figure 4.3

Stochastic variation model of orofacial pain. The different plots are generated by the addition of random integers from 0 to 100. Plots A–C represent the 'nonpainful' outcomes since the summed scores never exceed an arbitrary threshold (400) for pain development. In contrast, plots D–F represent the 'painful condition' where the summed scores at some point exceed the threshold creating different trajectories based on stochastic variation.

pathophysiology and management and also to steer away from a univariate model and more towards a multivariate model.

Clinical implications

If orofacial pain clinicians think about their patients in a univariate model it is likely that they will not see the full picture and only address one factor in the treatment plan. Malocclusion as the source of TMD and orofacial pain is a good example of the aforementioned univariate thinking. In this way of thinking a straightforward approach to the problem, such as correcting the malocclusion through orthodontics, occlusal equilibration, and/or occlusal rehabilitation, is thought to be the cure. Unfortunately, this approach fails to address the many risk factors

that have been described above such as poor sleep and psychological issues. For an updated review, the reader is referred to recent articles in this field (Turp et al., 2008; Michelotti & Iodice, 2010). Based on the best epidemiological studies, occlusion continues to be a relatively low-risk factor and other risk factors are likely to be at play. This means that other therapeutic approaches should be used and studies have shown that patients may benefit from cognitive behavioral approaches (Dworkin et al., 1994; Dworkin et al., 2002). There are several types of cognitive behavioral therapies ranging from providing basic information and counseling the patient to hypnosis and mindfulness. Based on the stochastic model and the different types of risk and preventive factors, along with the evidence of neurobiological

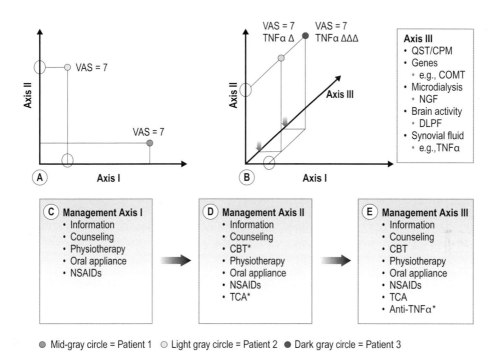

Mid-gray circle = Patient 1   ○ Light gray circle = Patient 2   ● Dark gray circle = Patient 3

Figure 4.4

Steps in individualized orofacial pain management. (A) The 'two-axes' approach according to Dworkin and LeResche (1992) for understanding orofacial pain. Axis I represents the physical symptoms and Axis II the psychosocial distress. Patient 1 (medium gray) may complain of pain reported on a 0–10 visual analog scale (VAS) as '7' which Patient 2 (light gray) may also do but with a significantly different combination of physical symptoms versus psychosocial distress. (B) It may also be timely to consider a third axis representing various biomarkers: quantitative sensory testing (QST, conditioned pain modulation [CPM]); genes, (catechol-O-methyltransferase (COMT)); microdialysis of, for example nerve growth factor (NGF); brain activity, for example in the dorsolateral-prefrontal cortex (DLPF) or synovial fluid (tumor necrosis factor alpha [TNFα]). Patient 3 (dark gray) may have the same Axis I and Axis II constitution as Patient 2 but may differ in one or more of the biomarkers identified in Axis III. In this example Patient 3 could have elevated levels of tumor necrosis factor alpha (TNFα) in the temporomandibular joint. (C) The therapeutic consequences of a simple Axis I approach would be that Patients 1 and 2 would be treated in a similar way with self-care approaches, oral appliances and nonsteroidal anti-inflammatory drugs (NSAIDs). (D) With the Axis II approach it becomes apparent that Patient 2, in addition to the prescribed treatment, would also benefit from more cognitive behavioral therapy (CBT) and perhaps low doses of tricyclic antidepressants (TCA) (indicated by *). (E) With the proposed Axis III, Patient 3 would, in addition to the management offered in the Axis II approach, also be considered for treatment with anti-TNFα medication (indicated by *).

mechanisms underlying most orofacial pain conditions, it may be appropriate to also consider pharmacological interventions. However, keep in mind that the efficacy of most medications used to manage chronic pain conditions has been quite modest (Finnerup et al., 2015). With the exception of triptans that are used for treating migraines, few true revolutionary pain medications have been developed in the last few years. It seems that a combined approach with cognitive behavioral therapies, physiotherapy, and pharmacology would be a feasible solution. With this in mind, if we can accurately phenotype and genotype patients, then individualized and poly-target pain management would be a logical next step. Finally, it should be stated that the intensity of the therapy required might vary during the timecourse due to the inherent dynamic nature of the interactions.

Conceptually the biopsychosocial or 'psychobio-social' pain model and the original RDC/TMD axes I and II approach has offered a logical approach to the management of chronic orofacial pain (Figure 4.4A,C,D). Most pain management programs are indeed building on this foundation with pharmacology, physiotherapy, self-care programs, and more cognitive behavioral therapy. This multimodality approach has been shown to be efficacious in managing pain but rarely does it completely cure the chronic pain patient (Figure 4.4C,D). Perhaps the most important lesson from the stochastic variation model would be that pain management needs to be individualized and in this quest for personalized treatments we may need to consider individual risk factors and biomarkers. As such, a third axis in addition to the two axes offered by the RDC/TMD and DC/TMD approaches may need to be considered. Figure 4.4B illustrates such an approach moving from a single axis approach to a three axes approach and the consequences for management

(Figure 4.4E). Since it seems that multimodal pain management strategies offer better results than single modality strategies, dentists and orofacial pain specialists should apply these more often and abandon old paradigms, such as emphasizing the need for permanent occlusal oriented-treatment. It is not just a future challenge for researchers to continue to unravel the complexity of chronic orofacial pain but also for clinicians to embrace new pain classifications, concepts and a comprehensive assessment of risk factors. It is with this hope that this chapter has outlined the current status of TMD pain mechanisms and research and in addition has suggested future avenues for the continued advancement of the field.

Conclusion

This chapter, in part based on a recent review (Svensson & Kumar, 2016), provides a short assessment of basic orofacial pain mechanisms and of a number of recently identified risk factors for development of TMD pain. The RADOP diagram is suggested as a way to provide an overview of the many risk factors for TMD in the clinical setting. Furthermore, a stochastic variation model is suggested as a way to account for the interactions between the many different risk and protective factors involved in the development and maintenance of orofacial pain. We believe this model may help us understand individual timecourses and pain trajectories in the onset of orofacial pain/TMDs. Finally, it is suggested that univariate thinking in conceptual models and management approaches should be replaced by a multivariate or a poly-target approach. There is a continued need not only for more orofacial/TMD pain research but also for better orofacial/TMD pain research before we reach our ultimate goals of accurate and mechanistic diagnostics followed by effective and rational management of the orofacial pain patient.

References

Akhter R, Morita M, Ekuni D, Hassan NM, Furuta M, Yamanaka R, Matsuka Y, Wilson D. Self-reported aural symptoms, headache and temporomandibular disorders in Japanese young adults. BMC Musculoskelet Disord 2013; 14: 58.

Alstergren P, Ernberg M, Kvarnstrom M, Kopp S. Interleukin-1beta in synovial fluid from the arthritic temporomandibular joint and its relation to pain, mobility, and anterior open bite. J Oral Maxillofac Surg 1998; 56: 1059–1065.

Ayesh EE, Jensen TS, Svensson P. Hypersensitivity to mechanical and intra-articular electrical stimuli in persons with painful temporomandibular joints. J Dental Res 2007; 86: 1187–1192.

Burstein R, Yarnitsky D, Goor-Aryeh I, Ransil BJ, Bajwa ZH. An association between migraine and cutaneous allodynia. Ann Neurol 2000; 47: 614–624.

Bushnell MC, Ceko M, Low LA. Cognitive and emotional control of pain and its disruption in chronic pain. Nat Rev Neurosci 2013; 14: 502–511.

Cairns B. Pathophysiology of TMD pain: basic mechanisms and their implications for pharmacotherapy. J Oral Rehabil 2010; 37: 391–410.

Ceusters W, Nasri-Heir C, Alnaas D, Cairns BE, Michelotti A, Ohrbach R. Perspectives on next steps in classification of oro-facial pain – Part 3: biomarkers of chronic orofacial pain – from research to clinic. J Oral Rehabil 2015; 42: 956–66.

Chang TH, Yuh DY, Wu YT, Cheng WC, Lin FG, Shieh YS, Fu E, Huang RY. The association between temporomandibular disorders and joint hypermobility syndrome: a nationwide population-based study. Clin Oral Investig 2015; 19: 2123–2132.

Chiang CY, Dostrovsky JO, Iwata K, Sessle BJ. Role of glia in orofacial pain. Neuroscientist 2011; 17: 303–320.

Chichorro JG, Porreca F, Sessle B. Mechanisms of craniofacial pain. Cephalalgia 2017; 37: 613–626.

Choi YS, Choung PH, Moon HS, Kim SG. Temporomandibular disorders in 19-year-old Korean men. J Oral Maxillofac Surg 2002; 60: 797–803.

Denk F, McMahon SB, Tracey I. Pain vulnerability: a neurobiological perspective. Nat Neurosci 2014; 17: 192–200.

Drummond PD. Sensory-autonomic interactions in health and disease. Handb Clin Neurol 2013; 117: 309–319.

Dworkin SF, LeResche L. Research diagnostic criteria for temporomandibular disorders: review, criteria, examinations and specifications, critique. J Craniomandib Disord 1992; 6: 301–355.

Dworkin SF, Turner JA, Wilson L et al. Brief group cognitive-behavioral intervention for temporomandibular disorders. Pain 1994; 59: 175–187.

Dworkin SF, Huggins KH, Wilson L et al. A randomized clinical trial using research diagnostic criteria for temporomandibular disorders-axis II to target clinic cases for a tailored self-care TMD treatment program. J Orofac Pain 2002; 16: 48–63.

Fernandes G, Franco AL, Siqueira JT, Gonçalves DA, Camparis CM. Sleep bruxism increases the risk for painful temporomandibular disorder, depression and non-specific physical symptoms. J Oral Rehabil 2012; 39: 538–544.

Fernández-de-las-Peñas C, Galán-del-Río F, Fernández-Carnero J, Pesquera J, Arendt-Nielsen L, Svensson P. Bilateral widespread mechanical pain sensitivity in women with myofascial temporomandibular disorder: evidence of impairment in central nociceptive processing. J Pain 2009; 10: 1170–1178.

Fillingim RB, Slade GD, Diatchenko L et al. Summary of findings from the OPPERA baseline case-control study: implications and future directions. J Pain 2011a; 12: T102–107.

Fillingim RB, Ohrbach R, Greenspan JD et al. Potential psychosocial risk factors for chronic TMD: descriptive data and empirically identified domains from the OPPERA case-control study. J Pain 2011b; 12: T46–60.

Finnerup NB, Attal N, Haroutounian S et al. Pharmacotherapy for neuropathic pain in adults: a systematic review and meta-analysis. Lancet Neurol 2015; 14: 162–173.

Garrett PH, Sarlani E, Grace EG, Greenspan JD. Chronic temporomandibular disorders are not necessarily associated with a compromised endogenous analgesic system. J Orofac Pain 2013; 27: 142–150.

Gonçalves MC, Florencio LL, Chaves TC, Speciali JG, Bigal ME, Bevilaqua-Grossi D. Do women with migraine have higher prevalence of temporomandibular disorders? Braz J Phys Ther 2013; 17: 64–68.

Graven-Nielsen T, Arendt-Nielsen L. Impact of clinical and experimental pain on muscle strength and activity. Curr Rheumatol Rep 2008; 10: 475–481.

Hodges PW, Smeets RJ. Interaction between pain, movement, and physical activity: short-term benefits, long-term consequences, and targets for treatment. Clin J Pain 2015; 31: 97–107.

Huang GJ, LeResche L, Critchlow CW, Martin MD, Drangsholt MT. Risk factors for diagnostic subgroups of painful temporomandibular disorders (TMD). J Dental Res 2002; 81: 284–288.

Hucho T, Levine JD. Signaling pathways in sensitization: toward a nociceptor cell biology. Neuron 2007; 55: 365–376.

Jordani PC, Campi LB, Circeli GZ, Visscher CM, Bigal ME, Gonçalves DA. Obesity as a risk factor for temporomandibular disorders. J Oral Rehabil 2017; 44: 1–8.

Lavigne GJ, Nashed A, Manzini C, Carra MC. Does sleep differ among patients with common musculoskeletal pain disorders? Curr Rheumatol Rep 2011; 13: 535–542.

Lei J, Ye G, Wu JT, Pertovaara A, You HJ. Role of capsaicin- and heat-sensitive afferents in stimulation of acupoint-induced pain and analgesia in humans. Neuroscience 2017; 358: 325–335.

Maixner W, Diatchenko L, Dubner R, Fillingim RB, Greenspan JD, Knott C, Ohrbach R, Weir B, Slade GD. Orofacial pain prospective evaluation and risk assessment study--the OPPERA study. J Pain 2011; 12: T1–2.

Manji F, Nagelkerke N. A stochastic model for periodontal breakdown. J Periodontal Res 1989; 24: 279–281.

Marchand F, Perretti M, McMahon SB. Role of the immune system in chronic pain. Nat Rev Neurosci 2005; 6: 521–532.

Marklund S, Wanman A. Risk factors associated with incidence and persistence of signs and symptoms of temporomandibular disorders. Acta Odontol Scand 2010; 68: 289–299.

Miamoto CB, Pereira LJ, Paiva SM, Pordeus IA, Ramos-Jorge ML, Marques LS. Prevalence and risk indicators of temporomandibular disorder signs and symptoms in a pediatric population with spastic cerebral palsy. J Clin Pediatr Dent 2011; 35: 259–263.

Michelotti A, Iodice G. The role of orthodontics in temporomandibular disorders. J Oral Rehabil 2010; 37: 411–429.

Michelotti A, Cioffi I, Festa P, Scala G, Farella M. Oral parafunctions as risk factors for diagnostic TMD subgroups. J Oral Rehabil 2010; 37: 157–162.

Millan MJ. Descending control of pain. Prog Neurobiol 2002; 66: 355–474.

Miyake R, Ohkubo R, Takehara J, Morita M. Oral parafunctions and association with symptoms of temporomandibular disorders in Japanese university students. J Oral Rehabil 2004; 31: 518–523.

Moriarty O, McGuire BE, Finn DP. The effect of pain on cognitive function: a review of clinical and preclinical research. Prog Neurobiol 2011; 93: 385–404.

Ohrbach R, Fillingim RB, Mulkey F et al. Clinical findings and pain symptoms as potential risk factors for chronic TMD: descriptive data and empirically identified domains from the OPPERA case-control study. J Pain 2011; 12: T27-45.

Pereira LJ, Pereira-Cenci T, Del Bel Cury AA, Pereira SM, Pereira AC, Ambosano GM, Gavião MB. Risk indicators of temporomandibular disorder incidences in early adolescence. Pediatr Dent 2010; 32: 324–328.

Pfau DB, Rolke R, Nickel R, Treede RD, Daublaender M. Somatosensory profiles in subgroups of patients with myogenic temporomandibular disorders and Fibromyalgia Syndrome. Pain 2009; 147: 72–83.

Pullinger AG, Seligman DA, Gornbein JA. A multiple logistic regression analysis of the risk and relative odds of temporomandibular disorders as a function of common occlusal features. J Dental Res 1993; 72: 968–979.

Ren K, Dubner R. Descending modulation in persistent pain: an update. Pain 2002; 100: 1–6.

Ren K, Dubner R. The role of trigeminal interpolaris-caudalis transition zone in persistent orofacial pain. Int Rev Neurobiol 2011; 97: 207–225.

Sanders AE, Maixner W, Nackley AG, Diatchenko L, By K, Miller VE et al. Excess risk of temporomandibular disorder associated with cigarette smoking in young adults. J Pain 2012; 13: 21–31.

Sanders AE, Slade GD, Bair E, Fillingim RB, Knott C, Dubner R et al. General health status and incidence of first-onset temporomandibular disorder: the OPPERA prospective cohort study. J Pain 2013; 14: T51-62.

Sarlani E, Grace EG, Reynolds MA, Greenspan JD. Evidence for up-regulated central nociceptive processing in patients with masticatory myofascial pain. J Orofac Pain 2004a; 18: 41–55.

Sarlani E, Grace EG, Reynolds MA, Greenspan JD. Sex differences in temporal summation of pain and aftersensations following repetitive noxious mechanical stimulation. Pain 2004b; 109: 115–123.

Sato J, Segami N, Kaneyama K, Yoshimura H, Fujimura K, Yoshitake Y. Relationship of calcitonin gene-related peptide in synovial tissues and temporomandibular joint pain in humans. Oral Surg Oral Med Oral Pathol Oral Radiol 2004; 98: 533–540.

Sato J, Segami N, Yoshitake Y, Kaneyama K, Yoshimura H, Fujimura K, Kitagawa Y. Specific expression of substance P in synovial tissues of patients with symptomatic, non-reducing internal derangement of the temporo-mandibular joint: comparison with clinical findings. Br J Oral Maxillofac Surg 2007; 45: 372–377.

Sessle BJ. Acute and chronic craniofacial pain: brainstem mechanisms of nociceptive transmission and neuroplasticity, and their clinical correlates. Crit Rev Oral Biol Med 2000; 11: 57–91.

Sessle BJ. Peripheral and central mechanisms of orofacial inflammatory pain. Int Rev Neurobiol 2011; 97: 179–206.

Slade GD, Fillingim RB, Sanders AE, Bair E, Greenspan JD, Ohrbach R et al. Summary of findings from the OPPERA prospective cohort study of incidence of first-onset temporomandibular disorder: implications and future directions. J Pain 2013a; 14: T116-124.

Slade GD, Sanders AE, Bair E et al. Preclinical episodes of orofacial pain symptoms and their association with health care behaviors in the OPPERA prospective cohort study. Pain 2013b; 154: 750–760.

Smith SB, Maixner DW, Greenspan JD et al. Potential genetic risk factors for chronic TMD: genetic associations from the OPPERA case control study. J Pain 2011; 12: T92-101.

Stohler CS, Zubieta JK. Pain imaging in the emerging era of molecular medicine. Methods Mol Biol 2010; 617: 517–537.

Stuginski-Barbosa J, Macedo HR, Bigal ME, Speciali JG. Signs of temporomandibular disorders in migraine patients: a prospective, controlled study. Clin J Pain 2010; 26: 418–421.

Svensson P, Kumar A. Trigeminal pain and sensitization: proposal of a new stochastic model. In: Kasch H, Turk D, Jensen T (eds) Whiplash injury: perspectives on the development of chronic pain. Philadelphia: Wolters Kluwer Health; 2015, pp. 77–88.

Svensson P, Kumar A. Assessment of risk factors for orofacial pain and recent developments in classification. Implications for management. J Oral Rehabil 2016; 43: 977–989.

Svensson P, List T, Hector G. Analysis of stimulus-evoked pain in patients with myofascial temporomandibular pain disorders. Pain 2001; 92: 399–409.

Szumilas M. Explaining Odds Ratios. J Can Acad Child Adolesc Psychiatry 2010; 19: 227–229.

Takahashi T, Kondoh T, Fukuda M, Yamazaki Y, Toyosaki T, Suzuki R. Proinflammatory cytokines detectable in synovial fluids from patients with temporomandibular disorders. Oral Surg Oral Med Oral Pathol Oral Radiol Endod 1998; 85: 135–141.

Takeuchi Y, Zeredo JL, Fujiyama R, Amagasa T, Toda K. Effects of experimentally induced inflammation on temporomandibular joint nociceptors in rats. Neurosci Lett 2004; 354: 172–174.

Tracey I, Mantyh PW. The cerebral signature for pain perception and its modulation. Neuron 2007; 55: 377–391.

Turp JC, Greene CS, Strub JR. Dental occlusion: a critical reflection on past, present and future concepts. J Oral Rehabil 2008; 35: 446–453.

Velly AM, Look JO, Carlson C et al. The effect of catastrophizing and depression on chronic pain–a prospective cohort study of temporomandibular muscle and joint pain disorders. Pain 2011; 152: 2377–2383.

Vierck CJ, Wong F, King CD, Mauderli AP, Schmidt S, Riley JL, 3rd. Characteristics of sensitization associated with chronic pain conditions. Clin J Pain 2014; 30: 119–128.

Woda A. Pain in the trigeminal system: from orofacial nociception to neural network modeling. J Dental Res 2003; 82: 764–768.

Woolf CJ. Central sensitization: implications for the diagnosis and treatment of pain. Pain 2011; 152: S2-15.

Woolf CJ, Bennett GJ, Doherty M et al. Towards a mechanism-based classification of pain? Pain 1998; 77: 227–229.

Yarnitsky D, Granot M, Granovsky Y. Pain modulation profile and pain therapy: between pro- and antinociception. Pain 2014; 155: 663–665.

You HJ, Lei J, Sui MY et al. Endogenous descending modulation: spatiotemporal effect of dynamic imbalance between descending facilitation and inhibition of nociception. J Physiol 2010; 588: 4177–4188.

Chapter 5

Musculoskeletal referred pain to the craniofacial region

Thomas Graven-Nielsen, César Fernández-de-las-Peñas, Megan McPhee, Lars Arendt-Nielsen

Introduction

Pain in the craniofacial region can have multiple sources. Obviously, pain may arise from trauma or noxious stimulation of particular structures, for example skin, muscle, joint, tendon, bone, or teeth, resulting in localized pain. However, extrasegmental structures may also induce craniofacial pain. 'Referred tenderness' was originally used in the first reports of referred sensations (Head, 1893), but this is now known as referred pain. In the spinal system, clinical examples of pain perceived in the knee or thigh may arise from an arthritic hip joint, and often distant pain is perceived due to palpation of myofascial trigger points (TrPs) (Simons et al., 1999). In visceral pain conditions, referred pain (and not localized pain) is frequently felt in somatic structures distant from the affected visceral organs. Although known for many years, the definition of referred pain as felt away from the pain locus is not fully operational when it comes to pain spreading from a structure; for example, pain from the trapezius muscle may be perceived as a large area covering the trapezius muscle and also the neck and head. In this chapter, pain felt both distant from and outside of the pain origin is defined as referred pain.

The purpose of this chapter is to present the nociceptive capacity of various structures and their capability to mediate pain referral and cause sensitization. Major findings on the topic of pain referral mechanisms originate from studies on extremity muscles, which will be presented together with specific examples of referred pain in the craniofacial region.

Pain in the craniofacial region from myofascial trigger points

Definition

Although there are different definitions of myofascial trigger points (TrPs), the most accepted defines a TrP as 'a hyper-irritable spot within a taut band of a skeletal muscle that is painful on compression, stretch, overload or contraction, which causes a referred pain pattern and autonomic phenomena' (Simons et al., 1999). Clinically, TrPs are classified as active and latent. Active TrPs are those in which local and referred pain reproduces any sensory or motor symptoms reported by the patient and the symptoms are recognized by the patient as his or her usual pain (Simons et al., 1999). Latent TrPs are those in which local and referred pain does not reproduce any familiar or usual symptoms in the patient (Simons et al., 1999). The relevance of 'pain recognition' is discussed in the current Diagnostic Criteria for Temporomandibular Disorders (DC/TMD) (Peck et al., 2014; Schiffman et al., 2014). It has been clinically observed that active TrPs induce a larger referred pain area and higher pain intensity than latent TrPs (Hong et al., 1997). In addition, this clinical distinction has been substantiated by a study showing higher levels of chemical mediators and other proinflammatory substances, for example substance P, bradykinin, and serotonin, in the vicinity of active TrPs compared with latent TrPs (Shah et al., 2005).

Sensitization mechanisms of trigger points

The referred pain evoked by TrPs is most likely mediated by a central mechanism (see the section below), whereas TrPs per se likely result from peripheral mechanisms where sensitizing agents cause increased pain sensitivity in very localized points (Shah et al., 2005). Findings also indicate the presence of nociceptive and non-nociceptive hypersensitivity at TrPs (Li et al., 2009; Wang et al., 2010b) in which a spinal dorsal horn mechanism may be involved (Kuan et al., 2007). Obviously, active TrP pain is processed at supraspinal levels and TrP hyperalgesia has been demonstrated to excite various brain areas associated with the pain experience (Niddam et al., 2008; Niddam, 2009). A recent study found that individuals with TrPs exhibited microstructural brain abnormalities mainly distributed in the limbic system and the brain areas involved in the pain neuromatrix (Xie et al., 2016).

Trigger points in temporomandibular disorders

Pain patterns in TMDs can be composed of referred pain patterns from muscle TrPs located in the neck, shoulder, and masticatory muscles. Simons et al. (1999) described the referred pain pattern from several muscles and also how referred pain can spread to the head or face (see the illustrations of referred pain patterns in Chapter 8 of this textbook). Although these muscles refer pain to the face (trigeminal innervated area), they can also refer to the head and neck (cervically innervated area), mimicking headaches. It has therefore been suggested that a number of different muscles are involved in the pathophysiology of TMDs (the masseter), and headaches (upper trapezius and suboccipital muscles) (Conti et al., 2016; Svensson, 2007).

Few clinical studies have investigated the presence of TrPs in patients with TMDs. Wright (2000) reported that the upper trapezius, lateral pterygoid, and masseter muscles were the most common sources of referred pain into the neck and craniofacial regions. Nevertheless, this study did not include a control group and patients were not examined in a blinded fashion (Wright, 2000). Fernández-de-las-Peñas et al. (2010) conducted a blinded, controlled study, where patients with myalgic TMD and healthy controls were examined for TrPs in the neck, shoulder, and head musculature. This study found that TrPs in the masticatory muscles (the masseter and temporalis), were more prevalent than TrPs within the neck and shoulder muscles (the upper trapezius, suboccipital and sternocleidomastoid muscles) (Fernández-de-las-Peñas et al. 2010). These findings support the notion that masticatory muscle TrPs are more likely to play a role in TMDs, whereas neck and shoulder TrPs are more likely to play a greater role in headaches. This hypothesis was confirmed by a clinical study showing that referred pain was more pronounced in the orofacial region in patients with TMDs, whereas in female patients with fibromyalgia it was more pronounced in the cervical spine (Alonso-Blanco et al., 2012). Experimental pain studies also support this notion (see the next section).

Experimental musculoskeletal referred pain

Intramuscular injections of hypertonic saline have been widely used to study referred pain from muscles (Graven-Nielsen, 2006) (Figure 5.1). Other deep structures, such as tendon, ligament, intervertebral disc, periosteum and joint structures, may also evoke referred pain but have been less extensively investigated. In contrast to the superficial pain experienced

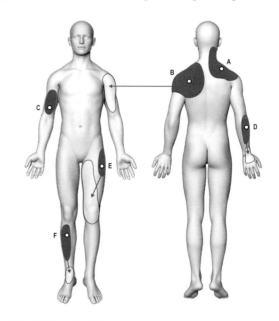

Figure 5.1

Typical enlarged local pain areas (shown in dark gray) and distinct referred pain areas (shown in white) experienced after intramuscular hypertonic saline injection (site denoted by white dot) into the trapezius (A), infraspinatus (B), biceps brachii (C), brachioradialis (D), vastus lateralis (E) and tibialis anterior muscles (F).

with visceral pain referral (Ness et al., 1990), muscle or deep tissue pain often evokes referred pain also perceived in deep structures (Kellgren, 1938). This can make it difficult to separate out which deep structures are the sources of pain and which are merely exhibiting referred symptoms.

Experimental investigations of pain in the pericranial muscles and nearby joints, ligaments, and muscles in the cervical spine have revealed that these structures are able to produce various patterns of referred pain. For example, early pioneering work has shown that injection of hypertonic saline into both the suboccipital muscles (Kellgren, 1938) and the cervical paravertebral muscles (Feinstein et al., 1954) is able to evoke a deep pain in the forehead region, similar to a headache. Similarly, hypertonic saline-induced pain from the atlanto-occipital joint (Campbell & Parsons, 1944), splenius capitis (Falla et al., 2007), and sternocleidomastoid muscle is also commonly felt about the cranium, in the parietofrontal, oculofrontotemporal, and occipitoparietal regions respectively.

Interestingly, however, there are clear differences between muscles in the extent of referred pain, with some muscles, for example the tibialis anterior and infraspinatus, giving rise to very distinct areas of pain, while other muscles, for example the biceps brachii, primarily give rise to local pain (Graven-Nielsen, 2006). This is also true in the craniofacial region, as was demonstrated when Schmidt-Hansen et al. (2006) systematically mapped saline-induced pain from muscles with trigeminal (masseter, anterior temporalis, posterior temporalis), and/or cervical (trapezius, splenius capitis and sternocleidomastoid) innervation (Figure 5.2). This study observed that the masseter and anterior temporalis muscles commonly produced trigeminal referral of pain to the face, jaw and parietofrontal region; whereas the posterior temporalis muscle also referred pain into cervical territories, such as the occipitotemporal region and occasionally the upper cervical region. The trapezius muscle almost exclusively produced pain in upper cervical regions; whereas splenius and sternocleidomastoid muscles produced referred

pain both in the craniocervical region and into the ophthalmic trigeminal territory, as previously purported to be comparable to headache pain. These findings are consistent with prior investigations of experimental pain in pericranial musculature (Jensen & Norup, 1992; Svensson & Graven-Nielsen, 2001). Hence there appears to be a clear distinction between trigeminally and cervically innervated muscles with only limited functional overlap observed, despite the extensive convergence between these systems reported in animal studies (Sessle et al., 1986).

Originally, it was reported that referred pain followed a segmental pattern (Kellgren, 1938) and was thus restricted to the dermatome, myotome or sclerotome of the spinal segment innervating the painful

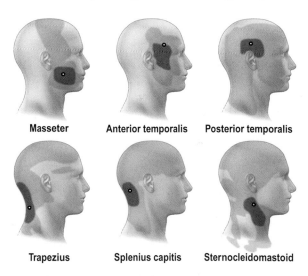

Masseter   **Anterior temporalis**   **Posterior temporalis**

Trapezius   **Splenius capitis**   **Sternocleidomastoid**

Figure 5.2

Pain distribution, as drawn on a body chart, following hypertonic saline injections into the masseter, anterior and posterior parts of the temporalis, trapezius, splenius capitis, and sternocleidomastoid muscles. Dark gray shapes represent the most commonly drawn pain areas (>5 subjects), light gray shapes represent the combined extent of the pain areas (≥1 subject), and white dots denote the injection sites. Based on original data from 20 subjects presented in Schmidt-Hansen et al. (2006).

structure. However, this is no longer considered to be accurate. The distribution of both clinical and experimentally induced referred pain does not always follow a strict segmental pattern. In fact, referred pain in areas three segments distant to an electrically stimulated lumbar dorsal root segment has been reported (Bogduk, 1980). Consistent with this, TrPs in the temporalis muscle (mandibular division of the trigeminal nerve) can refer pain to the teeth (maxillary division of trigeminal nerve), and TrPs within the suboccipital (C1) and splenius capitis (C2–C4) muscles can result in referred pain in the trigeminally innervated temple region (Simons et al., 1999). Thus, referred pain from muscle tissue most likely extends into the territories innervated by neighboring segments to the afferent nerve supplying the painful structure.

Another interesting feature of referred pain is the semidirectionality of its occurrence, with referral toward the distal joint being most common in the extremities. For example, inducing experimental pain in the tibialis anterior muscle will commonly evoke referred pain in the ankle, but strong experimental pressure-induced pain at the ankle will not evoke pain in the tibialis anterior muscle (Graven-Nielsen, 2006). In contrast, there are some examples of bidirectional referred pain from muscle (Feinstein et al., 1954), which are certainly well-illustrated in the craniofacial region. Here, experimental jaw-muscle (masseter) pain can refer pain to the teeth (Svensson et al., 1998), and odontogenic (tooth) pain can often mimic jaw-muscle and facial pain (Falace et al., 1996). Similarly, as already highlighted, temporomandibular structures can give rise to neck pain and headache-like referred symptoms, and the temporalis and upper cervical muscles can give rise to referred jaw and facial symptoms.

Clinically, osteoarthritis in the hip joint is often accompanied by complaints of knee pain (and vice versa), which may in some cases be the only symptom and illustrates pain referral from a joint. Fairly localized pain is however induced by stimulation of the fat pad of the knee (Joergensen et al., 2013). In contrast, experimental electrical facet joint stimulation induces low back pain and pain referral into the anterior leg, ipsilaterally, proximal to the knee, similar to what is observed clinically in facet joint pain (O'Neill et al., 2009). Pain patterns from cervical joints have been extensively studied typically by joint provocation followed by recordings of the referred pain areas. As an example, the pain patterns from the cervical zygapophyseal joints were assessed by distending the joint capsule in healthy volunteers with injections of contrast medium under fluoroscopic control (Dwyer et al., 1990). The referred pain patterns that result from stimulation of the upper cervical spine zygapophyseal joints have also been described by Aprill et al. (2002). The opposite approach was used in patients where the referred pain areas from the zygapophyseal joint pain were eliminated by selective nerve blocks (Cooper et al., 2007). Cervical facet joints are therefore likely to be a source of headache pain, due to the characteristic pain referral pattern to the head and neck. Limited information exists from stimulating the TMJ. One study injected glutamate into the TMJ, producing pain that was fairly localized in the orofacial region with a few cases of pain being in the occipital region (Alstergren et al., 2010).

In addition to pain, the region of referral may also exhibit changes in sensitivity to cutaneous and deep mechanical stimuli. However, the direction of such changes is still debated, with the seminal experimental studies showing hyperalgesia in the region of referred pain (Feinstein et al., 1954; Kellgren, 1938) and later experimental studies showing hypoalgesia in the region of referral (Graven-Nielsen et al., 1998). Clinical studies are also difficult to interpret in this respect as often generalized hypersensitivity may exist, meaning both local and remote sites will be affected regardless of the presence of referred pain in the remote region.

Temporal and spatial characteristics of referred pain

The appearance of referred pain is commonly delayed in comparison to the appearance of local pain. When using single bolus hypertonic saline injections, referred pain occurs approximately 20 seconds after the relatively instant perception of local pain (Graven-Nielsen et al., 1997). Similarly, continuous intramuscular electrical stimulation induces immediate and constant local nociceptive activity, and hence relatively immediate local pain, but referred pain is again delayed, appearing approximately 40 seconds later (Laursen et al., 1997). Further to this, prolonged exposure to experimental muscle pain, from either hypertonic saline infusion (Graven-Nielsen et al., 1998) or painful mechanical stimulation (Gibson et al., 2006), produces referred pain more frequently than during the initial phase or during a briefer painful exposure period. Together this indicates that referred pain is, at least to some extent, a time-dependent process.

In addition, the occurrence and area of referred pain may be related to the intensity of overall pain (Graven-Nielsen, 2006; Jensen & Norup, 1992). Similarly when referred pain develops in addition to local pain, the local and referred pain intensities are clearly well correlated (Graven-Nielsen, 2006). Given the relationship between pain intensity and the size of the pain area, however, it is possible that local pain may expand into the area of referred pain. In this case there is no longer true referred pain according to the definition (that is, pain not confined to the local pain area), and hence the prevalence of referred pain may be underestimated. Consistent with this, less than half of the intramuscular hypertonic saline injections seem to provoke true referred pain, but many participants (more than 60%) develop pain far from the injection site, or pain that spreads from the injection site into typical regions of referral (Graven-Nielsen, 2006). The location of painful stimulation in a muscle may also play a role in the development and extent of referred pain, with higher pain intensity and larger referred pain areas observed following hypertonic saline injection into the motor endplate zone compared to a control site (Qerama et al., 2004). However, this difference was not observed when using capsaicin (Qerama et al., 2004) and may instead be due to the difference in evoked pain intensity between sites with hypertonic saline. Pain intensity would therefore appear to be the primary determinant for the induction of referred pain from muscle.

In some instances, participants develop only referred pain and not local pain. This is an interesting conundrum, similar to what is often seen with referred pain from the viscera (Ness & Gebhart, 1990), and it is not entirely clear why this occurs. Potentially it is the result of anatomical variation, the excitation of different intramuscular nociceptive groups, or differences in descending modulatory systems, but it is yet to be confirmed.

The need for afferent somatosensory information from the referred pain area

To induce referred pain, somatosensory input from the periphery is at least partly involved. Differential nerve block techniques have demonstrated this, showing reduced referred pain intensity following blockage of myelinated afferents in the referred pain area (Laursen et al., 1999). Interestingly, the blockage of unmyelinated afferents conferred no greater pain reduction, suggesting that the proprioceptive fibers may be the most important peripheral component for the development of referred pain (Laursen et al., 1999). However, referred pain has also been induced in regions of complete sensory loss, for example following spinal cord injury, nerve lesion, amputation or regional anesthetic, with unchanged or only slightly decreased pain intensity (Feinstein et al., 1954; Harman, 1948; Kellgren, 1938; Whitty & Willison, 1958). Hence, the amount of peripheral somatosensory input required for referred pain induction varies depending on the location, structure, and central facilitatory mechanisms.

Experimental pain referral in musculoskeletal pain and headache

The presence of chronic musculoskeletal pain and headache conditions changes the behavior of experimentally induced muscle pain. Hypertonic saline injections into the anterior temporalis muscle result in larger pain areas of referral in patients with chronic and episodic tension-type headaches when compared to healthy controls (Schmidt-Hansen et al., 2007). Larger areas also resulted from injections into

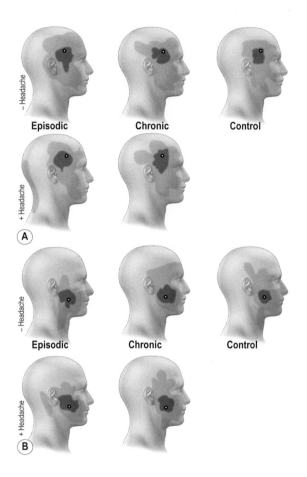

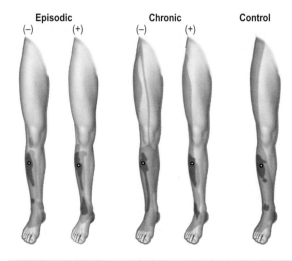

Figure 5.4

Pain areas induced by hypertonic saline injection (0.5 mL, 5.8%) into the tibialis anterior (TA) muscle in patients with headache and healthy participants. Patients with frequent episodic or chronic tension-type headache were assessed both during (+) and without (−) ongoing headache. Dark gray shapes represent the most commonly drawn pain areas (> 5 subjects), light gray shapes represent the combined extent of the pain areas (≥ 1 subject), and white dots denote the injection sites. Based on original data from Schmidt-Hansen et al. (2007).

Figure 5.3

Pain areas induced by hypertonic saline injection (0.5 mL, 5.8%) into the temporalis anterior (A) and masseter (B) muscles in patients with headache and healthy participants. Patients with frequent episodic or chronic tension-type headache were assessed both during (+) and without (−) ongoing headache, and were found to demonstrate larger pain areas than healthy participants, especially for the temporalis anterior muscle. Dark gray shapes represent the most commonly drawn pain areas (> 5 subjects), light gray shapes represent the combined extent of the pain areas (≥ 1 subject), and white dots denote the injection sites. Based on original data from Schmidt-Hansen et al. (2007).

adjacent and distant sites, for example the masseter (Figure 5.3) and tibialis anterior (Figure 5.4) muscles (Schmidt-Hansen et al., 2007), suggesting generalized sensitization in these patients. Such differences are also seen in widespread pain conditions, such as fibromyalgia, with higher pain intensity and larger referred pain areas in response to hypertonic saline injection than in matched healthy controls (Arendt-Nielsen & Graven-Nielsen, 2003). Fibromyalgia patients also commonly showed significant proximal referral of pain, unlike the predominantly distal referral patterns observed in healthy controls, which may also be indicative of sensitized central pain mechanisms. Larger areas of referred pain, following hypertonic saline injection into normally nonpainful muscles, have also been observed in patients with chronic whiplash-associated disorder (Johansen et al., 1999), TMD pain (Svensson et al., 2001), symptomatic knee osteoarthritis (Bajaj et al., 2001), and low back pain (O'Neill et al., 2007). These enlargements in referred pain areas suggest the presence of sensitized central pain processing or a loss of efficient descending inhibition, potentially as a consequence of the ongoing noxious input.

Mechanisms of referred pain

Animal experiments using single neuron recordings have shown extensive convergence in the caudal trigeminal sensory nucleus complex between cervical and trigeminal afferents (Sessle et al., 1986). This convergent-projection theory is one of the earliest neuroanatomical explanations for referred pain, suggesting that the convergence of multiple afferents onto the same spinal neuron gives rise to referred pain by precluding higher brain regions from accurately identifying the original source. However, this explanation fails to account for the delayed onset of referred pain. Instead, referred pain may be partly due to central hyperexcitability and the development of new receptive fields (Graven-Nielsen, 2006; Mense & Simons, 2001; Neugebauer & Schaible, 1990). The former, central hyperexcitability, is supported by findings of reduced frequency of referred pain in healthy subjects when treated with a low dose of ketamine (an NMDA-receptor antagonist) to antagonize central hyperexcitability (Schulte et al., 2003). The latter, development of new receptive fields, has been demonstrated in animal studies following noxious muscle stimulation (Hoheisel et al., 1993; Hu et al., 1992). There is assumed to be an extensive and complex network of collateral synaptic connections for each muscle afferent to different dorsal horn neurons (Mense & Simons, 2001), some of which are fully functional under normal conditions, and others which are latent. Ongoing strong noxious input may activate these latent synaptic connections, allowing for greater convergence of afferent inputs from nearby regions, and hence give rise to the delayed emergence of referred pain.

Sensitization of craniofacial pain mechanisms

Both peripheral and central sensitization processes are implicated in the development and maintenance of craniofacial pain conditions. Peripheral sensitization generally occurs with injury- or inflammation-related activation of muscle and/or joint nociceptive afferents (Cairns, 2010; Sessle 2011). Peripheral muscle nociceptors may be activated by a number of substances (Mense, 2009), but perhaps the two most important factors are the release of adenosine triphosphate (ATP) and protons (H+). The resulting neuronal activation stimulates neuropeptide release from the free nerve ending, termed neurogenic inflammation. Known substances involved in this process include substance P (SP), bradykinin (BK), calcitonin-gene-related peptide (CGRP), serotonin (5HT) and prostaglandin E2 (PGE2) (Xanthos & Sandkühler, 2014), and also tumor necrosis factor alpha (TNFα) and nerve growth factor (NGF) which can further sensitize muscle nociceptors (Mense, 2009).

Inflammation, caused by increased joint loading, remodeling and hence release of proinflammatory mediators (TNFα and interleukins [ILs]) may be the most potent driver of pain in some conditions (especially joint-related conditions). This up-regulation of proinflammatory mediators can then cause greater release of inflammatory substances, such as SP, BK, CGRP and PGE2, causing neurogenic inflammation and the hallmark inflammatory signs of redness, edema, warmth and pain (Takeuchi et al., 2004). Peripheral glial cells may also be involved in peripheral sensitization, as has been seen in some animal models of orofacial pain (Zhao et al., 2015). In these studies, satellite glial cells were activated in response to stress (a known contributor to many chronic orofacial conditions), which is associated with an over-release of proinflammatory mediators and the development of mechanical allodynia (Zhao et al., 2015). As may be expected, plasma levels of proinflammatory cytokines (such as IL-1β, IL-6, IL-10 and TNFα) have been demonstrated to be elevated in patients with TMD (Park & Chung, 2016;

Takahashi et al., 1998). Interestingly, the magnitude of cytokine elevation in these patients was associated with the level of disability and sleep disturbance (Park & Chung 2016), suggesting that TMD may be one condition where the inflammatory process is indeed a potent driver of pain and disability, and that this inflammation may be maintained or further exacerbated by factors such as sleep quality and stress.

Strong excitation of nociceptive-specific afferents (C fibers) from deep tissues can cause prolonged hyperexcitability of dorsal horn neurons that may be responsible for hyperalgesia (Woolf, 2011). If this hyperexcitability or sensitization is limited to second-order neurons, pain and hyperalgesia will be limited to the innervated field; but if such sensitization advances to third-order neurons, this may underlie the widespread pain reported by groups of patients with craniofacial pain conditions (Burstein et al., 2000). Consequently, the more widespread a musculoskeletal pain condition becomes, the more signs of generalized hypersensitivity are demonstrated (Carli et al., 2002).

For a range of TMDs, widespread changes in mechanical pain detection thresholds (Ayesh et al., 2007; Fernández-de-las-Peñas et al., 2009), along with enhanced temporal summation of pain (Maixner et al., 1995), and after-sensations (Sarlani et al., 2004) have been observed. Similar local and widespread changes in pain sensitivity, and facilitated temporal summation, have also been shown in patients with chronic tension-type headache (Abboud et al., 2013; Ashina et al., 2006), migraine (Burstein et al., 2000) cluster headache (Fernández-de-las-Peñas et al., 2011), and to a lesser extent in individuals with episodic tension-type headache (Bendtsen & Jensen, 2000). Such observations cannot solely be explained by peripheral sensitization or neurogenic inflammation and instead implicate central nociceptive processes, such as central hyperexcitability and a loss of descending inhibition. (See Chapters 4 and 6 of this textbook for further information on the effect of sensitization mechanisms on TMDs.)

Pain modulatory systems

Increasing evidence suggests that chronic pain conditions are associated with disturbed balance between descending pain inhibition and facilitation – a phenomenon which may play a role in maintaining the sensitization of central pain mechanisms (You et al., 2010). To quantify descending inhibitory function, a counterirritation analgesia paradigm is used, whereby a tonic painful stimulus is applied extrasegmentally to alter the perception of pain in response to a particular painful stimulus. The reduced pain sensitivity that is produced is thought to result from the activation of medullary inhibitory projections that act postsynaptically to inhibit spinal and trigeminal wide dynamic range neurons in the dorsal horn (Le Bars et al., 1975). This paradigm and the effect it produces is termed diffuse noxious inhibitory control (DNIC) in animals or conditioned pain modulation (CPM) in humans (Yarnitsky et al., 2010). CPM can be evoked experimentally by applying a tonic nociceptive conditioning stimulus (such as tonic pressure or submersion of an extremity into ice water) while concurrently or sequentially applying a segmentally distinct acute nociceptive test stimulus (such as a pressure or thermal pain detection threshold or defined supra-threshold stimulus). The magnitude of the CPM effect is then quantified as the difference between the acute nociceptive stimulus rating with and without conditioning, with an improvement during conditioning normally expected (that is, increased pain detection threshold or lowered evoked pain). However, as the CPM effect reflects the net sum of descending pain inhibition and facilitation, in many patients with chronic pain there tends to be a reduced inhibitory effect (Yarnitsky, 2015).

Interestingly, the ability of the craniofacial region to drive CPM has not been extensively investigated. It is clear that spinal nociceptive systems can produce inhibitory effects on pain perception in the craniofacial region, and it seems that the reverse is also possible, despite it often being overlooked. One conditioning model that has been used is compression-induced head pain, which effectively modulates pain perception at the masseter and tibialis anterior muscles (Sowman et al., 2011). Similarly cold-induced head pain has also been used to effectively modulate pain perception at the masseter, neck, elbow, and finger (Wang et al., 2010a). Hence, it seems as though CPM mechanisms can operate effectively across trigeminal and spinal nociceptive systems.

Dysfunctional descending pain modulation has been implicated as a pertinent mechanism in a number of craniofacial pain conditions, mostly in tension-type headache and migraine (Drummond & Knudsen, 2011; Sandrini et al., 2006). Although it is unclear if such a mechanism is involved in the etiology of these pain conditions, dysfunctional descending pain modulation likely contributes to the magnitude of symptoms experienced. In other craniofacial conditions, such as TMDs, alterations in CPM are not consistently demonstrated, with some studies showing comparable CPM to controls and others showing impairments (Garrett et al., 2013; Kothari et al., 2015; Oono et al., 2014). However, these inconsistencies may be due to differences in CPM methodology or heterogeneity in the etiologies of TMDs tested (Kothari et al., 2015). Nevertheless, dysfunctional descending pain modulation may be a common mechanism across various craniofacial and other musculoskeletal pain conditions, potentially contributing to the spreading of pain hypersensitivity. There are known to be overlaps between painful TMDs and headache disorders, as well as a high prevalence of TMDs in individuals with fibromyalgia syndrome, whiplash-associated disorder and other chronic pain disorders, for which dysfunctional descending pain modulation may provide a mechanistic link.

Conclusion

Referred craniofacial pain from musculoskeletal tissues can be experimentally assessed. Such investigations have shown distinct pain distributions for different individual muscles, which may be relevant to the perception of pain in the craniofacial region. Expanded referral patterns, facilitated temporal pain summation, and enhanced pain sensitivity, have been observed in craniofacial disorders and other musculoskeletal pain conditions. Similarly, an impairment of descending pain inhibition has also been demonstrated across different craniofacial pain disorders. Together, these mechanisms may drive the development, maintenance and/or progression of chronic craniofacial pain states, and hence should be a target for the development of rational treatment strategies.

Acknowledgments

Center for Neuroplasticity and Pain (CNAP) is supported by the Danish National Research Foundation (DNRF121).

References

Abboud J, Marchand AA, Sorra K, Descarreaux M. Musculoskeletal physical outcome measures in individuals with tension-type headache: a scoping review. Cephalalgia 2013; 33: 1319–1336.

Alonso-Blanco C, Fernández-de-las-Peñas C, de-la-Llave-Rincón AI, Zarco-Moreno P, Galán-del-Río F, Svensson P. Characteristics of referred muscle pain to the head from active trigger points in women with myofascial temporomandibular pain and fibromyalgia syndrome. J Headache Pain 2012; 13: 625–637.

Alstergren P, Ernberg M, Nilsson M, Hajati AK, Sessle BJ, Kopp S. Glutamate-induced temporomandibular joint pain in healthy individuals is partially mediated by peripheral NMDA receptors. J Orofac Pain 2010; 24: 172–180.

Aprill C, Axinn MJ, Bogduk N. Occipital headaches stemming from the lateral atlanto-axial (C1–2) joint. Cephalalgia 2002; 22: 15–22.

Arendt-Nielsen L, Graven-Nielsen T. Central sensitization in fibromyalgia and other musculoskeletal disorders. Curr Pain Headache Rep 2003; 7: 355–361.

Ashina S, Bendtsen L, Ashina M, Magerl W, Jensen R. Generalized hyperalgesia in patients with chronic tension-type headache. Cephalalgia 2006; 26: 940–948.

Ayesh EE, Jensen TS, Svensson P. Hypersensitivity to mechanical and intra-articular electrical stimuli in persons with painful temporomandibular joints. J Dent Res 2007; 86: 1187–1192.

Bajaj P, Bajaj P, Graven-Nielsen T, Arendt-Nielsen L. Osteoarthritis and its association with muscle hyperalgesia: an experimental controlled study. Pain 2001; 93: 107–114.

Bendtsen L, Jensen R. Amitriptyline reduces myofascial tenderness in patients with chronic tension-type headache. Cephalalgia 2000; 20: 603–610.

Bogduk N. Lumbar dorsal ramus syndrome. Med J Aust 1980; 2: 537–541.

Burstein R, Cutrer MF, Yarnitsky D. The development of cutaneous allodynia during a migraine attack: clinical evidence for the sequential recruitment of spinal and supraspinal nociceptive neurons in migraine. Brain 2000; 123: 1703–1709.

Cairns BE. Pathophysiology of TMD pain—basic mechanisms and their implications for pharmacotherapy. J Oral Rehabil 2010; 37: 391–410.

Campbell DG, Parsons CM. Referred head pain and its concomitants. J Nerv Mental Dis 1944; 99: 544–551.

Carli G, Suman AL, Biasi G, Marcolongo R. Reactivity to superficial and deep stimuli in patients with chronic musculoskeletal pain. Pain 2002; 100: 259–269.

Conti PC, Costa YM, Gonçalves DA, Svensson P. Headaches and myofascial temporomandibular disorders: overlapping entities, separate managements? J Oral Rehabil 2016; 43: 702–715.

Cooper G, Bailey B, Bogduk N. Cervical zygapophysial joint pain maps. Pain Med 2007; 8: 344–353.

Drummond PD, Knudsen L. Central pain modulation and scalp tenderness in frequent episodic tension-type headache. Headache 2011; 51: 375–383.

Dwyer A, Aprill C, Bogduk N. Cervical zygapophyseal joint pain patterns. I: A study in normal volunteers. Spine 1990; 15: 453–457.

Falace DA, Reid K, Rayens MK. The influence of deep (odontogenic) pain intensity, quality, and duration on the incidence and characteristics of referred orofacial pain. J Orofac Pain 1996; 10: 232–239.

Falla D, Farina D, Dahl MK, Graven-Nielsen T. Muscle pain induces task-dependent changes in cervical agonist/antagonist activity. J Appl Physiol 2007; 102: 601–609.

Feinstein B, Langton JNK, Jameson RM, Schiller F. Experiments on pain referred from deep somatic tissues. J Bone Joint Surg Am 1954; 36A: 981–997.

Fernández-de-las-Peñas C, Galán-del-Río F, Fernández-Carnero J, Pesquera J, Arendt-Nielsen L, Svensson P. Bilateral widespread mechanical pain sensitivity in women with myofascial temporomandibular disorder: evidence of impairment in central nociceptive processing. J Pain 2009; 10: 1170–1178.

Fernández-de-las-Peñas C, Galán-del-Río F, Alonso-Blanco C, Jímenez-García R, Arendt-Nielsen L, Svensson P. Referred pain from muscle trigger points in the masticatory and neck-shoulder musculature in women with temporomandibular disorders. J Pain 2010; 11: 1295–1304.

Fernández-de-Las-Penas C, Ortega-Santiago R, Cuadrado ML, López-de-Silanes C, Pareja JA. Bilateral widespread mechanical pain hypersensitivity as sign of central sensitization in patients with cluster headache. Headache 2011; 51: 384–391.

Garrett PH, Sarlani E, Grace EG, Greenspan JD. Chronic temporomandibular disorders are not necessarily associated with a compromised endogenous analgesic system. J Orofac Pain 2013; 27: 142–150.

Gibson W, Arendt-Nielsen L, Graven-Nielsen T. Referred pain and hyperalgesia in human tendon and muscle belly tissue. Pain 2006; 120: 113–123.

Graven-Nielsen T. Fundamentals of muscle pain, referred pain, and deep tissue hyperalgesia. Scand J Rheumatol 2006; 35: S1-S43.

Graven-Nielsen T, Arendt-Nielsen L, Svensson P, Jensen TS. Stimulus-response functions in areas with experimentally induced referred muscle pain: a psychophysical study. Brain Res 1997; 744: 121–128.

Graven-Nielsen T, Babenko V, Svensson P, Arendt-Nielsen L. Experimentally induced muscle pain induces hypoalgesia in heterotopic deep tissues, but not in homotopic deep tissues. Brain Res 1998; 787: 203–210.

Harman JB. The localization of deep pain. Br Med J 1948; 188–192.

Head H. On disturbances of sensation with especial reference to the pain of visceral disease. Brain 1893; 16: 1–133.

Hoheisel U, Mense S, Simons DG, Yu XM. Appearance of new receptive fields in rat dorsal horn neurons following noxious stimulation of skeletal muscle: a model for referral of muscle pain? Neurosci Lett 1993; 153: 9–12.

Hong CZ, Kuan TS, Chen JT, Chen SM. Referred pain elicited by palpation and by needling of myofascial trigger points: a comparison. Arch Phys Med Rehabil 1997; 78: 957–960.

Hu JW, Sessle BJ, Raboisson P, Dallel R, Woda A. Stimulation of craniofacial muscle afferents induces prolonged facilitatory effects in trigeminal nociceptive brain-stem neurones. Pain 1992; 48: 53–60.

Jensen K, Norup M. Experimental pain in human temporal muscle induced by hypertonic saline, potassium and acidity. Cephalalgia 1992; 12: 101–106.

Joergensen TS, Henriksen M, Danneskiold-Samsoee B, Bliddal H, Graven-Nielsen T. Experimental knee pain evoke [sic] spreading hyperalgesia and facilitated temporal summation of pain. Pain Med 2013; 14: 874–883.

Johansen MK, Graven-Nielsen T, Olesen AS, Arendt-Nielsen L. Generalised muscular hyperalgesia in chronic whiplash syndrome. Pain 1999; 83: 229–234.

Kellgren JH. Observations on referred pain arising from muscle. Clin Sci 1938; 3: 175–190.

Kothari SF, Baad-Hansen L, Oono Y, Svensson P. Somatosensory assessment and conditioned pain modulation in temporomandibular disorders pain patients. Pain 2015; 156: 2545–2555.

Kuan TS, Hong CZ, Chen JT, Chen SM, Chien CH. The spinal cord connections of the myofascial trigger spots. Eur J Pain 2007; 11: 624–634.

Laursen RJ, Graven-Nielsen T, Jensen TS, Arendt-Nielsen L. Quantification of local and referred pain in humans induced by intramuscular electrical stimulation. Eur J Pain 1997; 1: 105–113.

Laursen RJ, Graven-Nielsen T, Jensen TS, Arendt-Nielsen L. The effect of compression and regional anaesthetic block on referred pain intensity in humans. Pain 1999; 80: 257–263.

Le Bars D, Menétrey D, Conseiller C, Besson JM. Depressive effects of morphine upon lamina V cells activities in the dorsal horn of the spinal cat. Brain Res 1975; 98: 261–277.

Li LT, Ge HY, Yue SW, Arendt-Nielsen L. Nociceptive and non-nociceptive hyper-sensitivity at latent myofascial trigger points. Clin J Pain 2009; 25: 132–137.

Maixner W, Fillingim R, Booker D, Sigurdsson A. Sensitivity of patients with painful temporomandibular disorders to experimentally evoked pain. Pain 1995; 63: 341–351.

Mense S. Algesic agents exciting muscle nociceptors. Exp Brain Res 2009; 196: 89–100

Mense S, Simons DG. Muscle Pain: Understanding its Nature, Diagnosis, and Treatment. Philadelphia, USA: Lippincott Williams & Wilkins; 2001.

Ness TJ, Gebhart GF. Visceral pain: A review of experimental studies. Pain 1990; 41: 167–234.

Ness TJ, Metcalf AM, Gebhart GF. A psychophysiological study in humans using phasic colonic distension as a noxious visceral stimulus. Pain 1990; 43: 377–386.

Neugebauer V, Schaible HG. Evidence for a central component in the sensitization of spinal neurons with joint input during development of acute arthritis in cat's knee. J Neurophysiol 1990; 64: 299–311.

Niddam DM. Brain manifestation and modulation of pain from myofascial trigger points. Curr Pain Headache Rep 2009; 13: 370–375.

Niddam DM, Chan RC, Lee SH, Yeh TC, Hsieh JC. Central representation of hyperalgesia from myofascial trigger point. Neuroimage 2008; 39: 1299–1306.

O'Neill S, Manniche C, Graven-Nielsen T, Arendt-Nielsen L. Generalized deep-tissue hyperalgesia in patients with chronic low-back pain. Eur J Pain 2007; 11: 415–420.

O'Neill S, Graven-Nielsen T, Manniche C, Arendt-Nielsen L. Ultrasound guided, painful electrical stimulation of lumbar facet joint structures: an experimental model of acute low back pain. Pain 2009; 144: 76–83.

Oono Y, Wang K, Baad-Hansen L, Futarmal S, Kohase H, Svensson P, Arendt-Nielsen L. Conditioned pain modulation in temporomandibular disorders (TMD) pain patients. Exp Brain Res 2014; 232: 3111–3119.

Park JW, Chung JW. Inflammatory cytokines and sleep disturbance in patients with temporomandibular disorders. J Oral Facial Pain Headache 2016; 30: 27–33.

Peck CC, Goulet JP, Lobbezoo F et al. Expanding the taxonomy of the diagnostic criteria for temporomandibular disorders. J Oral Rehabil 2014; 41: 2–23.

Qerama E, Fuglsang-Frederiksen A, Kasch H, Bach FW, Jensen TS. Evoked pain in the motor endplate region of the brachial biceps muscle: an experimental study. Muscle Nerve 2004; 29: 393–400.

Sandrini G, Rossi P, Milanov I, Serrao M, Cecchini AP, Nappi G. Abnormal modulatory influence of diffuse noxious inhibitory controls in migraine and chronic tension-type headache patients. Cephalalgia 2006; 26: 782–789.

Sarlani E, Grace EG, Reynolds MA, Greenspan JD. Sex differences in temporal summation of pain and aftersensations following repetitive noxious mechanical stimulation. Pain 2004; 109: 115–23.

Schiffman E, Ohrbach R, Truelove E et al. Diagnostic Criteria for Temporomandibular Disorders (DC/TMD) for Clinical and Research Applications: recommendations of the International RDC/TMD Consortium Network and Orofacial Pain Special Interest Group. J Oral Facial Pain Headache 2014; 28: 6–27.

Schmidt-Hansen PT, Svensson P, Jensen TS, Graven-Nielsen T, Bach FW. Patterns of experimentally induced pain in pericranial muscles. Cephalalgia 2006; 26: 568–577.

Schmidt-Hansen PT, Svensson P, Bendtsen L, Graven-Nielsen T, Bach FW. Increased muscle pain sensitivity in patients with tension-type headache. Pain 2007; 129: 113–121.

Schulte H, Graven-Nielsen T, Sollevi A, Jansson Y, Arendt-Nielsen L, Segerdahl M. Pharmacological modulation of experimental phasic and tonic muscle pain by morphine, alfentanil and ketamine in healthy volunteers. Acta Anaesthesiol Scand 2003; 47: 1020–1030.

Sessle BJ. Peripheral and central mechanisms of orofacial inflammatory pain. Int Rev Neurobiol 2011; 97: 179–206.

Sessle BJ, Hu JW, Amano N, Zhong G. Convergence of cutaneous, tooth pulp, visceral, neck and muscle afferents onto nociceptive and non-nociceptive neurones in trigeminal subnucleus caudalis (medullary dorsal horn) and its implications for referred pain. Pain 1986; 27: 219–235.

Shah JP, Phillips TM, Danoff JV, Gerber LH. An in vivo microanalytical technique for measuring the local biochemical milieu of human skeletal muscle. J Appl Physiol 2005; 99: 1977–1984.

Simons DG, Travell JG, Simons L. Myofascial Pain and Dysfunction: The Trigger Point Manual. Philadelphia, USA: Lippincott Williams & Wilkins; 1999.

Chapter 5

Sowman PF, Wang K, Svensson P, Arendt-Nielsen L. Diffuse noxious inhibitory control evoked by tonic craniofacial pain in humans. Eur J Pain 2011; 15: 139–145.

Svensson P. Muscle pain in the head: overlap between temporomandibular disorders and tension-type headaches. Curr Opin Neurol 2007; 20: 320–325.

Svensson P, Graven-Nielsen T. Craniofacial muscle pain: review of mechanisms and clinical manifestations. J Orofac Pain 2001; 15: 117–145.

Svensson P, De Laat A, Graven-Nielsen T, Arendt-Nielsen L. Experimental jaw-muscle pain does not change heteronymous H-reflexes in the human temporalis muscle. Exp Brain Res 1998; 121: 311–318.

Svensson P, List T, Hector G. Analysis of stimulus-evoked pain in patients with myofascial temporomandibular pain disorders. Pain 2001; 92: 399–409.

Takahashi T, Kondoh T, Fukuda M, Yamazaki Y, Toyosaki T, Suzuki R. Proinflammatory cytokines detectable in synovial fluids from patients with temporomandibular disorders. Oral Surg Oral Med Oral Pathol Oral Radiol Endod 1998; 85: 135–141.

Takeuchi Y, Zeredo JL, Fujiyama R, Amagasa T, Toda K. Effects of experimentally induced inflammation on temporomandibular joint nociceptors in rats. Neurosci Lett 2004; 354: 172–174.

Wang K, Svensson P, Sessle BJ, Cairns BE, Arendt-Nielsen L. Painful conditioning stimuli of the craniofacial region evokes diffuse noxious inhibitory controls in men and women. J Orofac Pain 2010a; 24: 255–261.

Wang YH, Ding XL, Zhang Y, Chen J, Ge HY, Arendt-Nielsen L, Yue SW. Ischemic compression block attenuates mechanical hyperalgesia evoked from latent myofascial trigger points. Exp Brain Res 2010b; 202: 265–270.

Whitty CWM, Willison RG. Some aspects of referred pain. Lancet 1958; 2: 226–231.

Woolf CJ. Central sensitization: implications for the diagnosis and treatment of pain. Pain 2011; 152: S2-S15.

Wright EF. Referred craniofacial pain patterns in patients with temporomandibular disorder. J Am Dent Assoc 2000; 131: 1307–1315.

Xanthos DN, Sandkühler J. Neurogenic neuroinflammation: inflammatory CNS reactions in response to neuronal activity. Nat Rev Neurosci 2014; 15: 43–53.

Xie P, Qin B, Song G et al. Microstructural abnormalities were found in brain gray matter from patients with chronic myofascial pain. Front Neuroanat 2016; 10: 122.

Yarnitsky D. Role of endogenous pain modulation in chronic pain mechanisms and treatment. Pain 2015; 156: S24-S31.

Yarnitsky D, Arendt-Nielsen L, Bouhassira D et al. Recommendations on terminology and practice of psychophysical DNIC testing. Eur J Pain 2010; 14: 339.

You HJ, Lei J, Sui MY, Huang L, Tan YX, Tjølsen A, Arendt-Nielsen L. Endogenous descending modulation: spatiotemporal effect of dynamic imbalance between descending facilitation and inhibition of nociception. J Physiol 2010; 588: 4177–4188.

Zhao YJ, Liu Y, Zhao YH, Li Q, Zhang M, Chen YJ. Activation of satellite glial cells in the trigeminal ganglion contributes to masseter mechanical allodynia induced by restraint stress in rats. Neurosci Lett 2015; 602: 150–155.

Chapter 6

Quantitative sensory testing in temporomandibular disorders

César Fernández-de-las-Peñas, Peter Svensson, Lars Arendt-Nielsen

Sensitization mechanisms in temporomandibular disorders

Temporomandibular disorder (TMD) is a major clinical health problem for which the identification of peripheral and central sensitization has improved understanding, diagnosis, and management. There is an ongoing debate as to the role of peripheral and central sensitization mechanisms; it is likely that the two mechanisms are interconnected in TMD and both to some degree contribute to its clinical manifestations.

Peripheral sensitization is defined as an increased responsiveness and a reduced threshold of peripheral nociceptors to stimulation of their receptive fields, and it is mainly characterized by increased spontaneous activity, decreased response threshold to noxious stimuli, increased responsiveness to the same noxious stimuli, and/or increased receptive field sizes. This applies to neuropathic pain (Meacham et al., 2017), musculoskeletal pain (Mense et al., 2001; Arendt-Nielsen et al., 2011) and visceral pain (Gebhart & Bielefeldt, 2016). The clinical manifestation of peripheral sensitization is deep tissue hyperalgesia at the area of the injury or painful area, that is, increased pain sensitivity to painful stimuli (Graven-Nielsen & Mense, 2001; Graven-Nielsen & Arendt-Nielsen, 2010). It seems that different substances can sensitize primary nociceptive fibers. Particularly effective stimulants for muscle nociceptors are endogenous substances such as substance P, glutamate, bradykinin, serotonin, histamine or prostaglandins in animals (Mense et al., 2001) and humans (Babenko et al., 1999). The release of these substances causes antidromic release of other neuropeptides such as calcitonin gene-related peptide or neurokinin A from nerve endings which will lower pH and will activate the arachidonic acid cascade (Mense et al., 2001). In fact, the excitatory amino acid glutamate has been found in primary afferent fibers from deep craniofacial tissues (for example masseter or temporalis muscles, temporomandibular joint) in both animals (Cairns et al., 2003) and humans (Cairns et al., 2007).

Central sensitization is defined in animals as increased response to painful stimulation mediated by amplification of signaling to the central nervous system (CNS) and can occur through increased excitation (sensitization) or decreased pain inhibition. In humans CNS activity cannot be directly recorded and hence proxies have to be used. Central sensitization can occur within minutes in the presence of peripheral nociception; however, long-lasting stimuli are able to induce prolonged plastic changes in the CNS. Interestingly, it seems that sensitization can also be reversed within a few minutes. In fact, nociceptive input from deep tissues (muscles) is more effective for inducing prolonged changes in the dorsal horn neurons than input from superficial tissues (skin) (Wall & Woolf, 1984). During central sensitization, the dorsal horn will become hyperexcitable in response to noxious stimulation generating new receptive fields at a distance from the origin of pain promoting the development of referred pain in musculoskeletal animal models (Mense et al., 2001). Therefore, the expansion or creation of receptive fields of central neurons explains the underlying referred pain associated with deep-tissue injury. In the context of orofacial pain, it is important to note that second dorsal horn neurons are integrated into the trigeminocervical nucleus caudalis, that is, the convergence of trigeminal and cervical afferents onto neurons in the brainstem (Goadsby & Bartsch, 2010). A recent study has found that chronic TMD is associated with alterations in the anatomy of the medullary dorsal horn, as well as its afferent and efferent projections (Wilcox et al., 2015). Nociceptive input from spinal dorsal horn neurons reaches the supraspinal structures resulting in increased excitability of these cortical neurons, decreased central pain inhibition or increased facilitation of nociceptive transmission in the dorsal horn. The sensitization of supraspinal structures will be clinically manifested as increased sensitivity over distant pain-free areas, that is, generalized or widespread pain hypersensitivity.

As mentioned previously, central sensitization is induced by prolonged, long-lasting nociceptive stimulation or by decreased pain inhibition, that is, impairment in diffuse noxious inhibitory control (DNIC) in animals, now known as conditioning pain modulation (CPM). In fact, current evidence supports that both increased pain facilitation and ineffective pain inhibition represent a predisposition to chronic pain in humans (Staud, 2012). Proper activation of CPM modulates CNS excitability at both dorsal horn and supraspinal levels by promoting temporary hypoalgesia in the presence of nociceptive stimulus. There is evidence suggesting less efficient CPM in several pain conditions involving the head, such as TMD (King et al., 2009), tension-type headache (Pielstickera et al., 2005), and migraine (Sandrini et al., 2006). However, other studies have not found differences in CPM between patients with TMD and healthy controls (Kothari et al., 2015).

Finally, imaging techniques have also contributed to better understanding of central pain processing (May, 2008). Different studies have demonstrated the presence of altered brain morphology in areas related to pain in patients with TMD (Lin, 2014), tension-type headache (Schmidt-Wilcke et al., 2005), and migraine (Kim et al., 2008). In fact, independent of the exact nature of these brain changes, it is accepted that chronic pain patients exhibit a decrease in gray matter as a common feature, and, while the exact loci differ between groups, there seems to be overlap in some areas including the cingulate cortex, insula, and dorsolateral prefrontal cortex (May, 2008). In myofascial TMD, Younger et al. (2010) demonstrated changes in gray matter volume in several areas of the trigemino-thalamo-cortical pathway but also an increased gray matter volume in some limbic regions. These changes seem to be associated with the intensity and duration of pain symptoms suggesting that they may be a consequence of the pain (Apkarian et al., 2009).

Quantitative sensory testing

Quantitative sensory testing (QST) is usually applied for assessment of nociceptive gain or somatosensory loss and can include the assessment of vibration, thermal, electrical, and mechanical stimulus (Hansson et al., 2007). Although QST is not a diagnostic test for any particular disease entity, it has demonstrated diagnostic capabilities in patients with TMD, burning mouth syndrome, or atypical odontalgia (Svensson et al., 2011).

There are several protocols for assessing QST. The German Research Network on Neuropathic Pain (DFNS) has developed a standardized QST battery for testing sensory loss (small or large nerve fiber functions), gain (hyperalgesia, allodynia, hyperpathia), and cutaneous or deep pain sensitivity (Rolke et al., 2006a). This protocol is optimized for assessing neuropathic pain conditions and hence not optimal for assessing pain from deeper structures. In general, the QST protocol takes between 30–60 minutes for each patient. This protocol assesses somatosensory functions across the full spectrum of primary nerve-fiber afferents. The procedures can be used to assess:

- *Aβ fibers* using mechanical detection thresholds to von Frey hairs and vibration;

- *Aδ fibers* using a cold detection threshold and a mechanical pain threshold to pinprick stimuli;

- *C fibers* using heat detection and heat-pain thresholds; and,

- *Aδ cold fibers* for the presence of paradoxical heat sensations.

The intra- and inter-examiner reliability of the QST protocol ranges from acceptable to excellent (Geber et al., 2011) including the orofacial region (Pigg et al., 2010). Tests can be grouped as summarized in the sections below (Rolke et al., 2006a).

Thermal thresholds

The heat detection threshold is defined as the first slightest sensation of warmth whereas the cold detection threshold is defined as the first slightest sensation of cold perceived by the subject. Heat- and cold-pain thresholds are defined as the moment when the sensation changes from warmth or cold to heat pain or cold pain, respectively. Individuals are instructed to press a switch as soon they perceive a change in temperature.

Different equipment is used for assessing thermal thresholds depending on the area of the body being tested. For the orofacial area, the recommended contact thermode area is $4\,cm^2$ for the extraoral region and $0.81\,cm^2$ for the intraoral region (Pigg et al., 2010). Jääskeläinen (2004) recommends the use of a thermode of $9\,mm^2$ (Figure 6.1) for examining trigeminal nerve conduction. The mean of three to five tests in each region is generally calculated and used for data analysis. A rest of at least five seconds occurs between repeated measurements. Paradoxical heat sensations can be also assessed by questioning the individual during the thermal sensory limen (the difference in threshold for alternating cool and warm stimuli) procedure (Rolke et al., 2006a).

Vibration threshold

The VIBRAMETER® (SOMEDIC, Sweden) is the equipment most commonly used for assessing vibration threshold. The range of amplitude for the vibration stimulus ranges from 0.1–130 µm, with a rate of change of 0.5 µm/s. The patient has their eyes closed during the procedure (Figure 6.2). The vibration-detection threshold in the German QST protocol consists only of the disappearance-vibration threshold (Rolke et al., 2006a). However, several

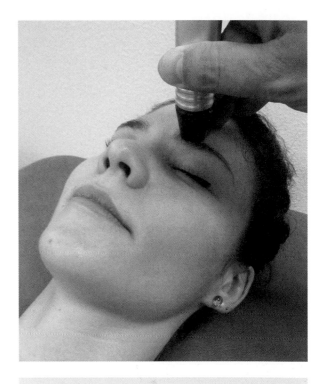

Figure 6.1
Assessment of thermal threshold over the supraorbital notch.

studies have used both the appearance and disappearance thresholds. Onset (appearance-ON) amplitude is defined as the amplitude (µm) at which subjects are able to perceive the vibration stimulus, while the offset (disappearance-OFF) amplitude is the amplitude at which the vibration sensation is no longer perceived by the subject. Both thresholds are repeated three times and the mean is calculated. The mean of both the onset and offset amplitudes is used to calculate the vibration threshold.

Mechanical detection threshold

The mechanical detection threshold is usually assessed with von Frey hairs (Semmes-Weinstein monofilaments, rounded tip, 0.5 mm in diameter). The filament is applied vertically on the area and

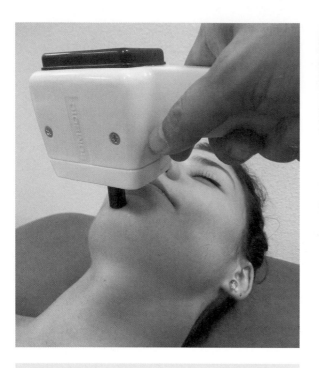

Figure 6.2
Assessment of vibration threshold over the chin.

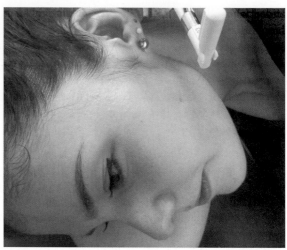

Figure 6.3
Assessment of mechanical detection threshold with von Frey hairs over the masseter muscle.

pressure is slowly applied until the filament bows (Figure 6.3). The stimulus is maintained for approximately 1.5 seconds and then it is removed slowly in 1.5 seconds. The subject is instructed to close the eyes during the test procedure and to raise the hand as soon as a stimulus in the test site is felt. The method of limits is the most common method used: different threshold determinations are made using a series of ascending and descending stimulus intensities.

Mechanical pain threshold

Mechanical pain threshold is assessed using custom-made weighted pinprick stimuli as a set of different pinprick mechanical stimulators with fixed stimulus intensities (contact area: 0.2 mm in diameter). The stimulators are applied at a rate of two seconds on, two seconds off in an ascending order until the first perception of sharpness is reached. The

final threshold is the geometric mean of five series of ascending and descending stimuli.

Pressure pain sensitivity

Mechanical pain sensitivity is generally assessed using a handheld pressure algometer (Figure 6.4). Different thresholds are usually assessed: the pressure pain threshold (PPT), which is the lowest pressure that is perceived as painful; and the pressure tolerance threshold (PPTo), which is the maximal pressure that is tolerated. The most common method of assessing mechanical pain sensitivity is with an electronic algometer (SOMEDIC, Sweden). Subjects are instructed to press the stop switch when the sensation changes from pressure to pain (PPT) or when they cannot tolerate more pressure (PPTo). The mean of three tests is usually calculated. A 30-second resting period is allowed between each measure to avoid temporal summation. The method has been found to have fair-to-excellent test-retest reliability for the mechanical somatosensory assessment of masticatory structures (Costa et al., 2017).

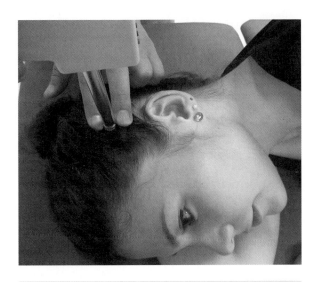

Figure 6.4
Assessment of pressure pain thresholds over the temporalis muscle.

Pressure algometry can be also used for determining the temporal summation of pain mimicking the initial phase of the wind-up process (Arendt-Nielsen & Graven-Nielsen, 2008). To elicit temporal summation, the mechanical stimulus is repeated at constant intervals, for example five times with a pre-determined frequency of 1 Hz at a constant intensity. The intensity of the five consecutive stimuli is gradually increased until the subject feels an increase in pain perception during the repeated stimulation.

Considerations for quantitative sensory testing

Women are generally more sensitive than men to many types of QST regardless of ethnicity (Komiyama et al., 2007), anatomical site of assessment (Matos et al., 2011) or age (Rolke et al., 2006b). Secondly, older subjects tend to be less sensitive than younger subjects (Rolke et al., 2006b; Blankenburg et al., 2010). Thirdly, ethnicity can determine the response to painful stimuli (Campbell et al., 2005) since Caucasians have demonstrated higher

thresholds than Asians and Africans (Komiyama et al., 2007). In fact, Caucasians also exhibit lower electrical exteroceptive suppression reflex thresholds in the trigeminal region than Japanese (Komiyama et al., 2009).

Finally, sensitivity varies depending on the area of the body being assessed. Several studies demonstrate that the face is more sensitive (exhibits lower thresholds) to thermal and mechanical stimuli than the hand or foot (Rolke et al., 2006b; Blankenburg et al., 2010). Further to this, sensitivity is higher on the face and tongue than on the gingiva (Pigg et al., 2010). Interestingly, pain sensitivity to different stimuli is also different depending on the territory of the trigeminal nerve (Matos et al., 2011; Yekta et al., 2010). Yang et al. (2014) demonstrated that somatosensory variability was region- and stimulus-dependent with some body areas being more sensitive to certain stimuli and other body areas being more sensitive to different stimuli. Contributing factors to site-dependent sensitivity include differences in innervation density, overlap of receptor fields, reaction time artifacts related to the distance of the brain, and environmental thickening of the epidermis.

Quantitative sensory testing for temporomandibular disorders

The use of QST has helped to better understand the mechanism-based diagnosis of orofacial pain. Several studies investigating different QST in patients with TMD and orofacial pain suggest the presence of sensitization mechanisms (La Touche et al., 2017). In fact, 85 per cent of TMD patients exhibit at least one or more somatosensory abnormalities (Kothari et al., 2015).

There is evidence indicating the presence of both peripheral and central sensitization in individuals with TMD (see Chapter 4). Briefly, this is supported by the presence of pressure pain hyperalgesia within the trigeminal area, particularly in the masticatory muscles (Maixner et al., 1998; Farella et al., 2000), and the association between widespread pressure pain hypersensitivity (Fernández-de-las-Peñas et al., 2009) or gray matter changes (Younger et al., 2010) with the intensity and duration of the TMD symptoms. Several studies have also reported that patients with TMD exhibit widespread pressure-pain hypersensitivity (Maixner et al., 1995; Svensson et al., 2001; Sarlani & Greenspan, 2003; Fernández-de-las-Peñas et al., 2009) as a sign of central sensitization; nevertheless, the magnitude of this sensitization seems to be higher within the trigeminal area. In fact, the largest case-control study including 185 patients with TMD and 1,633 healthy controls found that the highest differences were observed PPT at both trigeminal and nontrigeminal sites (Greenspan et al., 2011). Additionally, some authors have proposed PPTs cut-off values for identification of patients with TMD and orofacial pain (Cunha et al., 2014). Others have proposed the use of sustained mechanical pain sensitization (significant linear decrements in PPTs across the consecutive testing sessions) in the masseter muscle to discriminate between individuals with TMD and healthy people (Quartana et al., 2015). Nevertheless, although at the first onset of symptoms PPTs are modest predictors of persistent TMD, they are poor predictors of the incidence of TMD (Slade et al., 2014).

Importantly, the presence of comorbid neck pain symptoms (Muñoz-García et al., 2017), migraine (Pinto Fiamengui et al., 2013) or widespread symptoms (Chen et al., 2012), but not TMD-associated headache (Costa et al., 2016), is associated with higher pressure pain hyperalgesia in the trigeminal and extratrigeminal regions. This may be related to the fact that chronic pain results in apparently phenotypically different pain syndromes depending on the tissue affected, possibly reflecting a common contribution of central sensitization (Woolf, 2011). This is supported by a study showing that the pain profiles including somatosensory function were significantly different between patients with TMJ arthralgia and OA patients reflecting that, although they exhibit similar sensitization mechanisms, different orofacial pain conditions have differential pain mechanisms (Kothari et al., 2016)

Some studies have reported that individuals with myofascial TMD exhibit abnormal thermal thresholds and thermal temporal summation over the masticatory muscles (Maixner et al., 1998; Fernández-de-las-Peñas et al., 2010a; Carvalho et al., 2016; Janal et al., 2016), whereas others did not find such differences (Svensson et al., 2001; Raphael, 2009). Thermal hyperalgesia has been also found in patients with orofacial pain of arthrogenous origin (Park et al., 2010).

Finally, it should be considered that the presence of somatosensory disturbances is heterogeneous in individuals with orofacial pain. Pfau et al. (2009) described two subgroups of patients with TMD, sensitive and insensitive, based on a greater fibromyalgia tender point count. The sensitive TMD group was more sensitive to pressure and thermal stimuli than the nonsensitive TMD and control groups (Pfau et al., 2009). These authors suggested that TMD may act as precursor of fibromyalgia in a continuous spectrum sharing the same underlying pathology, supporting common nociceptive pain pathways in chronic pain conditions. However, it may be useful for identification of specific subtypes of TMD pain patients to use the somatosensory profile which may have potential implications for the management strategy and prognosis. Future studies will be needed to test this proposal but it is important to emphasize that the current knowledge and technology (QST) will allow such prospective studies to really advance and optimize care of TMD pain patients. Below is a brief review of the clinical applications of QST in TMD pain.

Clinical applications

Clinical identification of central sensitization

Although QST research suggests the presence of central sensitization in patients with TMD, identification of sensitization mechanisms in the clinical setting represents a challenge for clinicians (Nijs et al., 2010). In fact, identification of central sensitization can determine some treatment parameters, for example intensity, amplitude and frequency, of the therapeutic interventions and also the necessity of multimodal treatments including physical therapy, pain neuroscience education, cognitive behavioral therapy, and exercises (Nijs et al., 2014a). The main concern for clinicians is that no clear clinical symptom and/or sign with a strong diagnostic value for central sensitization exist and that not all patients with the same condition will exhibit central sensitization. It has been proposed that classification of central sensitization entails two major steps: the exclusion of neuropathic pain and the differential classification of nociceptive versus central sensitization pain (Nijs et al., 2014b). Therefore, identification of sensitization mechanisms in a clinical setting should be based on a cluster of symptoms and signs (Nijs et al., 2016).

Firstly, the clinical history provides a number of clues that potentially point toward the presence of central sensitization. For instance, the presence of hypersensitivity to bright light, sound or smell, abnormal thermal sensations, pressure hyperalgesia or allodynia are associated with central sensitization. Several of these features are present in different headaches explaining the overlap between symptoms in patients with TMD and tension-type headache or migraine (Svensson, 2007). In fact, the presence of larger spontaneous symptomatic areas is correlated with some measures of central sensitization, at least, in individuals with knee osteoarthritis (Lluch-Girbés et al., 2016). Larger pain areas have also been observed in the sensitive TMD group (Pfau et al., 2009).

Secondly, physical examination of a patient with TMD should include symptomatic and non-symptomatic areas for determining the presence of generalized sensitivity to manual palpation. Some authors have proposed that the presence of enlarged referred pain areas during palpation of muscle tissues is a sign of central sensitization

(Graven-Nielsen & Arendt-Nielsen, 2010). A study found that patients with myofascial TMD exhibited larger referred pain areas elicited by TrPs as compared to healthy controls (Fernández-de-las-Peñas et al., 2010b).

Management considerations and central sensitization

The challenge facing clinicians is how to select the proper treatment approach for patients with TMD whose individual clinical presentations with potential complex nociceptive pain mechanisms are likely to be somewhat different. In fact, the selection of a proper multimodal approach should consider the manifestations of peripheral and central sensitization (Nijs et al., 2010). For instance, it is commonly observed in the clinical setting that patients exhibiting a lower degree of central sensitization need fewer treatments to obtain positive outcomes.

It is important to remember that an ongoing source of peripheral nociception is usually required before a peripheral nociceptive input can promote central sensitization (Woolf, 2011). Therefore, it is crucial to limit the time course of afferent stimulation of peripheral nociceptors and early therapeutic programs would be theoretically crucial to prevent central sensitization (Arendt-Nielsen et al., 2011).

Clinical identification of the predominant sensitization process, peripheral or central, should orient the therapeutic program. In those patients mediated by peripheral nociceptive mechanisms (peripheral sensitization), treatment of the symptomatic tissues and application of appropriate exercises and functional activity should be encouraged. In patients mediated by central processes (central sensitization), a multimodal pharmacological, physical and cognitive approach should be encouraged.

Chapter 6

Finally, an abnormal response to exercise observed in subjects with central sensitization should also be considered. In healthy people, exercise usually exerts related hypoalgesia by activating the descending inhibitory mechanisms. In individuals with orofacial pain exhibiting central sensitization, exercise induces hyperalgesia instead of hypoalgesia (Mohn et al., 2008). Current theories propose the inclusion of graded exposure principles during exercise therapy for targeting the brain circuitries orchestrated by the amygdala (the memory-of-fear center in the brain). It is important that the patient's exercise therapy takes into account an understanding of pain neuroscience, including central sensitization mechanisms (Nijs et al., 2015).

Conclusion

The use of quantitative sensory testing (QST) has permitted a better understanding of loss and gain of function in the nociceptive pathways in individual patients with TMD and orofacial pain. The presence of sensitization mechanisms in TMD can determine the clinical prognosis and therapeutic strategies applied to these patients. A cluster of signs and symptoms can indicate to clinicians the likely presence of central sensitization in orofacial pain patients. Clinical identification of these sensitization processes is crucial for providing a proper explanation to patients and also for managing their therapy.

References

Apkarian AV, Baliki MN, Geha PY. Towards a theory of chronic pain. Prog Neurobiol 2009; 87: 81–97.

Arendt-Nielsen L, Graven-Nielsen T. Translational aspects of musculoskeletal pain: from animals to patients. In Graven-Nielsen T, Arendt-Nielsen L, Mense S (eds). Fundamentals of Musculoskeletal Pain. Seattle: IASP Press; 2008: pp. 347–366.

Arendt-Nielsen L, Fernández-de-las-Peñas C, Graven-Nielsen T. Basic aspects of musculoskeletal pain: from acute to chronic pain. J Manual Manipul Ther 2011; 19: 186–193

Babenko VV, Graven-Nielsen T, Svensson P, Drewes AM, Jensen TS, Arendt-Nielsen L. Experimental human muscle pain induced by intramuscular injections of bradykinin, serotonin, and substance P. Eur J Pain 1999; 3: 93–102.

Blankenburg M, Boekens H, Hechler T et al. Reference values for quantitative sensory testing in children and adolescents: developmental and gender differences of somatosensory perception. Pain 2010; 149: 76–88.

Cairns BE, Wang K, Hu JW, Sessle BJ, Arendt-Nielsen L, Svensson P. The effect of glutamate-evoked masseter muscle pain on the human jaw-stretch reflex differs in men and women. J Orofac Pain 2003; 17: 317–325.

Cairns BE, Dong X, Mann MK, Svensson P, Sessle BJ, Arendt-Nielsen L, McErlane KM. Systemic administration of monosodium glutamate elevates intramuscular glutamate levels and sensitizes rat masseter muscle afferent fibers. Pain 2007; 132: 33–41.

Campbell CM, Edwards RR, Fillingim RB. Ethnic differences in responses to multiple experimental pain stimuli. Pain 2005; 113: 20–26.

Carvalho GF, Chaves TC, Florencio LL, Dach F, Bigal ME, Bevilaqua-Grossi D. Reduced thermal threshold in patients with temporomandibular disorders. J Oral Rehabil 2016; 43: 401–408.

Chen H, Slade G, Lim PF, Miller V, Maixner W, Diatchenko L. Relationship between temporomandibular disorders, widespread palpation tenderness, and multiple pain conditions: a case-control study. J Pain 2012; 13: 1016–1027.

Costa YM, Porporatti AL, Stuginski-Barbosa J, Bonjardim LR, Speciali JG, Conti PC. Headache attributed to masticatory myofascial pain: impact on facial pain and pressure pain threshold. J Oral Rehabil 2016; 43: 161–168.

Costa YM, Morita-Neto O, de Araújo-Júnior EN, Sampaio FA, Conti PC, Bonjardim L. Test-retest reliability of quantitative sensory testing for mechanical somatosensory and pain modulation assessment of masticatory structures. J Oral Rehabil 2017; 44: 197–204.

Cunha CO, Pinto-Fiamengui LM, Castro AC, Lauris JR, Conti PC. Determination of a pressure pain threshold cut-off value for the diagnosis of temporomandibular joint arthralgia. J Oral Rehabil 2014; 41: 323–329.

Farella M, Michelotti A, Steenks MH, Romeo R, Cimino R, Bosman F. The diagnostic value of pressure algometry in myofascial pain of the jaw muscles. J Oral Rehabil 2000; 27: 9–14.

Fernández-de-las-Peñas C, Galán del Río F, Fernández Carnero J, Pesquera J, Arendt-Nielsen L, Svensson P. Bilateral widespread mechanical pain sensitivity in myofascial temporomandibular disorder: Evidence of impairment in central nociceptive processing. J Pain 2009; 10: 1170–1178.

Fernández-de-las-Peñas C, Galán-del-Río F, Ortega-Santiago R, Jiménez-García R, Arendt-Nielsen L, Svensson P. Bilateral thermal hyperalgesia in trigeminal and extra-trigeminal regions in patients with myofascial temporomandibular disorders. Exp Brain Res 2010a; 202: 171–179.

Fernández-de-las-Peñas C, Galán-del-Río F, Alonso-Blanco C, Jiménez-García R,

Arendt-Nielsen L, Svensson P. Referred pain from muscle trigger points in the masticatory and neck-shoulder musculature in women with temporomandibular disorders. J Pain 2010b; 11: 1295–1304.

Geber C, Klein T, Azad S et al. Test-retest and inter-observer reliability of quantitative sensory testing according to the protocol of the German Research Network on Neuropathic Pain (DFNS): a multi-centre study. Pain 2011; 152: 548–556.

Gebhart GF, Bielefeldt K. Physiology of visceral pain. Compr Physiol 2016; 6: 1609–1633.

Goadsby PJ, Bartsch T. The anatomy and physiology of the trigeminocervical complex. In Fernández-de-las-Peñas C, Arendt-Nielsen L, Gerwin RD (eds). Tension-Type and Cervicogenic Headache: Pathophysiology, Diagnosis, and Management. Boston: Jones & Bartlett Publishers; 2010, pp. 109–116.

Graven-Nielsen T, Arendt-Nielsen L. Assessment of mechanisms in localized and widespread musculoskeletal pain. Nat Rev Rheumatol 2010; 6: 599–606.

Graven-Nielsen T, Mense S. The peripheral apparatus of muscle pain: evidence from animal and human studies. Clin J Pain 2001; 17: 2–10.

Greenspan JD, Slade GD, Bair E et al. Pain sensitivity risk factors for chronic TMD: descriptive data and empirically identified domains from the OPPERA case control study. J Pain 2011; 12: T61–74.

Hansson P, Backonja M, Bouhassira D. Usefulness and limitations of quantitative sensory testing: clinical and research application in neuropathic pain states. Pain 2007; 129: 256–259.

Jääskeläinen SK. Clinical neurophysiology and quantitative sensory testing in the investigation of orofacial pain and sensory function. J Orofac Pain 2004; 18: 85–107.

Janal MN, Raphael KG, Cook DB, Sirois DA, Nemelivsky L, Staud R. Thermal temporal summation and decay of after-sensations in temporomandibular myofascial pain patients with and without comorbid fibromyalgia. J Pain Res 2016; 9: 641–652.

King CD, Wong F, Currie T, et al. Deficiency in endogenous modulation of prolonged heat pain in patients with irritable bowel syndrome and temporomandibular disorder Pain 2009; 143: 172–178.

Kim JH, Suh SI, Seol HY et al. Regional grey matter changes in patients with migraine: a voxel-based morphometry study. Cephalalgia 2008; 28: 598–604.

Komiyama O, Kawara M, De Laat A. Ethnic differences regarding tactile and pain thresholds in the trigeminal region. J Pain 2007; 8: 363–369.

Komiyama O, Wang K, Svensson P, Arendt-Nielsen L, Kawara M, De Laat A. Ethnic differences regarding sensory, pain, and reflex responses in the trigeminal region. Clin Neurophysiol 2009; 120: 384–389.

Kothari SF, Baad-Hansen L, Oono Y, Svensson P. Somatosensory assessment and conditioned pain modulation in temporomandibular disorders pain patients. Pain 2015; 156: 2545–2555.

Kothari SF, Baad-Hansen L, Hansen LB et al. Pain profiling of patients with temporomandibular joint arthralgia and osteoarthritis diagnosed with different imaging techniques. J Headache Pain 2016; 17: 61.

La Touche R, Paris-Alemany A, Hidalgo-Pérez A, López-de-Uralde-Villanueva I, Angulo-Diaz-Parreño S, Muñoz-García D. Evidence for central sensitization in patients with temporomandibular disorders: a systematic review and meta-analysis of observational studies. Pain Pract 2017, May 29 [Epub ahead of print].

Lin C. Brain signature of chronic orofacial pain: a systematic review and meta-analysis on neuroimaging research of trigeminal neuropathic pain and temporomandibular joint disorders. PLoS One 2014; 9: e94300.

Lluch-Girbés E, Dueñas L, Barbero M, Falla D, Baert IAC, Meeus M, Sánchez-Frutos J, Aguilella L, Nijs J. Expanded distribution of pain as a sign of central sensitization in individuals with symptomatic knee osteoarthritis. Phys Ther 2016; 96: 1196–1207.

Maixner W, Fillingim R, Booker D, Sigurdsson A. Sensitivity of patients with painful temporo-mandibular disorders to experimentally evoked pain. Pain 1995; 63: 341–351.

Maixner W, Fillingim R, Sigurdsson A, Kincaid S, Silva S. Sensitivity of patients with painful temporomandibular disorders to experimentally evoked pain: evidence for altered temporal summation of pain. Pain 1998; 76: 71–81.

Matos R, Wang K, Jensen JD, Jensen T, Neuman B, Svensson P, Arendt-Nielsen L. Quantitative sensory testing in the trigeminal region: site and gender differences. J Orofac Pain 2011; 25: 161–169.

May A. Chronic pain may change the structure of the brain. Pain 2008; 137: 7–15.

Meacham K, Shepherd A, Mohapatra DP, Haroutounian S. Neuropathic pain: central vs. peripheral mechanisms. Curr Pain Headache Rep 2017; 21: 28.

Mense S, Simons DG, Russell IJ. Muscle Pain: Understanding its Nature, Diagnosis and Treatment. Philadelphia: Lippincott, Williams & Wilkins; 2001.

Mohn C, Vassend O, Knardahl S. Experimental pain sensitivity in women with temporomandibular disorders and pain-free controls: the relationship to orofacial muscular contraction and cardiovascular responses. Clin J Pain 2008; 24: 343–352.

Muñoz-García D, López-de-Uralde-Villanueva I, Beltran-Alacreu H, La Touche R, Fernández-Carnero J. Patients with concomitant chronic neck pain and myofascial pain in masticatory muscles have more widespread pain and distal hyperalgesia than patients with only chronic neck pain. Pain Med 2017; 18: 526–537.

Nijs J, Van Houdenhove B, Oostendorp RA. Recognition of central sensitization in patients with musculoskeletal pain: application of pain neurophysiology in manual therapy practice. Man Ther 2010; 15: 135–141.

Nijs J, Malfliet A, Ickmans K, Baert I, Meeus M. Treatment of central sensitization in patients with unexplained chronic pain: an update. Expert Opin Pharmacother 2014a; 15: 1671–1683.

Nijs J, Torres-Cueco R, van Wilgen CP et al. Applying modern pain neuroscience in clinical practice: criteria for the classification of central sensitization pain. Pain Physician 2014b; 17: 447–457.

Nijs J, Lluch Girbés E, Lundberg M, Malfliet A, Sterling M. Exercise therapy for chronic musculoskeletal pain: Innovation by altering pain memories. Man Ther 2015; 20: 216–220.

Nijs J, Goubert D, Ickmans K. Recognition and treatment of central sensitization in chronic pain patients: not limited to specialized care. J Orthop Sports Phys Ther 2016; 46: 1024–1028.

Park JW, Clark GT, Kim YK, Chung JW. Analysis of thermal pain sensitivity and psychological profiles in different subgroups of TMD patients. Int J Oral Maxillofac Surg 2010; 39: 968–974.

Pfau DB, Rolke R, Treede RD, Daublaender M. Somato-sensory profiles in subgroups of patients with myogenic temporomandibular disorders and fibromyalgia syndrome. Pain 2009; 147: 72–83.

Pielstickera A, Haagc G, Zaudigh M, Lautenbachera S. Impairment of pain inhibition in chronic tension-type headache. Pain 2005; 118: 215–223.

Pigg M, Baad-Hansen L, Svensson P, Drangsholt M, List T. Reliability of intraoral quantitative sensory testing (QST). Pain 2010; 148: 220–226.

Pinto Fiamengui LM, Freitas de Carvalho JJ, Cunha CO, Bonjardim LR, Fiamengui Filho JF, Conti PC. The influence of myofascial temporomandibular disorder pain on the pressure pain threshold of women during a migraine attack. J Orofac Pain 2013; 27: 343–349.

Quartana PJ, Finan PH, Smith M. Evidence for sustained mechanical pain sensitization in women with chronic temporomandibular disorder versus healthy female participants. J Pain 2015; 16: 1127–1135.

Raphael KG. Temporal summation of heat pain in temporomandibular disorder patients. J Orofac Pain 2009; 23: 54–64.

Rolke R, Andrews Campbell K, Magerl W, Birklein F, Treede RD. Quantitative sensory testing: a comprehensive protocol for clinical trials. Eur J Pain 2006a; 10: 77–88.

Rolke R, Baron R, Maier C et al. Quantitative sensory testing in the German Research Network on Neuropathic Pain (DFNS): standardized protocol and reference values. Pain 2006b; 123: 231–243.

Sandrini G, Rossi P, Milanov L, Serrao M, Cecchini AP, Nappi G. Abnormal modulatory influence of diffuse noxious inhibitory controls in migraine and chronic tension-type headache patients. Cephalalgia 2006; 26: 782–789.

Sarlani E, Greenspan J. Evidence for generalized hyperalgesia in temporomandibular disorders patients. Pain 2003; 10: 221–226.

Schmidt-Wilcke T, Leinisch E, Straube A, Kampfe N, Draganski B, Diener HC, Bogdahn U, May A. Gray matter decrease in patients with chronic tension type headache. Neurology 2005; 65: 1483–486.

Slade GD, Sanders AE, Ohrbach R, et al. Pressure pain thresholds fluctuate with, but do not usefully predict, the clinical course of painful temporomandibular disorder. Pain 2014; 155: 2134–2143.

Staud R. Abnormal endogenous pain modulation is a shared characteristic of many chronic pain conditions. Expert Rev Neurother 2012; 12: 577–585.

Svensson P. Muscle pain in the head: overlap between temporomandibular disorders and tension-type headaches Curr Opin Neurol 2007; 20: 320–325.

Svensson P, List T, Hector G. Analysis of stimulus-evoked pain in patients with myofascial temporomandibular pain disorders Pain 2001; 92: 399–409.

Svensson P, Baad-Hansen L, Pigg M et al. Guidelines and recommendations for assessment of somato-sensory function in orofacial pain conditions: a taskforce report. J Oral Rehabil 2011; 38: 366–394.

Wall PD, Woolf CJ. Muscle but not cutaneous C-afferent input produces prolonged increases in the excitability of the flexion reflex in the rat. J Physiol 1984; 356: 443–458.

Wilcox SL, Gustin SM, Macey PM, Peck CC, Murray GM, Henderson LA. Anatomical changes within the medullary dorsal horn in chronic temporomandibular disorder pain. Neuroimage 2015; 117: 258–266.

Woolf CJ. Central sensitization: implications for the diagnosis and treatment of pain. Pain 2011; 152: S2–15.

Yang G, Baad-Hansen L, Wang K, Xie QF, Svensson P. A study on variability of quantitative sensory testing in healthy participants and painful temporomandibular disorder patients. Somatosens Mot Res 2014; 31: 62–71.

Yekta SS, Smeets R, Stein JM, Ellrich J. Assessment of trigeminal nerve functions by quantitative sensory testing in patients and healthy volunteers. J Oral Maxillofac Surg 2010; 68: 2437–2451.

Younger JW, Shen YF, Goddard G, Mackey SC. Chronic myofascial temporomandibular pain is associated with neural abnormalities in the trigeminal and limbic systems. Pain 2010; 149: 222–228.

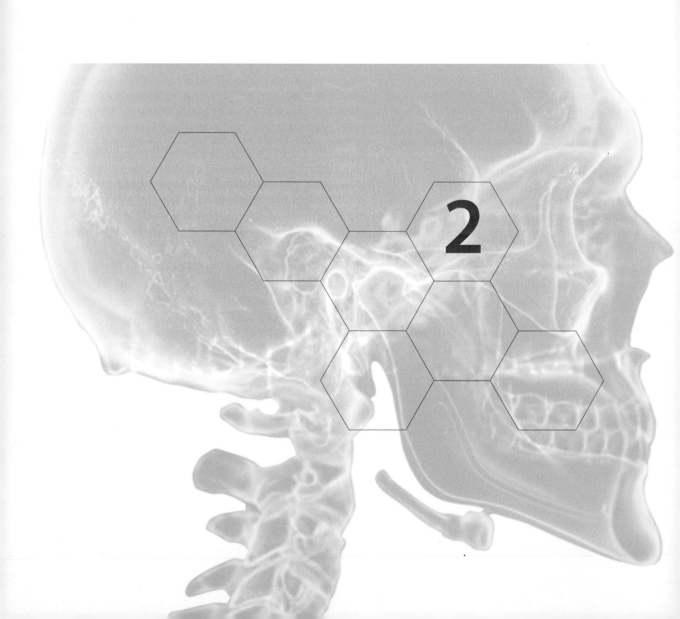

PART 2
Examining for temporomandibular disorders

Chapter 7

Clinical history in temporomandibular disorders and orofacial pain

Gary M. Heir, José L. de-la-Hoz

'When you have eliminated the impossible, whatever remains, however improbable, must be the truth.'

— **Arthur Conan Doyle, 1890**

Introduction

The orofacial pain clinician is often called upon to deduce the cause of a hidden malady, often after a series of ineffective treatments. Differential diagnosis of orofacial pain requires the same deductive and inductive analytical processes as might be employed by Sherlock Holmes, the fictional detective. This chapter will approach the complex, chronic orofacial pain patient in a similar manner as might be considered by an effective detective.

Diagnostic detective work should follow a regimen of obtaining facts, observation of clues, and processing of the information prior to coming to a first conclusion. An important feature of the diagnostic paradigm is found in the admonition from William Osler (1849–1919), considered by many as the father of modern medical education and one of the founders of Johns Hopkins University. He instructed us to:

'Observe, record, tabulate, communicate. Use your five senses. [...] Learn to see, learn to hear, learn to feel, learn to smell, and know that by practice alone you can become expert ... Listen to your patient, he is telling you the diagnosis.'

—**William Osler (quoted in Bryan, 1997)**

We must assemble the clues, define the problem, think the case through to a differential diagnosis and effect the appropriate treatment.

'Without an accurate diagnosis, treatment may only be successful with good luck.'

—**Weldon Bell, circa 1980**

The discipline of orofacial pain

The International Association for the Study of Pain (IASP) defines orofacial pain as pain perceived in the face and/or oral cavity, caused by diseases or disorders of regional structures, dysfunction of the nervous system, or through referral from distant sources (IASP, 2016).

Treatment of orofacial pain is a specialty in dentistry in many parts of the world and an emerging area of specialization in others. Orofacial pain is typically diagnosed and treated by the dental practitioner who is routinely confronted by patients with pain. While the majority of facial pain may be of an odontogenic cause, not all orofacial pain is of dental origin. Therefore, 'Never assume the obvious is true' (Safire, n.d.). Simply because there is facial pain, and there are teeth in the area of the pain, do not assume that one has anything to do with the other until proven. Failure to understand pain etiologies and mechanisms can lead to inaccurate diagnoses, ineffective and harmful treatment, or, more importantly, misdiagnosis of otherwise ominous conditions. It is the responsibility of the dental practitioner treating orofacial pain to achieve an accurate diagnosis and to treat odontogenic and nonodontogenic causes of facial pain appropriately.

Proper understanding of clinical examination

There is increasing recognition of epidemiology, pain mechanisms, and etiologies which fill the peer-reviewed literature. Safe and effective, evidence-based protocols for diagnosis and treatment strategies for chronic temporomandibular and orofacial pain disorders are widely accepted. With the increasing use of the Internet as a source of information, patients often come with voluminous information, whether correct or not, convinced of a diagnosis and anticipated treatment. We must remain vigilant. The approach to every patient, whether performing a routine dental examination or comprehensive orofacial pain evaluation, must include listening for signs and symptoms, and looking for clues and observation of the patient as routine rather than the exception. At minimum is a screening evaluation for all patients.

Screening evaluation

It is the responsibility of dental healthcare providers to satisfy the minimal medical–dental healthcare requirements when examining each dental patient. Every new or recall patient should be screened for temporomandibular disorders (TMDs) and other orofacial pain conditions as part of comprehensive orodental examination. This screening will guide the clinician to a more comprehensive and detailed examination when necessary. Ideally, the screening evaluation should consist of a brief questionnaire such as the TMD pain screener (Table 7.1), or the more detailed Diagnostic Criteria for Temporomandibular Disorders Symptom Questionnaire as shown in Appendix 7.1 (International RDC/TMD Consortium Network, 2013a).

A physical examination should follow the intake of the history. A detailed screening examination is provided in Appendix 7.2 (International RDC/TMD Consortium Network, 2013b). It should include observation of the active and passive mandibular range of motion (ROM), lateral and protrusive movements, deflections or deviations, palpation and auscultation of the temporomandibular joints (TMJs) and palpation of the masticatory musculature (superficial and deep masseter, temporalis). If any abnormal finding is detected, a more extensive examination is indicated.

Comprehensive examination

The first step for providing effective treatment is an accurate diagnosis. Assemble the clues and begin with a differential diagnosis. Before instituting any treatment, the prudent clinician must stop, look, and listen.

Table 7.1

TMD pain screener (International RDC/TMD Consortium Network, 2011).

1. In the last 30 days, how long did any pain last in your jaw or temple area on either side?
   a. No pain
   b. Pain comes and goes
   c. Pain is always present

2. In the last 30 days, have you had pain or stiffness in your jaw on awakening?
   a. No
   b. Yes

3. In the last 30 days, did the following activities change any pain (that is, make it better or make it worse) in your jaw or temple area on either side?
   A. Chewing hard or tough food.
      a. No
      b. Yes
   B. Opening your mouth or moving your jaw forward or to the side
      a. No
      b. Yes
   C. Jaw habits such as holding teeth together, clenching, grinding, or chewing gum
      a. No
      b. Yes
   D. Other jaw activities such as talking, kissing or yawning
      a. No
      b. Yes

Items 1 through 3A constitute the short version of the screening instrument, and items 1 through 3D constitute the long version. An **a** response receives 0 points, a **b** response 1 point and a **c** response 2 points.

Recognizing problematic diagnostic habits

The seasoned practitioner acquires a habitual routine when examining patients. As we become more experienced there is a tendency to skip through some of the diagnostic steps when presented with clinically obvious conditions. However, orofacial pain disorders often require a more in-depth analysis. Some of the problems and pitfalls to avoid include the following:

1. Adhering to a preconceived diagnosis

'If the only tool you have is a hammer, you treat everything as if it were a nail.'

—(Attributed to Mark Twain)

If we are accustomed to seeing orofacial pain as odontogenic in origin, despite a lack of clinical or radiographic evidence, many patients may undergo unnecessary endodontic therapy for conditions such as trigeminal neuralgia and cluster headache.

2. Inadequate or excessive history

Patients with chronic orofacial pain have typically been seeking relief for as long as four to five years, have spent thousands of dollars, and may have undergone multiple procedures without benefit. They have a story to tell, and the clinician must listen. Allowing the patient to discuss his or her problem in detail can be therapeutic. Many times, patients will comment, 'No one listens to me.' However, care must be taken to focus on the history of the current problem and the relevant facts. Collecting excessive and superfluous data may be as detrimental as collecting inadequate data.

3. 'Doctors think, machines don't.' (Weldon Bell, circa 1980)

There are numerous diagnostic aids available for measuring and monitoring physiologic parameters. When incorporating diagnostic aids, they should be utilized only to supply information not otherwise available through the history and physical examination. Adjunctive diagnostic testing may be considered appropriate to collect data that are otherwise unavailable, and which are necessary to arrive at, confirm or refute a diagnosis, or necessary to formulate a treatment plan. Adjunctive diagnostic testing may also be appropriate in cases of ineffective treatment where additional testing may be necessary for reconsideration of the diagnosis or alteration of the treatment plan. The results of any diagnostic test should correlate with clinical findings, and not be used as stand-alone diagnostic tools. Always take into account the sensitivity and specificity of the diagnostic aids utilized.

4. Never make decisions based on incomplete information

Avoid the tendency to accept the first positive finding as the cause of the problem. Always take a complete history and perform a physical examination. Premature conclusions based on incomplete data stop subsequent thinking.

'The temptation to form premature theories upon insufficient data is the bane of our profession.'

—Arthur Conan Doyle, 1914

Collecting the clues and analyzing a case

Specific components must be assembled. The following steps are recommended for every orofacial pain patient, from what might appear a simple case to the most complex.

1. Questionnaires

Provide the patient with a general health and orofacial pain questionnaire for completion prior to the initial evaluation. This questionnaire serves several purposes. It allows the patient to adequately describe clinical complaints, and may assist in recalling additional features or conditions that could play a role in recalling complaints of which the patient might not otherwise be aware. The questionnaire also acts as a guide for the history intake. This process is best accomplished by mailing the questionnaires to the patient prior to the initial visit. If this is not possible, the form could be provided by the reception desk upon arrival prior to the appointment. Delivery in advance of the initial evaluation is preferable as this allows the patient to complete the questionnaire at home without external pressure or distractions.

2. Patient observation

These steps should be followed during the clinical evaluation:

- observe the patient
- obtain an accurate and detailed history
- perform a comprehensive physical assessment
- utilize appropriate adjunctive testing when necessary
- arrive at a differential diagnosis
- effect a focused and goal-oriented treatment plan.

The history

'If you have one hour to spend with the patient, spend 59 minutes on the history.'

—Weldon Bell, circa 1980

It is important to recognize that the orofacial pain patient, especially the chronic orofacial pain patient, may be frustrated and/or depressed, if not despondent, over the lack of efficacy of prior treatment. Establishing a good relationship with the patient is essential. Begin the history by facing the patient at eye level to aid in observation of asymmetries of form and function. Ask: 'How can I help you? *What do you think the problem is?*' In these days of managed care, patients often feel rushed through a physical examination with little opportunity to elucidate their complaints or history. Giving this opportunity, even for a few minutes, demonstrates empathy and will facilitate future treatment. Nevertheless, the professional must control the interview and avoid including non-related details that may confuse the history, thus preventing deviation from the primary goal. The essential points to keep in mind when taking the history are outlined below.

1. Chief complaint

The primary symptoms or conditions for which the patient is seeking the consultation. Let the patient present, in a brief and orderly manner, the complaint that brought him or her to the examination. For that purpose, ask the patient to describe the primary reason for seeking a consultation. Let the patient know that this is only the starting point, and that the rest of his or her story will be developed during the history and examination.

Intent: It is important to identify what brought the patient to seek an orofacial pain evaluation. There can only be one chief complaint. All other problems are secondary to the primary reason for the patient's visit. Secondary complaints should be listed and documented in the order of severity and described in detail.

A detailed description of the chief complaint or chronic illness includes: chronology of the problem, location, duration, quality, intensity, frequency, precipitating and ameliorating factors, past medical history, past treatment, past and current medications, and review of psychosocial history.

Chronology

'Tell me how your problem began?' Allow the patient to tell his or her story. Control the interview. In general, ask open-ended questions that allow the patient to offer additional information. Closed-ended questions allowing only 'yes' or 'no' answers may exclude important details.

Intent: Determine if the onset of the problem was spontaneous or secondary to an illness or injury.

Location

'Where is your pain?' 'Does the location change?' 'Is there a dermatomal or nondermatomal distribution?' 'Is it unilateral or bilateral?' Ask the patient to identify the exact location of the pain, either with a finger or hand, describing both the primary location and possible radiation and/or referral.

Intent: To identify dermatomal or pain patterns with no specific correlation. This information may aid in differentiation of peripheral versus central pain.

Duration

'How long does the pain last?'

Intent: Necessary information to determine if pain is continuous or episodic. If continuous, does pain wax and wane in intensity? How long do exacerbations last? If episodic, what is the duration of each episode?

Questions to consider: 'Does it hurt all day?' 'Does it hurt when you are asleep?' 'Does the pain awaken you?' 'Does it hurt when you are awake?' 'Is it worse in the morning, during the day or in the evening?'

Intent: Various conditions have characteristic temporal behavior that may be identified by the duration of attacks.

Quality

'Describe your pain?' Orofacial pain may be classified as arising from musculoskeletal, neurogenic, or neurovascular etiologies, each of which may have a characteristic quality of pain.

- Musculoskeletal – typically aching or sore:
  - ▶ The response to provocation is graded, the greater the provocation, the more pain there is;
  - ▶ May be associated with dysfunction.
- Neuropathic – sensory distortions:
  - ▶ dysesthesia
  - ▶ allodynia
  - ▶ hyperalgesia
  - ▶ hypoalgesia, etc.
- Vascular – may have a pulsatile or throbbing component.

Intent: To aid in identifying the system or source of pain.

Intensity

'How strong is your pain or how strong are your painful episodes?'

Intent: Different pain disorders may present with varying intensities. Assessing intensity, along with the quality and duration, will aid in identifying the source.

It may be useful to offer hints, for example, 'mild' indicates no need for analgesic medication, 'moderate' pain may require the occasional use of a mild analgesic, while 'severe' means the patient requires repeated and strong analgesic medications.

Frequency

'How frequently does your pain occur?' 'How long are periods between attacks?' 'If your pain is constant, does it wax and wane?'

Intent: Many pain conditions have characteristic durations and frequencies which help to guide the diagnostic process.

Precipitating and ameliorating factors

'What makes your pain better or worse?'

Questions to consider: Is pain precipitated or made better by cold, heat, movement, for example of the joints, speaking, yawning, clenching, touching the area, physical exercise, sleep, changes in the weather, standing, lying down, stress, loud noise, fatigue, or menstruation?

Intent: Learning what affects the pain, or which past treatment or medications have not been effective, can often help in identifying the source or eliminating the improbable to focus on the possible.

2. Past medical history

Knowledge of the patient's current health status, history of past illnesses or trauma, prior hospitalizations, and current and past medications is essential. If the patient received treatment for the current complaint, a review of attempted treatment and its outcome is necessary. It is essential to collect details on any treatment for the chief complaint. Appropriate medications may have been given at a subclinical dose or for too short a period to have any effect. The patient may have been noncompliant. Other forms of therapy may not have been applied appropriately, for example, over-aggressive physical therapy, etc. The past use of some medications may identify prior attempts at diagnosis, such as the use of carbamazepine which suggests a diagnosis of trigeminal neuralgia. If medications or treatments were provided appropriately, at the correct dose, and for appropriate periods of time without effect, the diagnosis must be reassessed. In addition, current medications may play a role in precipitating or perpetuating symptoms. Selective serotonin reuptake inhibitors (SSRIs) may induce or exacerbate bruxism. Serotonin and norepinephrine reuptake inhibitors (SNRIs) have been associated with headache. Angiotensin-converting-enzyme (ACE) inhibitors and statins may result in muscle and joint pain as well as intraoral burning. Taking a detailed history may reveal which medications should be discontinued, rather than which medications might be added.

Review of systems

A review of systems requires a history of any prior or current complaints related to the head, ears, nose or throat, cardiovascular system, respiratory system, gastrointestinal system, genitourinary system, musculoskeletal system, dermatologic disorders, endocrine problems, blood disorders or immunological problems.

Review of the psychosocial history

Be aware of possible psychological embellishment. Important factors include:

- marital status
- family illnesses or family history
- changes in personal or professional life
- history of physical, sexual or substance abuse
- reports of habits, for example clenching, bruxism, nail biting
- potential for addictive behavior, prior use of medications not prescribed by a physician, family members with potential abuse of medications, etc.

Screening for obstructive sleep apnea

The patient should be screened for:

- snoring
- multiple awakenings from sleep due to gasping
- poor sleep latency
- daytime somnolence.

The clinical examination

The essential components of a clinical examination include:

- observation
- postural evaluation
- head and neck inspection
- cervical range of motion
- intraoral examination
- muscle palpation of upper quarter
- mandibular range of motion
- temporomandibular joint noises

- temporomandibular joint palpation and loading

- sleep-disordered breathing screening examination

- cranial nerve screening, and

- neurologic screening.

Observation

The clinical examination begins with observation in the waiting room. How does your patient sit, stand and ambulate? Check posture, gait and balance as he or she enters the examination room or operatory. Is there an impaired gait, does the patient lean to one side or the other? Does the patient appear to have discomfort or pain? Does any movement suggest protection of a painful area? Record all findings.

Once the patient is seated in the examination chair, sit at eye level facing the patient and observe for facial symmetry of coloration and muscle tone, muscle tics and symmetrical movements. Subtle weakness of the facial or oculomotor nerves affecting blink reflex may be better observed when the patient does not suspect you are formally examining him or her.

The neurological evaluation includes the patient's ability to communicate. Assess the ability to construct sentences and give complete answers. Is it necessary to repeat questions several times before receiving a response? Is there short- or long-term memory dysfunction? Is the patient easily confused? If there was a history of stroke or other intracranial pathology, it may be necessary to include a family member in the examination process.

Another essential component of the observation portion of the examination is the patient's posture and cervical range of motion. While this will be tested formally, observing how the patient was standing in the waiting room, walking to the examination room, or sitting in the examination chair may reveal abnormal or protective upper-quarter posturing or head positioning consistent with musculoskeletal pain or other craniocervical disorders. Observe if the head is in a forward position, side-bent and/or rotated. Is there posterior cranial rotation? One technique, while conversing with the patient, is to move from side to side, forcing the patient to turn the head to the left and right. The unsuspecting patient, not realizing this is part of the examination may favor one side or the other, and move the entire upper quarter to one side while rotating the head easily to the other. It is not within the scope of this chapter to discuss the meaning of restricted cervical range of motion, but this observation may be extremely useful during the latter portions of the clinical evaluation.

Intraoral examination

Once the patient is seated, the examination must include a dental evaluation. Many facial pain disorders are of odontogenic origin. Therefore, it is essential to perform a complete dental examination. This should include dental radiographs when indicated, thermal testing, percussion of teeth, etc. Dental pathology must be eliminated as primary source of orofacial pain prior to pursuing nonodontogenic causes. If dental or periodontal is suspected, the use of anesthetic diagnostic infiltration or blocks to isolate primary dental pain is strongly recommended.

The intraoral examination must include an evaluation of the soft tissues. The gingiva, ventral and dorsal surfaces of the tongue, floor of the mouth and buccal mucosa must be inspected for lesions, ulcerations, or infections. In addition, a prominent linea alba, tongue scalloping, and a high Mallampati score suggest the need for referral for polysomnography in the presence of a history of disturbed sleep.

Musculoskeletal evaluation

The musculoskeletal evaluation of the head, neck and orofacial region must include:

- TMJ
  - ▸ palpation
    - ◆ TMJ
    - ◆ masticatory musculature
  - ▸ mandibular range of motion
  - ▸ auscultation
- evaluation of posture and cervical range of motion
- evaluation of the muscles of the upper quarter.

Cranial nerve screening exam

The cranial nerve examination is essential for orofacial pain patients, as neuropathic or pain of neurologic origin is the third most common complaint among patients seeking treatment in an orofacial pain clinic. Cognition and recall have been described above as part of this examination. The mechanics of the cranial nerve examination are not within the scope of this chapter, but a complete cranial nerve exam should take less than two minutes to accomplish, and must be considered essential to any orofacial pain evaluation. Abnormal findings require referral for further evaluation.

Adjunctive testing

The use of adjunctive testing should be secondary to a well taken history and thorough clinical examination. These tests should be used judiciously by the clinician. The type of adjunctive diagnostic testing employed must be individualized for the specific needs of the patient. Consideration of adjunctive testing should depend upon the potential for adding necessary information required for determining a diagnosis and treatment plan. This may include:

- imaging
- serology or genetics
- indomethacin trials
- diagnostic anesthesia.

Diagnosis

Diagnosis is the recognition of a disease or condition by its outward signs and symptoms. It includes analysis of the underlying physiological or biochemical cause(s) of a disease or condition. To recognize the abnormal, the clinician must have a clear understanding of what is normal.

Differential diagnosis

Differential diagnosis is the determination of which disease the patient is suffering from, by the systematic comparison and contrasting of clinical findings of two or more diseases with similar symptoms.

Treatment

Effective treatment must be based on an accurate diagnosis. Treatment should be evidence based and as minimally invasive as possible, especially for temporomandibular disorders, which tend to gravitate toward the mean. Keep in mind that often the best treatment may not be another medication or procedure, but knowing when not to treat, or which treatment or medication to discontinue.

Differential diagnosis and appropriate and effective treatment depend on identification of the source, after obtaining a history as described above. If pain is not of odontogenic origin, the next most common source for orofacial pain is the musculoskeletal system.

- Identify the source by the clinical characteristics.
- Listen to the history.
- Observe body language.
- Think of possibilities.
- Refine the list.

Intent: Don't assume, prove. Know normal in order to assess abnormal.

Case report

The following is an example of a sequential collection of data, analysis of the data, use of adjunctive testing, formulation of a differential diagnosis and treatment for a combined neuropathic and musculoskeletal case report. The techniques employed in this example can be applied to every case of chronic orofacial pain.

Main symptom

The patient is a 43-year-old male who presents with a complaint of chronic pain in the area of teeth #15–16. The patient comes on referral from an endodontist for, '… a chronic pain or orofacial pain component. A radiograph of tooth #14 suggests there may be some indication to retreat the palatal and distal buccal canals: however, his complaints are not consistent or typical of endodontic pain.'

Past medical history

The past medical history includes renal calculi, tuberculosis 30 years ago, and an injury to the left eye resulting in removal and the placement of a prosthesis five years ago.

Detailed description of the chief complaint or chronic illness

Chronology of the problem: At the age of approximately 15 to 16 years, the patient became aware of a dull achy pain, which he described as 'like a toothache.' He stated it was pressure-like pain and worsened by chewing. He could not recall any tenderness of the teeth or thermal sensitivity. He stated that the pain fluctuated in intensity and radiated to his temple. This pain continued relatively unchanged until at the age of approximately 21 years when he underwent an endodontic procedure of tooth #14 followed by a post, core and crown restoration. He reported short-term relief, but complaints soon returned. Over the following few years the patient admitted to 'spotty dental treatment.' Approximately 9 years ago he underwent three endodontic procedures including retreatment of #14, and endodontic procedures of #15 and #16, with no relief. The following year he underwent extractions of #15 and #16. Again there was no relief. This was followed by periodontal procedures and equilibrations, which seemed to have reduced the complaint, but still the dull achy pain persisted. Two years prior to this evaluation he underwent a bone graft in the area of #14 and #15 with no change in symptoms. He was told he had an exostosis in the area and had 'the bump off.' Despite these procedures pain continued.

Location: upper jaw left spreading to the temple.

Duration: constant.

Frequency: continuous.

Quality: achy, like a toothache.

Intensity: 3/10 to 9/10.

Exacerbating factors: physical pressure, resting position, tension or stress and fatigue, touching the area with his tongue provokes pain.

Ameliorating factors: not known.

Past medical history: see Chronology above.

Past treatment: see Chronology above.

Past and current medications: The patient is not taking any medication, but states for years, 'I would chew on aspirin before that I usually would take ibuprofen.'

Review of psychosocial history: The patient is a cable and telephone lineman, married, with two young children. He denies the use of alcohol and nonprescription medications. He takes three caffeinated beverages per day and an occasional glass of beer or wine.

The clinical exam

Observation: The patient appears in good health, with a positive outlook. He has a normal gait when walking into the operatory. Facial form is symmetrical regarding coloration, muscle tone and function, with the exception of blinking of the left eye due to the placement of the prosthesis.

Postural evaluation: There is no postural dysfunction.

Head and neck inspection: No gross abnormalities are observed except for the left eye.

Cervical ROM: No restrictions of movement in extension, flexion, side-bending, or left and right rotation are detected.

Intraoral examination: A clinical examination finds that the patient is missing #15 and #16; otherwise the occlusion is intact and stable. There is significant incisal guidance with a 15 per cent overlap, anterior attrition and evidence of bruxism and clenching, to which the claimant admits. Intraorally, all structures appear to be within normal limits and the extraction site is well-healed.

Mandibular ROM: The mandibular range of movement is 55 mm of opening which is smooth and coordinated, with 12 mm of lateral movements.

Muscle palpation of the upper quarter: Mild tenderness bilaterally, with no referral patterns or reproduction of familiar pain.

TMJ noises: There is a left-sided midrange opening click of the joint.

TMJ palpation and loading: A palpatory evaluation of the masticatory musculature was performed with positive findings and reproduction of the patient's familiar pain. Provocation of the left temporalis in the area consistent with the deep masseter and the body of the superficial masseter was locally tender, and referred pain to the patient's edentulous area reproducing the primary complaint. Palpation of the TMJs was equally tender, and when provoked, produced pain similar to but not exactly consistent with the chief complaint. Provocation of the medial and lateral pterygoids was also capable of reproducing the primary familiar pain.

Sleep-disordered breathing screening examination: The patient's Epworth Sleepiness Scale score was 4, and he denies snoring. The Mallampati score is 2. The neck circumference is 14½ inches. There is no indication for a sleep-breathing disorder.

Cranial nerve screening: A cranial nerve screening evaluation, except for the territory of the right prosthetic eye and intraorally in the upper left posterior quadrant, found all cranial nerves intact. The exceptions will be noted below when describing diagnostic testing in the clinical examination section.

Neurologic screening: The neurologic screening examination begins with the interview and includes a cranial nerve exam. No abnormalities were detected.

Focused clinical examination: The area of the extractions and multiple surgeries was examined. Using a blunt probe in the form of a cotton stick applicator, light stroking produced a response consistent with allodynia and firm pressure, which may have been possibly uncomfortable, produced pain of a greater response than would be expected, consistent with hyperalgesia. Firm palpation along the scar from the prior surgery produced sharp, tingling electric-like pain consistent with that detected by Tinel's sign which may represent small neuroma formation along the course of the scar tissue.

Adjunctive testing

A diagnostic anesthetic infiltration was used to isolate the source of pain. A small amount was injected into the hyperalgesic areas, which eliminated the continuous pain radiating from the upper left posterior quadrant. There was no effect on the pain emanating from the masseter and temporalis muscles.

Differential diagnosis

- Painful post-traumatic trigeminal neuropathy of the upper left quadrant.

- Myofascial pain of the left masticatory musculature.

Treatment

- Repeat injections incorporating dexamethasone 4 mg/mL.

- Provide an intraoral orthotic to protect the dentition from bruxism and, combined with physical therapy, to facilitate treatment of myofascial pain of the masticatory musculature.

Treatment outcome

Neuropathic pain was reduced to 0/10. Myofascial pain was reduced to 1–2/10 within four weeks.

Conclusion

Comparisons of the diagnostic process to the techniques of fastidious detective work have been suggested, but this is not a new concept. 'Observe, record, tabulate, communicate. Use your five senses. Learn to see, learn to hear, learn to feel, learn to smell, and know that by practice alone you can become expert.' (William Osler, as quoted by Bryan, 1997). Always consider that the patient may present with more than one malady. Especially in the aging population, we will see medically compromised patients with numerous comorbidities and possibly taking multiple medications. The successful detective and excellent clinician will sort out the clues, assemble a timeline, connect or discard facts, and arrive at a conclusion. The detective will solve the mystery, the adept clinician will diagnose the patient in a similar fashion.

In conclusion, if a dental source of facial pain is not obvious, no dental treatment should be initiated until a full assessment has been carried out and a diagnosis is achieved. Orofacial pain disorders mimicking dental pathology can be ominous. Plan treatment carefully based on an accurate diagnosis.

Diagnostic Criteria for Temporomandibular Disorders
Symptom Questionnaire

Patient name _____   Date (mm-dd-yyyy) ☐☐ ☐☐ ☐☐☐☐

PAIN

		NO	YES
1	Have you ever had pain in your jaw, temple, in the ear, or in front of the ear on either side?	☐	☐

If you answered NO, then skip to question 5

| **2** | How many years and months ago did your pain in the jaw, temple, in the ear, or in front of the ear begin? | ☐ Years ☐ Months |

3 In the last 30 days, which of the following best describes any pain in your jaw, temple, in the ear, or in front of the ear on either side?

Select ONE response

If you answered NO to question 3, then skip to question 5

☐ No pain
☐ Pain comes and goes
☐ Pain is always present

4 In the last 30 days, did the following activities change any pain (that is, make it better or make it worse) in your jaw, temple, in the ear, or in front of the ear on either side?

		NO	YES
A	Chewing hard or tough food	☐	☐
B	Opening your mouth, or moving your jaw forward or to the side	☐	☐
C	Jaw habits such as holding teeth together, clenching/grinding teeth, or chewing gum	☐	☐
D	Other jaw activities such as talking, kissing, or yawning	☐	☐

HEADACHE

		NO	YES
5	In the last 30 days, have you had any headaches that included the temple areas of your head?	☐	☐

If you answered NO to question 5, then skip to question 8

| **6** | How long ago did your temple headache first begin? | ☐ Years ☐ Months |

7 In the last 30 days, did the following activities change any pain (that is, make it better or make it worse) in your temple area on either side?

		NO	YES
A	Chewing hard or tough food	☐	☐
B	Opening your mouth, or moving your jaw forward or to the side	☐	☐
C	Jaw habits such as holding teeth together, clenching/grinding, or chewing gum	☐	☐
D	Other jaw activities such as talking, kissing, or yawning	☐	☐

		NO	YES	Office use		
				R	L	DNK
JAW JOINT NOISES						
8	In the last 30 days, have you had any jaw joint noise(s) when you moved or used your jaw?	☐	☐	☐	☐	☐
CLOSED LOCKING OF THE JAW						
9	Have you ever had your jaw lock or catch, even for a moment, so that it would not open ALL THE WAY?	☐	☐	☐	☐	☐
	If you answered NO to question 9, then skip to question 13					
10	Was your jaw lock or catch severe enough to limit your jaw opening and interfere with your ability to eat?	☐	☐	☐	☐	☐
11	In the last 30 days, did your jaw lock so you could not open ALL THE WAY, even for a moment, and then unlock so you could open ALL THE WAY?	☐	☐	☐	☐	☐
	If you answered NO to question 11, then skip to question 13					
12	Is your jaw currently locked or limited so that your jaw will not open ALL THE WAY?	☐	☐	☐	☐	☐
OPEN LOCKING OF THE JAW						
13	In the last 30 days, when you opened your mouth wide, did your jaw lock or catch even for a moment such that you could not close it from this wide open position?	☐	☐	☐	☐	☐
	If you answered NO to question 13, then you are finished					
14	In the last 30 days, when your jaw locked or caught wide open, did you have to do something to get it to close including resting, moving, or maneuvering it?	☐	☐	☐	☐	☐

Appendix 7.1 continued

105

DC/TMD examination form

Date completed (mm-dd-yyyy)

Patient _____ Examiner _____ [ ][ ][ ][ ][ ][ ][ ][ ]

1A Location of pain: last 30 days (select all that apply)

Right pain				**Left pain**			
☐ None	☐ Temporalis	☐ Other M muscles	☐ Non-mast. structures	☐ None	☐ Temporalis	☐ Other M muscles	☐ Non-mast. structures
	☐ Masseter	☐ TMJ			☐ Masseter	☐ TMJ	

1B Location of headache: last 30 days (select all that apply)

☐ None   ☐ Temporal   ☐ Other   ☐ None   ☐ Temporal   ☐ Other

---

2 Incisal relationships

Reference tooth   ☐ FDI #11   ☐ FDI #21   ☐ Other

Right Left N/A

Horizontal incisal overjet ☐ If negative [ ][ ] mm   Vertical incisal overlap ☐ If negative [ ][ ] mm   Midline deviation ☐ ☐ ☐ [ ][ ] mm

---

3 Opening pattern (supplemental; select all that apply)

☐ Straight   ☐ Corrected deviation   Uncorrected deviation   Right ☐   Left ☐

---

4 Opening movements

A Pain-free opening [ ][ ] mm

Right side	Pain		Familiar pain		Familiar headache		Left side	Pain		Familiar pain		Familiar headache	
Temporalis	N	Y	N	Y	N	Y	Temporalis	N	Y	N	Y	N	Y
Masseter	N	Y	N	Y			Masseter	N	Y	N	Y		
TMJ	N	Y	N	Y			TMJ	N	Y	N	Y		
Other M muscle	N	Y	N	Y			Other M muscle	N	Y	N	Y		
Non-mast.	N	Y	N	Y			Non-mast.	N	Y	N	Y		

B Maximum unassisted opening [ ][ ] mm

C Maximum assisted opening [ ][ ] mm

D Terminated? [Y] [N]

Right side	Pain		Familiar pain		Familiar headache		Left side	Pain		Familiar pain		Familiar headache	
Temporalis	N	Y	N	Y	N	Y	Temporalis	N	Y	N	Y	N	Y
Masseter	N	Y	N	Y			Masseter	N	Y	N	Y		
TMJ	N	Y	N	Y			TMJ	N	Y	N	Y		
Other M muscle	N	Y	N	Y			Other M muscle	N	Y	N	Y		
Non-mast.	N	Y	N	Y			Non-mast.	N	Y	N	Y		

---

5 Lateral and protrusive movements

A Right lateral [ ][ ] mm

Right side	Pain		Familiar pain		Familiar headache		Left side	Pain		Familiar pain		Familiar headache	
Temporalis	N	Y	N	Y	N	Y	Temporalis	N	Y	N	Y	N	Y
Masseter	N	Y	N	Y			Masseter	N	Y	N	Y		
TMJ	N	Y	N	Y			TMJ	N	Y	N	Y		
Other M muscle	N	Y	N	Y			Other M muscle	N	Y	N	Y		
Non-mast.	N	Y	N	Y			Non-mast.	N	Y	N	Y		

B Left lateral [ ][ ] mm

Right side	Pain		Familiar pain		Familiar headache		Left side	Pain		Familiar pain		Familiar headache	
Temporalis	N	Y	N	Y	N	Y	Temporalis	N	Y	N	Y	N	Y
Masseter	N	Y	N	Y			Masseter	N	Y	N	Y		
TMJ	N	Y	N	Y			TMJ	N	Y	N	Y		
Other M muscle	N	Y	N	Y			Other M muscle	N	Y	N	Y		
Non-mast.	N	Y	N	Y			Non-mast.	N	Y	N	Y		

C Protrusion [ ][ ] mm

☐ If negative

Right side	Pain		Familiar pain		Familiar headache		Left side	Pain		Familiar pain		Familiar headache	
Temporalis	N	Y	N	Y	N	Y	Temporalis	N	Y	N	Y	N	Y
Masseter	N	Y	N	Y			Masseter	N	Y	N	Y		
TMJ	N	Y	N	Y			TMJ	N	Y	N	Y		
Other M muscle	N	Y	N	Y			Other M muscle	N	Y	N	Y		
Non-mast.	N	Y	N	Y			Non-mast.	N	Y	N	Y		

6 TMJ noises during open and close movements

	Right TMJ							
	Examiner Open	Close	Patient		Pain with click		Familiar pain	
Click	N Y	N Y	N Y	→	N Y		N Y	
Crepitus	N Y	N Y	N Y					

	Left TMJ							
	Examiner Open	Close	Patient		Pain with click		Familiar pain	
Click	N Y	N Y	N Y	→	N Y		N Y	
Crepitus	N Y	N Y	N Y					

7 TMJ noises during lateral and protrusive movements

	Right TMJ					
	Examiner	Patient		Pain with click		Familiar pain
Click	N Y	N Y	→	N Y		N Y
Crepitus	N Y	N Y				

	Left TMJ					
	Examiner	Patient		Pain with click		Familiar pain
Click	N Y	N Y	→	N Y		N Y
Crepitus	N Y	N Y				

8 Joint locking

Right TMJ	Locking	Reduction Patient	Examiner
While opening	N Y	N Y	N Y
Wide open position	N Y	N Y	N Y

Left TMJ	Locking	Reduction Patient	Examiner
While opening	N Y	N Y	N Y
Wide open position	N Y	N Y	N Y

9 Muscle and TMJ pain with palpation

Right side (1Kg)	Pain	Familiar pain	Familiar headache	Referred pain
Temporalis (posterior)	N Y	N Y	N Y	N Y
Temporalis (middle)	N Y	N Y	N Y	N Y
Temporalis (anterior)	N Y	N Y	N Y	N Y
Masseter (origin)	N Y	N Y		N Y
Masseter (body)	N Y	N Y		N Y
Masseter (insertion)	N Y	N Y		N Y

Left side (1Kg)	Pain	Familiar pain	Familiar headache	Referred pain
Temporalis (posterior)	N Y	N Y	N Y	N Y
Temporalis (middle)	N Y	N Y	N Y	N Y
Temporalis (anterior)	N Y	N Y	N Y	N Y
Masseter (origin)	N Y	N Y		N Y
Masseter (body)	N Y	N Y		N Y
Masseter (insertion)	N Y	N Y		N Y

TMJ	Pain	Familiar pain	Referred pain
Lateral pole (0.5 Kg)	N Y	N Y	N Y
Around lateral pole (1 Kg)	N Y	N Y	N Y

TMJ	Pain	Familiar pain	Referred pain
Lateral pole (0.5 Kg)	N Y	N Y	N Y
Around lateral pole (1 Kg)	N Y	N Y	N Y

10 Supplemental muscle pain with palpation

Right side	Pain	Familiar pain	Referred pain
Posterior mandibular region	N Y	N Y	N Y
Submandibular region	N Y	N Y	N Y
Lateral pterygoid area	N Y	N Y	N Y
Temporalis tendon	N Y	N Y	N Y

Left side	Pain	Familiar pain	Referred pain
Posterior mandibular region	N Y	N Y	N Y
Submandibular region	N Y	N Y	N Y
Lateral pterygoid area	N Y	N Y	N Y
Temporalis tendon	N Y	N Y	N Y

11 Diagnoses

Pain disorders	Right TMJ disorders	Left TMJ disorders
☐ None	☐ None	☐ None
☐ Myalgia	Disc displacement (select one)	Disc displacement (select one)
☐ Myofascial pain with referral	☐ ... with reduction	☐ ... with reduction
☐ Right arthralgia	☐ ... with reduction, with intermittent locking	☐ ... with reduction, with intermittent locking
☐ Left arthralgia	☐ ... without reduction, with limited opening	☐ ... without reduction, with limited opening
☐ Headache attributed to TMD	☐ ... without reduction, without limited opening	☐ ... without reduction, without limited opening
☐	☐ Degenerative joint disease	☐ Degenerative joint disease
☐	☐ Dislocation	☐ Dislocation

Chapter 7

References

Bell W. Private communication with author, circa 1980.

Bryan CS. Osler: Inspirations from a Great Physician. New York & London: Oxford University Press, 1997.

Doyle AC. The Sign of the Four, 1890.

Doyle AC. The Strand Magazine, London, September 1914 and May 1915.

International Association for the study of pain (IASP), orofacial pain special interest group 2016 Available: https://www.iasp-pain.org/SIG/OrofacialHeadPain [Oct 8, 2017].

International RDC/TMD Consortium Network. TMD pain screener, 2011. Available: https://ubwp.buffalo.edu/rdc-tmdinternational/wp-content/uploads/sites/58/2017/01/TMD-Pain-Screener_revised-10Aug2011.pdf [Oct 8, 2017].

International RDC/TMD Consortium Network. Diagnostic criteria for temporomandibular disorders: symptom questionnaire, 2013a. Available: https://ubwp.buffalo.edu/rdc-tmdinternational/wp-content/uploads/sites/58/2017/01/DC-TMD_SQ_shortform_2013-05-12.pdf [Oct 1, 2017].

International RDC/TMD Consortium Network. Clinical examination form, 2013b. Available: https://ubwp.buffalo.edu/rdc-tmdinternational/wp-content/uploads/sites/58/2017/01/DC-TMD_examform_international_2013-05-12.pdf [Oct 1, 2017].

Safire: William Safire, American author 1929–2009 [n.d.].

Chapter 8

Clinical examination of the temporomandibular joint and masticatory muscles

Mariano Rocabado, César Fernández-de-las-Peñas

Manual examination of the temporomandibular joint

Mandibular range of motion

Clinical examination of the temporomandibular joint (TMJ) begins with the patient history and interview (see Chapter 7), examination of range of motion, and evaluation of clicking sounds. Mandibular range of motion assessment includes unassisted mouth opening without pain (pain free), maximum unassisted opening (even if pain is felt), maximum assisted opening (overpressure by the clinician even if pain is felt), lateral deviations, and protrusive excursion. The quantity and

quality of the jaw movement should be assessed. The cut-off limits (normative values) are 35 or 40 mm for pain-free active mouth opening and 7 mm for lateral deviations (Schiffman et al., 2014). Clinicians should note that mandible range of motion is age dependent, so normative values will tend to be lower (Hassel et al., 2006). Intrarater reliability of mandibular range of motion ranges from moderate (ICC: 0.6) to excellent (ICC: 0.90) depending on the movement (de Wijer et al., 1995; List et al., 2006). The reliability was lower in those mandibular movements with the presence of pain (κ: 0.47–0.59). The clinician can use a movement diagram to record the quantity and quality of mandible movements (Figure 8.1A). In fact, deviation of the

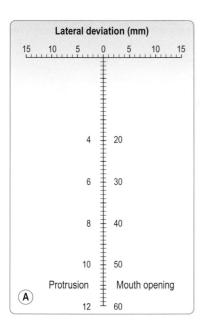
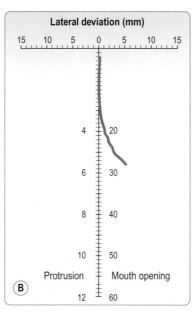
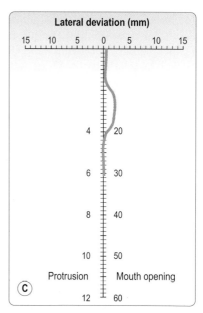

Figure 8.1

(A) Movement diagram for assessing mandibular range of motion. (B) Diagram recording a patient with limited mouth opening at 30 mm and a lateral deviation from the midrange of motion to the final position of mouth opening. (C) Diagram recording a patient with limited mouth opening at 30 mm and a lateral deviation at the midrange of motion that is corrected at the end of the movement.

mandible to either side during active mouth opening should be assessed. This lateral deviation of the mandible can occur at the end of mouth opening without correction (Figure 8.1B) or can occur at the midrange of movement but it is corrected during the movement (Figure 8.1C). A 4:1 ratio should be mantained during mouth opening: for every 1mm of lateral deviation of the mandible, 4mm of mouth opening should be mantained in the contra- lateral joint.

Temporomandibular joint clicking sounds

Another important assessment is to evaluate the presence of TMJ clicking sounds during mouth movements, that is, joint clicking during opening, closing, lateral deviation to the same side, lateral deviation to the opposite side, or protrusion, or reciprocal clicking eliminated in opening from a protruded position. Reciprocal clicking of the TMJ is indicative of reduced disc displacement since the disc snaps in and out of this position during an open–close cycle, causing an opening and/or closing click. The reliability of identification of TMJ clicking sound ranges from fair (κ: 0.40) to good (κ: 0.70) (List et al., 2006). Hassel et al. (2006) reported an overall percentage agreement of 83 per cent for TMJ clicking sounds during mouth opening and/or closing, 65 per cent during lateral deviations, and 76 per cent during protrusions. Other authors have reported good reliability values (κ: >0.75) for examination of TMJ clicking sounds (Gallo et al., 2000). Interestingly, the presence of TMJ clicking sounds is not age dependent (Hassel et al., 2006). Huddleston Slater et al. (2004) have reported an excellent reliability (κ: 0.86) for recognition of internal derangements based on clinical findings, particularly the presence of TMJ clicking sounds during the examination.

Compression (overpressure) tests to the temporomandibular joint

The clinician can increase the overload on the TMJ with overpressure during the evaluation of the mandibular range of motion. In fact, different compressive

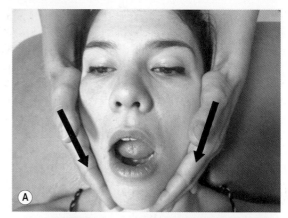

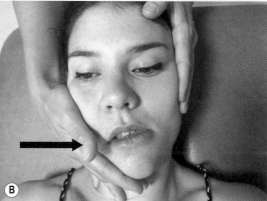

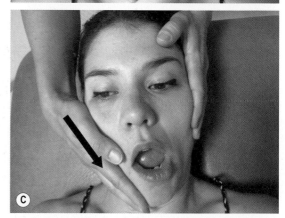

Figure 8.2

Overpressure during mandibular range of motion in mouth opening (A), lateral deviation (B) or combined motion C).

loads (toward cranial, dorsal, or dorsocranial) can be applied (Figure 8.2). The application of overpressure will increase the compressive forces over the disc and TMJ stimulating the nociceptors and evidencing the presence of tissue irritability. Of particular relevance is the application of compressive forces to the retrodiscal tissue since it is highly sensitive to sustained compression (Langendoen et al., 1997). De Wijer et al. (1995) reported substantial (κ: 0.60) interexaminer reliability for compression tests in individuals with TMD pain.

Palpation of the temporomandibular joint

Palpation of the TMJ is probably the most relevant clinical examination test (Sipilä et al., 2011). The prevalence of local-induced pain with palpation of the TMJ has been found to be 58 per cent in patients with post-traumatic stress disorder (Uhac et al., 2011) and 45 per cent in patients with rheumatoid arthritis (Witulski et al., 2014). Among these patients, the posterior pole of the TMJ was the most sensitive area in around 40 per cent of cases (Uhac et al., 2011; Witulski et al., 2014). In fact, the prevalence of

induced pain with palpation on the posterior pole of the TMJ has increased its prevalence between 1993 and 2003 (Köhler et al., 2013). It is interesting to note that pain on palpation of the TMJ was significantly associated with TMD severity in a sample of elderly patients (Camacho et al., 2014).

An important topic for discussion with regard to manual palpation is how much pressure should be applied and for how long, particularly since the TMJ can be very sensitive in individuals with arthrogenous TMD (Benoliel & Sharav, 2009). Cunha et al. (2014) found 89.7 per cent specificity and 70 per cent sensitivity when 1.36 Kg/cm^2 pressure was applied during palpation of the TMJ. This value was considered to be the most appropriate threshold at which to diagnose moderate to severe TMJ arthralgia. How long the pressure should be maintained has not been determined.

The entire TMJ should be palpated to get an impression of the presence of joint inflammatory pain. One of the most expanded protocols for TMJ palpation has been described by Rocabado (personal

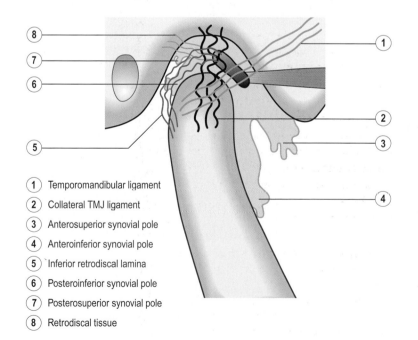

Figure 8.3

Anatomical points for manual examination of TMJ irritability proposed by Rocabado. © Mariano Rocabado.

1. Temporomandibular ligament
2. Collateral TMJ ligament
3. Anterosuperior synovial pole
4. Anteroinferior synovial pole
5. Inferior retrodiscal lamina
6. Posteroinferior synovial pole
7. Posterosuperior synovial pole
8. Retrodiscal tissue

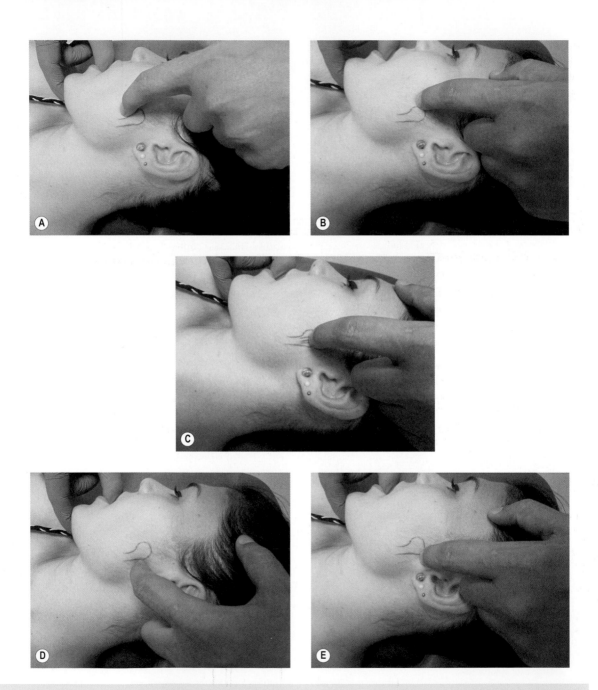

Figure 8.4
Palpation of the anteroinferior synovial pole (A); anterosuperior synovial pole (B); collateral TMJ ligament (C); posteroinferior synovial pole (D); and, posterosuperior synovial pole (E).

communication; Figure 8.3). This protocol consists of palpation of five connective tissue structures and three manual maneuvers for testing the temporomandibular ligament, the inferior retrodiscal lamina, and the retrodiscal tissue. For palpation of the TMJ, the patient lies in supine with the head slightly turned to the opposite side. The mouth is slightly opened (10 mm) and slightly protruded. From that position, the clinician can palpate the anteroinferior synovial pole (Figure 8.4A), the anterosuperior synovial pole (Figure 8.4B), the collateral TMJ ligament (Figure 8.4C); the posteroinferior synovial pole (Figure 8.4D), and the posterosuperior synovial pole (Figure 8.4E) of the TMJ.

Since the temporomandibular ligament has dense connective tissue (Cuccia et al., 2011), it needs a manual maneuver to assess its irritability. The clinician places the thumb of the first hand on top of the last upper mandibular molars and the index finger on the inferior portion of the mandible. The other hand stabilizes the patient's head and the index and middle fingers palpate the ligament (see Figure 11.7). From that position, the clinician applies an inferior and posterior force through the thumb (Figure 8.5).

The retrodiscal tissue attaches to the disc posteriorly and is divided into two laminae: the superior lamina which is attached to the squamotympanic fissure of the temporalis bone and is composed of fibroelastic tissue; and the inferior lamina, which is attached to the back of the mandible condyle and is composed of nonelastic, rigid collagen fibers. The region between both laminae contains highly vascular and neural tissue (Langendoen et al., 1997). The posterior part of the TMJ and the retrodiscal tissue receive an extensive innervation from free nerve endings (Langendoen et al., 1997). It has been observed that the retrodiscal tissue signal intensity is higher in abnormal TMJs, suggesting an increased vascularity in the tissue (Lee & Yoon 2009). Therefore, examination of the retrodiscal tissue consists of two maneuvers. First, the inferior retrodiscal lamina is assessed. With one hand the same position as used for the temporomandibular ligament (Figure 8.5) but with the other hand placed at the angle of the mandible, a posterior and superior (compressive) force through the thumb should be applied by the clinician (Figure 8.6). To assess the retrodiscal tissue, a posterior, superior, and finally an anterior force through the thumb is applied by the clinician (Figure 8.7).

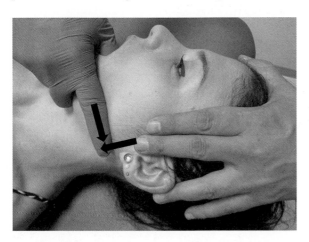

Figure 8.5
Maneuver for assessing the irritability of the temporomandibular ligament.

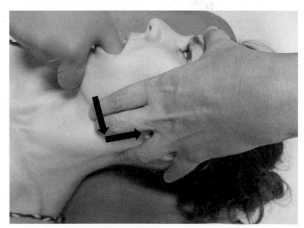

Figure 8.6
Maneuver for assessing the irritability of the inferior retrodiscal lamina.

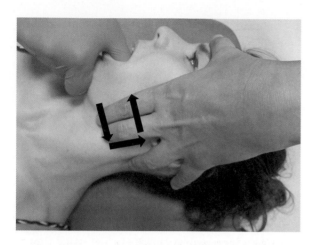

Figure 8.7
Maneuver for assessing the irritability of the retrodiscal tissue.

All these maneuvers should be considered positive when the patient experiences pain (local and/or referred) and, most importantly, when the elicited pain reproduces any of the patient's symptoms, such as pain recognition.

Manual examination of the masticatory musculature

Tenderness or painful palpation of the masticatory musculature

As has been described in Chapter 2, the current diagnostic criteria classification for TMD (DC/TMD) includes the subtypes local myalgia and myofascial pain in the Axis I category (Peck et al., 2014; Schiffman et al., 2014). It is important to clarify that local myalgia or myofascial pain in this case means local pain during palpation without pain referral (see the subsequent section).

Local pain during palpation of masticatory muscles occurs in 57–97 per cent of patients with TMD as opposed to 10–29 per cent of patients without TMD (Ohrbach et al., 2011). Camacho et al. (2014) reported locally induced pain during palpation of the masticatory musculature in 78 per cent of elderly patients (over 60 years of age) with TMD and also that there was a significant association between the severity of TMD and palpation of the masticatory muscles.

In addition, palpation-induced pain in the masticatory muscles may play a role in the differential diagnosis between painful TMD and some primary headaches (Costa et al., 2016). In this study, palpation-induced local pain in the masseter muscle was associated with myogenous TMD, whereas palpation-induced local pain in the anterior temporalis muscle was observed in patients with TMD but also in primary headaches such as tension-type headache or migraine (Costa et al., 2016). These results accord with the research carried out by Sales Pinto et al. on the influence of myofascial pain on the pressure pain threshold of masticatory muscles in patients with migraine (Sales Pinto et al., 2013).

It seems that the masseter is one of the most significant muscles in TMD since pain on palpation of this muscle has been associated with ipsilateral arthrogenous TMD, for example disc displacement (Inoue et al., 2010; da Silva Parente Macedo et al., 2015). In fact, patients exhibiting palpation-induced local pain in the masseter muscle showed a threefold increased risk for the presence of arthrogenous TMD (da Silva Parente Macedo et al., 2015).

This subdivision proposed in the DC/TMD (Peck et al., 2014; Schiffman et al., 2014) highlights the relevance of manual palpation of the masticatory musculature; however, the reliability of the data on manual palpation is debatable. Gomes et al. (2008) reported moderate to good reliability values for palpation of the masticatory muscles in patients with TMD and healthy people, whereas Chaves et al. (2010) showed moderate to poor intrarater and inter-rater reliability in both children with TMD symptoms and healthy children (Chaves et al., 2010). However, reliability depends on the muscle examined as extraoral muscles (masseter or temporalis) exhibit better reliability than intraoral muscles (lateral or medial pterygoid).

One of the most important questions to consider here is how much pressure should the clinician apply and for how long (Benoliel & Sharav, 2009). It has been suggested that palpation pressure should be 1 Kg for intraoral structures and 1.5–2.0 Kg for extraoral structures (Goulet et al., 1998). Some devices have been developed with the aim of standardizing the pressure applied by clinicians. For instance, a pressure algometer for palpation and a fingertip adjustable palpometer have shown similar excellent interexaminer reliability to a conventional algometer (Bernhardt et al., 2007). Other authors developed a new mechanical palpometer for assessing deep-pain sensitivity, which also had excellent reliability (Futarmal et al., 2011). However, it should be noted that manual assessment without the use of any device is the most common method used in clinical practice.

On the question of how long the pressure should be maintained, it has been suggested that two to five seconds is enough to elicit a local pain response or pain referral, respectively. It is important to note that the subdivision of myalgia into local myalgia, myofascial pain, and myofascial pain with referral was proposed as a possible temporal progression of muscle pain from a localized myalgia to more widespread or spreading pain. The clinical distinction between localized muscle pain and pain referral is similar to the distinction between tender point (local pain) and trigger point (referred pain). Readers are referred to other literature for more on this subject (Fernández-de-las-Peñas & Arendt-Nielsen, 2016). In fact, palpation of the masticatory muscles is considered positive when a patient recognizes the palpation-induced local pain as a familiar pain (pain recognition) (Peck et al., 2014; Schiffman et al., 2014), since just the presence of tenderness in a muscle could reflect hyperalgesia or allodynia.

Visscher et al. (2004) observed that manual palpation was as reproducible as pressure algometry for pain recognition in patients with TMD.

Pain referral on palpation of the masticatory muscles: myofascial trigger points

The third subtype of myalgia described in Axis I of the DC/TMD is myofascial pain with referral, that is myalgia with report of pain at a site beyond the boundary of the muscle being palpated (Peck et al., 2014; Schiffman et al., 2014). This type of TMD pain has a sensitivity of 0.86, and a specificity of 0.98. It is interesting to note that this diagnosis has similar clinical features to muscle trigger points (TrPs), although this particular term is not used in the DC/TMD as has been commented on in Chapter 2.

TrPs are characterized by referred pain during palpation. Simons et al. (1999) described several head and neck muscles, in which referred pain could contribute to TMD pain symptoms. For instance, TrPs in masticatory muscles can refer pain to the TMJ simulating arthralgia. Clinically, if the pain referral elicited by a TrP reproduces any symptoms experienced by the patient, such as pain recognition, it is considered to be an active TrP. If the elicited referred pain does not reproduce any symptoms experienced by the patient, it is considered to be a latent TrP (Simons et al., 1999). It is important to consider that TrPs exhibit an important motor component, since they can also provoke muscle weakness, muscle inhibition, increased motor irritability, muscle imbalance, accelerated fatigability, or altered motor recruitment (Ge & Arendt-Nielsen, 2011).

Competent TrP diagnosis requires adequate training, skill development, and clinical practice to develop a high degree of reliability in the examination. Simons et al. (1999) described several signs and symptoms that may be used for the TrP diagnosis including a palpable taut band in a skeletal muscle, presence of a hypersensitive spot within the taut band, local twitch response on snapping palpation of the TrP, pain referral with stimulation or palpation of the hyperirritable spot, muscle weakness, pain on contraction in the shortened or lengthening position, or a jump sign. However, the reliability of each of these signs or symptoms in isolation is questioned (Rathbone et al., 2017). Readers are referred to other texts for discussion on the reliability of diagnosing TrPs (Myburgh et al. 2008; Lucas et al. 2009; Bron & Dommerholt 2012). New imaging modalities are being explored to better diagnose TrPs. For instance, in the masticatory muscles, infrared imaging could be useful as it is able to indicate the difference between referred and local pain within TrPs at 0.5°C (Haddad et al., 2012). Haddad et al. found sensitivity and specificity data of 62.5 per cent and 71.3 per cent respectively for the presence of referred pain, and 43.6 per cent and 60.6 per cent respectively for the presence of local pain (Haddad et al., 2012).

In clinical practice, Simons et al. (1999) and Gerwin et al. (1997) recommend that the minimum acceptable criteria for TrP diagnosis are the presence of a hypersensitive spot within a palpable taut band of a skeletal muscle combined with the patient's recognition of the referred pain elicited by the TrP. When applied by an experienced assessor, these criteria have obtained good interexaminer reliability (κ: 0.84 to 0.88). In fact, localized tenderness and pain recognition were the most reliable criteria (κ: 0.676 and κ: 0.575, respectively) observed in the meta-analysis conducted by Rathbone et al. (2017). Similarly, pain referral has also shown moderate (κ: 0.57) to excellent (κ: 0.84) reliability, depending on the muscle assessed (Gerwin et al., 1997).

Surprisingly, few clinical studies have investigated the presence of TrP referred pain in TMD. Two studies reported that the masseter, temporalis, upper trapezius, and lateral pterygoid muscles were the most common sources of referred pain in the neck and craniofacial regions in individuals with myogenous TMD (Wright, 2000; Fernández-de-las-Peñas et al., 2010). It is interesting to note that patients with TMD not only exhibited active TrPs in the masticatory muscles, but also in the neck and shoulder muscles. In addition, the opposite has also been observed in patients with mechanical neck pain exhibiting more latent TrPs (not spontaneously symptomatic) in the masseter and temporalis muscles and reduced jaw opening compared to healthy controls (De-la-Llave-Rincon et al., 2012). It appears that TrP-associated referred pain can play a relevant role in TMD pain.

Manual exploration of the masticatory musculature

Clinical history, examination of active and passive jaw movement patterns, quality and extension of pain area and associated symptoms, and consideration of referred pain patterns assist the clinician in determining which muscles may be clinically relevant for patients with TMD. TrP palpation starts with the identification of a taut band within the skeletal muscle by palpating perpendicular to the fiber direction. Patients may be asked to contract the muscle to better locate the fibers. Muscles may be placed in a relaxed or slightly prestretched position for palpation depending on the clinical presentation of the patient. Once the taut band is located, a hypersensitive spot within that taut band is identified. Manually strumming the taut band can elicit a local twitch response, which is a sudden involuntary contraction of the taut band, in superficial muscles. Manual strumming of the taut band can be done with a flat palpation, for example of the temporalis muscle, during which the therapist applies finger or thumb pressure to the muscle against the underlying bone tissue, or with a pincer palpation, for example of the superficial masseter, where the muscle is rolled between the tips of the digits.

The clinician should be wary of preconceived expectations of the location and referred pain patterns of TrPs, although most textbooks use some kind of standard marks for didactic purposes (Simons et al., 1999). Here we describe the referred pain from masticatory muscles most commonly involved in the genesis of TMD pain.

Masseter muscle

The masseter muscle is probably the muscle most commonly involved in TMDs. The referred pain, either experimentally induced or TrP-associated referred pain, is able to mimic sensory symptoms experienced by patients with TMDs (Svensson, 2007; Fernández-de-las-Peñas et al., 2010). TrPs in the superficial portion of this muscle refer pain to the eyebrow, the maxilla, the mandible, and to the teeth, whereas TrPs in the deep layer refer pain deep into the ear and to the TMJ

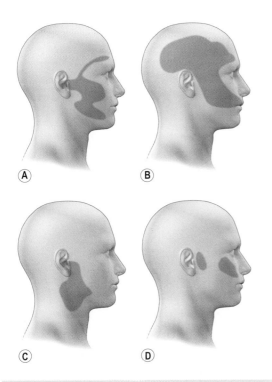

Figure 8.8
Referred pain elicited by trigger points within the masseter (A), temporalis (B), medial pterygoid (C), and lateral pterygoid (D) muscles.

(Simons et al., 1999) (Figure 8.8A). TrPs in this muscle usually restrict jaw opening. In fact, unilateral masseter TrPs tend to deviate the mandible toward the affected side, although deviation can be also associated with a unilateral TMJ internal derangement, which may cause the mandible to deviate toward the affected side (see Figures 8.1B and C). Symptoms are exacerbated by mouth opening, parafunctional habits such as chewing, and lying on the affected side. Since it is a superficial muscle, it can be palpated with a flat and/or pincer palpation depending on the irritability of the patient. Crossfiber palpation is used to locate taut bands in the superficial layer of the masseter and the pain referral can be easily elicited with a small amount of pressure.

Temporalis muscle

The temporalis is another commonly affected muscle in patients with TMD (Fernández-de-las-Peñas et al., 2010). In fact, palpation of the masseter and temporalis muscles is considered within the current version of the DC/TMD (Peck et al., 2014; Schiffman et al., 2014). Further to this, the temporalis has also been found to be involved in tension-type headache (Fernández-de-las-Peñas et al., 2007). This may be related to the fact that the referred pain from TrPs in the temporalis muscle can produce tooth pain or head pain, depending on the clinical presentation of the patient (Simons et al., 1999) (Figure 8.8B). Symptoms are exacerbated by dysfunctional habits such as bruxism, chewing gum, biting fingernails, and chewing ice. Palpation of the temporalis often reveals very painful TrPs even when palpation is conducted smoothly. Clinically, this muscle usually exhibits multiple TrPs (Fernández-de-las-Peñas et al., 2009). Since it is a superficial muscle, crossfiber flat palpation of the temporalis usually discloses multiple taut bands in the muscle.

Medial pterygoid muscle

The medial pterygoid is the 'mirror' intraoral muscle of the masseter, since both are able to suspend the angle of the mandible. Symptoms from this muscle are more diffuse compared with other masticatory muscles. TrPs in the medial pterygoid refer diffuse pain to the maxilla, mandible, teeth, mouth, ear, and TMJ (Simons et al., 1999) (Figure 8.8C). Masseter TrPs can promote activity of TrPs in this agonist muscle, so examination of both muscles is usually needed. Manual examination of the middle part of this muscle involves intraoral palpation. The pad of the index finger faces outward and slides over the molars until it encounters the bony anterior edge of the ramus of the mandible, which lies behind and lateral to the last molar. The middle part of the medial pterygoid muscle belly lies immediately beyond (posterior to) this bony edge (see Figure 12.10). Palpation will elicit exquisite tenderness in the patient with medial pterygoid TrPs, so this procedure should be conducted with extreme caution.

Lateral pterygoid muscle

The lateral pterygoid is one of the most important muscles in TMJ dynamics due to its anatomical relationship to the disc. The theory of internal derangement of the TMJ involves anterior displacement of the disc as a result of hyperactivity of the lateral pterygoid muscle. As the superior head of the muscle is attached to the disc, it may pull the disc in an anterior and superior-medial direction (Fujita et al., 2001). This hypothesis is supported by a biomechanical model showing that with prolonged increase in the force of the lateral pterygoid muscle, the disc was elongated anteriorly thus confirming that hyperactivity of this muscle could be involved in the progression of disc displacement (Tanaka et al., 2007). The referred pain from this muscle spreads to the maxilla and deep into the TMJ (Simons et al., 1999) (Figure 8.8D). Palpation of this muscle has been questioned in the literature, but a recent study has confirmed that palpation of the lateral pterygoid muscle can be attained (Stelzenmueller et al., 2016). A successful palpation of the lateral pterygoid can be conducted with mouth opening and lateral deviation to the examined side. The clinician's index finger palpates along the oral vestibule parallel to the upper section of the alveolar

process of the maxilla, onto the maxillary tuberosity, until the lateral plate of the pterygoid process is reached (see Figures 12.11 and 12.12).

Other muscles

There are other muscles, for example the sternocleidomastoid (Figure 8.9A), splenius capitis, (Figure 8.9B), suboccipital (Figure 8.9C), and upper trapezius (Figure 8.9D) in which referred pain can also contribute to the pain pattern observed in patients with TMDs (Fernández-de-las-Peñas et al., 2010). Readers are referred to other texts for

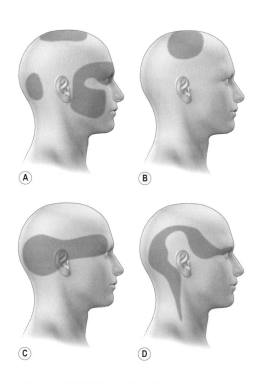

Figure 8.9

Referred pain elicited by trigger points within the sternocleidomastoid (A), splenius capitis (B), suboccipital (C), and upper trapezius (D) muscles.

more information on the examination of these muscles (Simons et al., 1999).

Conclusion

This chapter has described manual examination of the TMJ and its associated masticatory muscles focusing on TrPs and their referred pain that can contribute to the onset and continuation of symptoms in TMD patients. Clinicians should conduct a thorough examination of the masticatory system to determine clinically relevant findings to better characterize and manage TMD pain.

References

Benoliel R, Sharav Y. Tender muscles and masticatory myofascial pain diagnosis: how many or how much? J Orofac Pain 2009; 23: 300–301.

Bernhardt O, Schiffman EL, Look JO. Reliability and validity of a new fingertip-shaped pressure algometer for assessing pressure pain thresholds in the temporomandibular joint and masticatory muscles. J Orofac Pain 2007; 21: 29–38.

Bron C, Dommerholt JD. Etiology of myofascial trigger points. Curr Pain Headache Rep 2012; 16: 439–444.

Camacho JG, Oltramari-Navarro PV, Navarro Rde L et al. Signs and symptoms of temporomandibular disorders in the elderly. Codas 2014; 26: 76–80.

Chaves TC, Nagamine HM, de Sousa LM, de Oliveira AS, Grossi DB. Comparison between the reliability levels of manual palpation and pressure pain threshold in children who reported orofacial pain. Man Ther 2010; 15: 508–512.

Costa YM, Porporatti AL, Calderon PD, Conti PC, Bonjardim LR. Can palpation-induced muscle pain pattern contribute to the differential diagnosis among temporomandibular disorders, primary headaches phenotypes and possible bruxism? Med Oral Patol Oral Cir Bucal 2016; 21: e59–65.

Cuccia AM, Caradonna C, Caradonna D. Manual therapy of the mandibular accessory ligaments for the management of temporomandibular joint disorders. J Am Osteopath Assoc 2011; 111: 102–112.

Cunha CO, Pinto-Fiamenqui LM, Castro AC, Lauris JR, Conti PC. Determination of a pressure pain threshold cut-off value for the diagnosis of temporomandibular joint arthralgia. J Oral Rehabil 2014; 41: 323–329.

da Silva Parente Macedo LC, de Goffredo Filho GS, de Souza Tesch R, de Queiroz Farias Góes CP. Frequency of temporomandibular arthralgia among myofascial pain patients with pain on palpation of ipsilateral masseter. Cranio 2015; 33: 206–210.

De-la-Llave-Rincon AI, Alonso-Blanco C, Gil-Crujera A, Ambite-Quesada S, Svensson P, Fernández-de-las-Peñas C. Myofascial trigger points in the masticatory muscles in patients with and without chronic mechanical neck pain. J Manipulative Physiol Ther 2012; 35: 678–684.

de Wijer A, Lobbezoo-Scholte AM, Steenks MH, Bosman F. Reliability of clinical findings in temporomandibular disorders. J Orofac Pain 1995; 9: 181–191.

Fernández-de-las-Peñas C, Arendt-Nielsen L. Myofascial pain and fibromyalgia: two different but overlapping disorders. Pain Manag 2016; 6: 401–408.

Fernandez-de-las-Peñas C, Ge HY, Arendt-Nielsen L, Cuadrado ML, Pareja JA. The local and referred pain from myofascial trigger points in the temporalis muscle contributes to pain profile in chronic tension-type headache. Clin J Pain. 2007; 23: 786–792.

Fernández-de-las-Peñas C, Caminero AB, Madeleine P et al. Multiple active myofascial trigger points and pressure pain sensitivity maps in the temporalis muscle are related in chronic tension type headache. Clin J Pain 2009; 25: 506–512.

Fernández-de-las-Peñas C, Galán-Del-Río F, Alonso-Blanco C, Jiménez-García R, Arendt-Nielsen L, Svensson P. Referred pain from muscle trigger points in the masticatory and neck-shoulder musculature in women with temporomandibular disorders. J Pain 2010; 11: 1295–1304.

Fujita S, Iizuka T, Dauber W. Variation of heads of lateral pterygoid muscle and morphology of articular disc of human temporomandibular joint: anatomical and histological analysis. J Oral Rehabil 2001; 28: 560–571.

Futarmal S, Kothari M, Ayesh E, Baad-Hansen L, Svensson P. New palpometer with implications for assessment of deep pain sensitivity. J Dent Res 2011; 90: 918–922.

Gallo LM, Svoboda A, Palla S. Reproducibility of temporomandibular joint clicking. J Orofac Pain 2000; 14: 293–302.

Ge HY, Arendt-Nielsen L Latent myofascial trigger points. Curr Pain Head Reports 2011; 15: 386–392.

Gerwin RD, Shannon S, Hong CZ et al. Inter-rater reliability in myofascial trigger point examination. Pain 1997; 69: 65–73.

Gomes MB, Guimarães JP, Guimarães FC, Neves AC. Palpation and pressure pain threshold: reliability and validity in patients with temporomandibular disorders. Cranio 2008; 26: 202–210.

Goulet JP, Clark GT, Flack VF, Liu C. The reproducibility of muscle and joint tenderness detection methods and maximum mandibular movement measurement for the temporomandibular system. J Orofac Pain 1998; 12: 17–26.

Haddad DS, Brioschi ML, Arita ES. Thermographic and clinical correlation of myofascial trigger points in the masticatory muscles. Dentomaxillofac Radiol 2012; 41: 621–629.

Hassel AJ, Rammelsberg P, Schmitter M. Inter-examiner reliability in the clinical examination of temporomandibular disorder: influence of age. Community Dent Oral Epidemiol 2006; 34: 41–46.

Huddleston Slater JJ, Lobbezoo F, Chen YJ, Naeije M. A comparative study between clinical and instrumental methods for the recognition of internal derangements with a clicking sound on condylar movement. J Orofac Pain. 2004; 18: 138–147.

Inoue E, Maekawa K, Minakuchi H et al. The relationship between temporomandibular joint pathosis and muscle tenderness in the orofacial and neck/shoulder region. Oral Surg Oral Med Oral Pathol Oral Radiol Endod 2010; 109: 86–90.

Köhler AA, Hugoson A, Magnusson T. Clinical signs indicative of temporomandibular disorders in adults: time trends and associated factors. Swed Dent J 2013; 37: 1–11.

Langendoen J, Müller J, Jull GA Retrodiscal tissue of the temporomandibular joint: clinical anatomy and its role in diagnosis and treatment of arthropathies. Man Ther 1997; 2: 191–198.

Lee SH, Yoon HJ. The relationship between MRI findings and the relative signal intensity of retro- discal tissue in patients with temporomandibular joint disorders. Oral Surg Oral Med Oral Pathol Oral Radiol Endod 2009; 107: 113–115.

List T, John MT, Dworkin SF, Svensson P. Recalibration improves inter-examiner reliability of TMD examination. Acta Odontol Scand 2006; 64: 146–152.

Lucas N, Macaskill P, Irwig L et al. Reliability of physical examination for diagnosis of myofascial trigger points: a systematic review of the literature. Clin J Pain 2009; 25: 80–89.

Myburgh C, Larsen AH, Hartvigsen JA. systematic, critical review of manual palpation for identifying myofascial trigger points: evidence and clinical significance. Arch Phys Med Rehabil 2008; 89:1169–1176.

Ohrbach R, Fillingim RB, Mulkey F et al. Clinical findings and pain symptoms as potential risk factors for chronic TMD: descriptive data and empirically identified domains from the OPPERA case-control study. J Pain 2011; 12: S27-S45.

Peck CC, Goulet J-P, Lobbezoo F, et al. Expanding the taxonomy of the diagnostic criteria for temporomandibular disorders. J Oral Rehab 2014; 41: 2–23.

Rathbone ATL, Grosman-Rimon L, Kumbhare DA. Inter-rater agreement of manual palpation for identification of myofascial trigger points: A systematic review and meta-analysis. Clin J Pain 2017; 33: 715–729.

Sales Pinto LM, de Carvalho JJ, Cunha CO et al. Influence of myofascial pain on the pressure pain threshold of masticatory muscles in women with migraine. Clin J Pain 2013; 29: 362–365.

Schiffman E, Ohrbach R, Truelove E et al. Diagnostic criteria for temporomandibular disorders (DC/TMD) for clinical and research applications: Recommendations of the International RDC/TMD Consortium Network and Orofacial Pain Special Interest Group. J Oral Facial Pain Headache 2014; 28: 6–27.

Simons DG, Travell JG, Simons LS. Travell & Simons' Myofascial Pain and Dysfunction: The Trigger Point Manual. Vol. 1. 2nd ed.

Baltimore: Lippincott William & Wilkins; 1999.

Sipilä K, Suominen AL, Alanen P et al. Association of clinical findings of temporomandibular disorders (TMD) with self-reported musculoskeletal pains. Eur J Pain 2011; 15: 1061–1067.

Stelzenmueller W, Umstadt H, Weber D, Goenner-Oezkan V, Kopp S, Lisson J. The intraoral palpability of the lateral pterygoid muscle: A prospective study. Ann Anat 2016; 206: 89–95.

Svensson P. Muscle pain in the head: overlap between temporomandibular disorders and tension-type headaches. Curr Opin Neurol 2007; 20: 320–325.

Tanaka E, Hirose M, Inubushi T et al. Effect of hyperactivity of the lateral pterygoid muscle on the temporomandibular joint disk. J Biomech Eng 2007; 129: 890–897.

Uhac I, Tariba P, Kovac Z er al. Masticatory muscle and temporomandibular joint pain in Croatian war veterans with posttraumatic stress disorder. Coll Antropol 2011; 35: 1161–1166.

Visscher CM, Lobbezoo F, Naeije M. Comparison of algometry and palpation in the recognition of temporomandibular disorder pain complaints. J Orofac Pain 2004; 18: 214–219.

Witulski S, Vogl TJ, Rehart S, Ottl P. Evaluation of the TMJ by means of clinical TMD examination and MRI diagnostics in patients with rheumatoid arthritis. Biomed Res Int 2014; 2014: 328560.

Wright EF. Referred craniofacial pain patterns in patients with temporomandibular disorder. J Am Dent Assoc 2000; 131: 1307–1315.

Chapter 9

Clinical examination of the cervical and thoracic spine in patients with temporomandibular disorders

Michael C. O'Hara, Joe Girard, Bill Egan, Joshua A. Cleland

The cervical and thoracic spine in temporomandibular disorders

The cervical and thoracic spine should be considered as part of a comprehensive clinical assessment for individuals with temporomandibular disorders (TMDs). A functional relationship exists between the head, the cervical spine, the thoracic spine and the temporomandibular joint (TMJ) due to anatomical proximity and biomechanical interdependence (Corrêa & Bérzin, 2004; La Touche et al., 2011). The head, TMJ and cervical spine are neurologically linked via the trigeminal nerve. The trigeminal nerve has a complex arrangement that consists of a small motor component, which commands the muscles of mastication, and a larger sensory component, which is aligned from the midbrain to the upper cervical spinal cord (Bradnam & Barry, 2013). The trigeminal sensory complex receives and transmits proprioceptive, thermal, discriminatory and nociceptive information from associated structures of the head, TMJ and cervical spine (Bradnam & Barry, 2013). Further information can be found in Chapter 3 of this textbook.

Due to anatomical proximity, biomechanical relationships, and neurophysiological connection of the head, TMJ, cervical spine and thoracic spine, dysfunction of one region may affect the others. For example, forward head posture can contribute to biomechanical alterations of the TMJ, cervical, and thoracic spine (Ballenberger et al., 2012). Head position may affect the resting position of the mandible with possible alteration of muscle activity and tone, which may contribute to disorders of the TMJ (Olivo et al., 2006). In an experimental study, pressure pain thresholds of the muscles of mastication and maximal mouth opening have been reported to be influenced by the posture of the head and neck in patients with myofascial TMD (La Touche et al., 2011). It is

also plausible that TMD as well as the position of the tongue and mandible can potentially impact cervical range of motion (Grondin et al., 2017).

In recent research, cervical spine impairments in individuals with TMD have been observed (von Piekartz et al., 2016; Ballenburger et al., 2017). These impairments include limited and painful cervical range of motion, pain with upper cervical passive accessory motion testing, sensitivity to pressure of the cervical muscles, limitation in the cervical flexion-rotation test, and impairments during the craniocervical flexion test. These tests will all be described in detail below. Furthermore, patients with more severe TMD pain and disability, or TMD deemed to be of a mixed variety (both myogenic and arthrogenic), tend to have the greatest number of cervical spine impairments. At this time it is not certain whether these cervical spine impairments represent a coexisting cervical spine disorder or are due to secondary hyperalgesia as a result of central sensitization in individuals with TMD; nevertheless, its treatment may be beneficial for these patients.

It has been suggested that interventions targeting the TMJ may affect cervical pain and vice versa. Manual therapy and exercise directed at the cervical spine has been found to be effective in reducing pain and the pressure pain threshold of the masticatory muscles, and increasing pain-free mouth opening in individuals with TMD (La Touche et al., 2013). Additionally, treating patients with an occlusal splint was found to increase cervical spine range of motion and decrease cervical spine pain in a population of patients with TMD (Walczyńska-Dragon et al., 2014). Two studies reported superior outcomes for patients with cervicogenic headache, who also exhibited concomitant TMJ impairments, if they received manual therapy treatment directed to both the cervical spine and TMJ compared to the cervical spine alone (von Piekartz & Ludtke, 2011; von Piekartz & Hall, 2013).

There is no research detailing the coexistence of TMD in individuals with thoracic spine impairments or of the effects of treating TMD in patients with thoracic spine pain, or vice versa. However, there are studies suggesting clinically relevant relationships between TMD and posture as well as a dynamic relationship between the TMJ, cervical and thoracic spine in terms of breathing dynamics (Corrêa & Bérzin, 2004). Additionally, a case series illustrates positive, clinical benefit in treating TMD patients with a multimodal approach including the use of thoracic spine manipulation (González-Iglesias et al., 2013).

Preliminary evidence suggests that there are short-term benefits to treating the thoracic spine in individuals with neck pain (Cross et al., 2011). As treating the thoracic spine has been found to be beneficial in patients with neck pain and a link exists between the cervical spine and the TMJ, it is clinically reasonable to consider treating the thoracic spine in patients with TMD. For example, patients with TMD and concomitant forward head posture exhibit altered postural and anatomical changes, and among these changes are a hypomobile upper thoracic spine as well as significantly altered muscle length-tension dynamics (Corrêa & Bérzin, 2004). It is conceivable that addressing treatment to the thoracic spine, while addressing other impairments, may directly or indirectly benefit TMJ mechanics and function. Therefore, clinical assessment of the cervical and thoracic spines is essential when managing patients with TMD. The suggested examination procedures will be outlined in detail below.

Clinical examination of the cervical and thoracic spine

Individuals with TMD present with a variety of symptoms, including jaw pain, headache, and neck pain. Therefore, as part of a comprehensive examination for a patient with a TMD, the examiner should perform a clinical examination of the cervicothoracic region. The examination will attempt to reveal if the cervicothoracic region is associated with referred jaw pain, or if there are cervicothoracic region impairments relevant to the patient's chief complaint. The clinical examination of the cervicothoracic spine is comprised of a medical screening form as part of initial intake forms, several self-report questionnaires pertaining to pain and function, a patient interview, and a physical examination. Information obtained from intake forms and self-reported measures can give the clinician a general impression of a patient's health status and levels of pain and disability, as well as identify concerning items warranting follow-up questioning. The patient interview provides the clinician with information about potential involvement of the cervical or thoracic spine, in addition to screening for the presence of red flags. The physical examination is used to test hypotheses formed during the patient interview concerning the influence of the cervical and thoracic spine on the patient's current presentation.

Patient screening and historical information

Red flag items, including cancer, infection, visceral or general internal referral, cervical instability, fracture, and cardiopulmonary diagnoses, should be pursued further at this stage to rule out further medical pathologies. Yellow flags, such as cognitive or biopsychosocial factors, should be screened as well to determine how these may impact the patient's current symptoms. See Chapter 7 for details of how to assess the clinical history of a patient with TMD.

While obtaining the history, patients should be queried with respect to their age, occupation, duration of the current episode, mechanism of onset (gradual, sudden, or trauma), location and description of the most bothersome symptoms, positional ordering of symptoms (which posture is best and worst with regard to symptoms), aggravating and relieving factors, number and location of previous episodes if applicable, pattern of episodes, and response to previous interventions received. In particular, patients should be asked about symptoms in the cervical and/or thoracic region and, if present, the clinician should attempt to establish the aggravating and easing factors to each symptom. To ascertain the degree of irritability present, the examiner should ask about the severity of each symptom, how much activity it takes to provoke the symptoms, and how long it takes for the symptoms to settle to baseline after cessation of the activity. The examiner should also explore the relationship between the patient's different areas of symptoms. For example, if a patient reports both jaw and neck pain, the examiner should ask the patient if these symptoms are present simultaneously, separately, or if one precedes the other. It is important to note that some individuals with TMD may present with diffuse patterns of symptoms that could be a result of a more complex pain syndrome associated with central sensitization. These subjects may also present with comorbid mental health disorders, functional pain syndromes such as fibromyalgia, or other related disorders such as irritable bowel syndrome. At the end of the interview, the clinician should have an idea of the degree of complexity of the patient's disorder based on consideration of the multiple associated factors and should begin to not only formulate diagnostic hypotheses but also have a direction for the physical examination and treatment interventions.

Postural observation

The patient's posture should be assessed in standing and sitting, with as much of the upper quarter exposed to ensure appropriate viewing of the cervical and thoracic spine. Posture should be viewed from behind, the side, and in front.

Viewed sagittally, Kendall et al. (1993) described ideal alignment as occurring when the external auditory meatus aligns with the acromion process.

Griegel-Morris et al. (1992) found that the ability to identify abnormal postures (such as forward head, rounding of the right and left shoulder, and degree of thoracic kyphosis) against a plumb line was shown to have intrarater reliability of κ: 0.825 and inter-rater reliability of κ: 0.611. They also reported that chi-square analysis did not reveal significant increases in pain in patients with postural abnormalities (Griegel-Morris et al., 1992). Similar findings have been shown in other studies regarding cervico-thoracic posture and pain (Refshauge et al., 1995). Therefore, faulty postures should be considered in combination with all relevant findings and when the findings seem to correspond to the patient's symptom. Techniques to assess this link include symptom modification procedures, whereby active or passive (tape) modifications to encourage more neutral positions are provided to determine their effect on symptoms (Lewis, 2009).

Posteriorly, the position of the lumbar spine and thoracic spine is observed for the presence of scoliosis. The heights of the shoulders may be compared, along with the muscle bulk of the shoulder girdle. Disuse or nerve injury may feature muscle wasting, excessive bulk of accessory breathing muscles, and antalgic positioning of the neck. Here, the scapula should be observed, noting side-to-side differences in protraction and retraction, depression and elevation, and medial and lateral rotation. Abnormal features may indicate underlying pathologies, such as posterior protrusion of the medial border of the scapula for the long thoracic nerve injury or serratus anterior muscle weakness.

While in front of the patient, lateral flexion or rotation of the cervical spine can be noted. Shoulder-height symmetry and preferred carrying of either upper extremity can be observed. Muscle wasting of the anterior neck and trunk can be viewed anteriorly. Signs of intrinsic hand muscle wasting can be noted here, which may indicate the need for ruling out cervical myelopathy with subsequent examination.

Neurologic screening

A neurologic screen is designed to identify possible involvement of upper motor neuron or lower motor neuron pathology. Upper motor neuron signs include hyperreflexia, sensory changes in a nondermatomal pattern, clonus, positive Hoffmann or Babinski responses, general myotomal weakness below the suspected level of compression, and clumsy gait. Lower motor neuron signs feature diminished or absent deep tendon reflexes (DTR), decreased sensation to light touch in a dermatomal pattern, and muscle weakness along a specific myotome.

Light-touch sensation can be performed using a pinprick (end of paperclip) or tissue paper over corresponding C5–T1 dermatomes on each limb. Each area on each limb is tested simultaneously. Patients are instructed to identify sensation as appearing the same or different over each dermatome. Results are recorded as reduced, normal, or increased compared to the contralateral side. Sensory loss may be evident over one dermatome segment, which would require subsequent investigation. However, because areas of skin innervated by adjacent roots overlap, severance of an entire root does not produce a band of complete sensory loss. Generalized sensory loss may indicate a red flag feature of myelopathic conditions or yellow flag features of psychosocial distress.

Myotomal testing for muscle groups of the upper extremities is performed via manual muscle testing. For operational definitions for manual muscle testing, readers are referred to the textbook by Kendall et al. (1993). We recommend a truncated system for increased reliability for the purposes of neurologic screening: absent or markedly reduced (grade 0 out of 5), reduced (grades 1–4 out of 5), and normal (grade 5 out of 5). Muscle weakness of a particular dermatome may indicate nerve root compression, whereas a general pattern of weakness may indicate a serious neck condition or psychosocial distress.

Deep tendon reflexes can be assessed for the biceps brachii (C5), brachioradialis (C6 primarily) and triceps brachii (C7) muscles. The clinician strikes the tendon proximal to its corresponding insertion in the cubital fossa, distal aspect of the radius, and olecranon for the biceps brachii, brachioradialis, and triceps brachii, respectively. DTRs are traditionally graded as hyperactive indicative of upper motor neuron dysfunction (4+), hyperactive but within normal variation (3+), normal (2+), present but diminished (1+), or absent (0). A truncated system similar to myotomal assessment can be used by recording results as normal, increased, or absent/reduced compared to the contralateral side.

The inter-rater reliability of neurologic testing has been studied in populations with cervical spine pain (Viikari-Juntura, 1987). Sensation testing using three-level judgment (normal, hyperesthesia, hypoesthesia) yielded kappa values between 0.41–0.62. Strength testing using three-level judgment (normal, reduced, markedly reduced) yielded kappa values between 0.40–0.64. Viikari-Juntura et al. (1989) also assessed the validity of neurologic signs including diminished muscle strength, abnormal sensation, diminished reflexes, and visible atrophy, for predicting signs of nerve root compression on myelography. A sensitivity of 83 per cent and a specificity of 70 per cent were found when a positive neurologic screen featured one neurologic sign. If two or more signs defined a positive neurologic screen, sensitivity was found to decrease to 62 per cent and specificity increased to 78 per cent.

For patients whose history may indicate cervical myelopathy, Hoffmann and Babinski reflex testing should be completed. The Babinski reflex is tested with the patient in supine. The clinician supports the patient's foot in neutral and applies stimulation to the plantar aspect of the foot (lateral to medial from heel to metatarsal) with the blunt end of a reflex hammer. A positive test is defined by great toe extension and fanning of the second through fifth toes.

The Hoffmann reflex is tested with the patient sitting or standing with the head in neutral. The clinician stabilizes the proximal interphalangeal joint and flicks the distal phalanx into a flexed position. A positive test is defined by flexion of the interphalangeal joint of the thumb, with or without flexion of the index finger proximal or distal interphalangeal joints. In a study to determine reliability and diagnostic accuracy of examination measures for myelopathy performed by Cook et al. (2009), the Babinski sign demonstrated the highest positive likelihood ratio (LR + 4.0; 95%CI 1.1–16.6) and post-test probability (73 per cent) for diagnosis, but yielded only a moderate negative likelihood ratio (LR − 0.7; 95%CI 0.6–0.9). The Babinski and Hoffmann reflexes, along with gait deviation, an inverted supinator sign, and age greater than 45 years, have been included as part of a clinical prediction rule for the diagnosis of cervical myelopathy (Cook et al., 2010).

Ligamentous instability testing

Patients presenting with signs suggestive of central cord compression and who report a history of trauma and/or whiplash, or comorbidities such as rheumatoid arthritis or ankylosing spondylitis require testing for upper cervical spine ligament integrity. Despite a lack of research on the validity and accuracy of instability testing, it is important to include cervical ligament testing along with neurologic screening to better establish a clinical profile that would warrant appropriate referral for confirmatory imaging studies.

The Sharp–Purser test assesses the integrity of the transverse portion of the cruciform ligament, and attempts to identify subluxation of the atlas (C1) on the axis (C2) (Sharp & Purser, 1961). With the patient in a seated position, the examiner places one hand over the patient's forehead while the opposite hand stabilizes the spinous process of C2. The neck is then brought into 20 to 30 degrees of flexion. The examiner then provides a posteriorly directed shearing force with the hand on the patient's forehead. The test is considered positive if a sliding motion of the head posteriorly occurs. This is often accompanied by a reduction in symptoms. As studied by Uitvlugt and Indenbaum (1988), the diagnostic accuracy of this test was found to have a sensitivity of 0.69 and a specificity of 0.96.

The alar ligament stress test assesses the ligaments responsible for stability of the atlanto-occipital complex. The test is performed with the patient in supine or seated. The examiner stabilizes the axis by placing the left thumb adjacent to the left aspect of the spinous process of the axis. The examiner then side-bends the patient's head to the right with his or her right hand. In a stable spine, the examiner should feel the spinous process of the axis immediately move into the left thumb. A lag in movement of the spinous process of C2 with passive movement of the head is considered a positive test. The reliability or diagnostic accuracy of this test has not been studied.

Screening for cervical arterial dysfunction

Cervical arterial dysfunction is a term that broadly refers to any pathology or disease affecting either the carotid or vertebral arteries. This may include atherosclerosis, congenital vessel abnormalities, or cervical arterial dissection. Cervical arterial dissection is a vascular wall condition that typically involves a tear along the artery's lining and the formation of an intimal flap, which allows blood to penetrate into the muscular portion of the vessel wall. Blood flow between layers may cause layer separation, thus narrowing or completely obstructing vessel diameter. Accumulated blood in the vessel wall develops into a thrombus, obstructing blood flow to the vertebral or internal carotid artery, and emboli may detach from the thrombus (Haneline & Rosner, 2007). During end-range cervical range of motion, stress is placed on arterial structures and may be the primary source of patient complaints.

When obtaining a subjective history as a minimum the screening for cervical arterial dysfunction should include neck trauma, dizziness and/or nausea, visual disturbances (nystagmus), headache, paresthesias, and questions regarding comorbidities and steroid use. Initial signs indicative of cervical arterial dysfunction are headache and/or neck pain that is reported to be of an unusual quality. Additional risk factors and clinical features have been studied in the literature to identify dissection subjects from controls (Thomas et al., 2011). Red flag features derived by Kerry (2011) suggest screening for the '5 **Ds** And 3 **Ns**': dizziness, drop attacks, diplopia, dysphagia, dysarthria, ataxia, nystagmus, numbness, and nausea. Patients presenting with these features are likely to have a cervical dissection that has progressed to an ischemic brain event and should be referred for emergency medical treatment.

Assessing for possible cervical arterial dysfunction is essential given similar symptom referral patterns consistent with TMD (Kerry, 2011). Patients with risk factors or symptoms suggestive of cervical arterial dysfunction should undergo a systems based examination that sequentially assesses the cardiovascular, neurologic, and musculoskeletal systems. Neurologic examinations should include an upper quarter neurologic and cranial nerve examination. For the cardiovascular system, clinicians should take vital signs, including a baseline blood pressure, and consider palpating the carotid and vertebral pulses for any symptom reproduction of abnormality. For the musculoskeletal system, the guiding assumption for testing is that clinicians do not challenge cervical spine range of motion greater than that encountered during the typical cervical examination and treatment. In the absence of signs or symptoms indicative of cervical arterial dysfunction during the history and neurologic screen, the clinician may proceed with examination procedures. For patients who are post-trauma, upper cervical ligamentous stability assessment, as described above, should be considered. If the patient is determined to be appropriate for additional examination techniques, range of motion may be assessed. During examination procedures, the clinician watches the patient's eyes, and notes the presence of nystagmus, dizziness, lightheadedness, blurred vision, impaired sensation to the face, or other potential symptoms. Cardinal planes of motion as described later in this text should be assessed first followed by combined motions as a means to place incrementally greater degrees of stress on the neck and vasculature. In the absence of sinister signs, combined motions are performed by positioning the patient in sitting and asking the patient to look over his or her shoulder. The test is then repeated to the opposite side. This test has been colloquially named the seated extension-rotation test. In the presence of signs or symptoms suggestive of cervical arterial dysfunction, the patient is referred to an appropriate healthcare provider. Readers are referred to Rushton et al. (2014) for further details on this topic.

Range of motion testing

Active range of motion is assessed to establish limitations in motion and the patient's willingness to move through said range, and to identify the cervical range of movement that provokes any symptoms. With the patient positioned in an upright sitting position, baseline symptoms are established and will serve as a reference before proceeding to testing. To quantify motion in preparation for testing, use of a fluid-filled or bubble inclinometer is a clinically friendly and reliable means for measuring range of motion (Hole et al., 2000).

For each of the following motions, the patient's symptoms are assessed and compared to his or her baseline. The motions are recorded to have no effect, to increase symptoms, to decrease symptoms, to peripheralize (movement causes pain or paresthesia to travel distally), or centralize (movement causes pain or paresthesia to travel from a distal position to a proximal position). A comparable sign, or asterisk sign, can be established by clarifying motions that reproduce the patient's symptoms and can be reassessed following intervention. For those with TMD, the patient should be queried as to whether cervicothoracic motions affect jaw pain.

The assessment of cervical and thoracic range of motion is performed primarily in a sitting position, but alternative positioning in quadruped has been offered for measuring thoracic rotation (Johnson et al., 2012). Active range of motion of the thoracic spine should be assessed in addition to cervical or TMJ pain because thoracic spine dysfunction may directly influence movement and symptoms.

Thoracic spine active range of motion is performed with the patient seated with both arms crossed in front of the chest. The patient bends into forward flexion, backwards into extension, side-bends bilaterally, and rotates bilaterally. The clinician monitors the possible change in symptom behavior during and after each movement. Manual or verbal cueing can be useful to emphasize that motion is created at the thoracic versus the lumbar spine and pelvis. Overpressures in all cardinal planes may be provided if active range of motion is painless and to appreciate end feels. Combined movements, meaning flexion or extension with combined right or left rotation and side-bending, may be utilized if cardinal plane motions do not elicit symptoms.

Thoracic range of motion may be quantified via a fluid-filled inclinometer. Moderate reliability for inclinometer use of forward bending and bilateral side-bending has been reported (Molina et al., 2000). The examiner locates and marks the T1 spinous process and places the inclinometer at the mark and zeroes it. The inclinometer is stabilized against the patient's trunk using the thumb and index finger, while the remaining fingers rest on the upper trunk. After range of motion in all cardinal planes is complete, the sequence is repeated with the inclinometer at T12. Thoracic rotation can be reliably

measured using an inclinometer (Johnson et al., 2012). As demonstrated in the study, the patient is positioned quadruped with the knees and elbows at 90 degrees, sitting back on the heels, with the cervical spine in neutral, and the hand on the side being measured placed on top of the cervical spine. With an inclinometer at T1–T2, the patient rotates as far as possible. The standard error of measure is 2 degrees for this position, and the minimal detectable change is 6 degrees. Normative values for thoracic range of motion have not been determined.

Cervical spine range of motion can be assessed in a similar manner as previously discussed for the thoracic spine. Movement is completed in cardinal planes, appreciating possible changes in symptoms from the baseline and providing overpressures if motion is full and pain free. Combined motion testing, such as quadrant testing (i.e., right quadrant via extension, right rotation, and right side-bending), can be utilized to elicit symptoms if not provoked in cardinal plane testing.

Measuring cervical spine range of motion using an inclinometer has also been shown to be a valid, reliable means for assessment (Hole et al., 2000). For cervical flexion and extension, the inclinometer is placed on the top of the patient's head aligned with the external auditory meatus and then zeroed. The patient is then asked to flex the head forward as much as possible toward the chest. The degree of movement and possible contact of the chin to the chest is recorded. The patient follows this with extension by extending the neck backward as far as possible. The degree of extension is also recorded. Changes in symptoms should be assessed at this time, if not already completed.

For cervical side-bending, the inclinometer is placed on the top of the patient's head in alignment with the external auditory meatus while in the frontal plane. The patient is then cued to laterally flex the head by bringing the ear to the shoulder, and degree measurement is obtained. This is then repeated for the opposite side. Examiners must be cognizant of concomitant rotation or flexion with assessing bilateral side-bending, and provide corrective cueing.

Cervical rotation can be assessed using a universal goniometer or inclinometer. Using a goniometer, the patient is seated with the head positioned forward. The fulcrum of the goniometer is placed over the top of the head, with the stationary arm aligned with the acromion process and the mobile arm aligned to bisect the patient's nose. The patient is then asked to perform rotation by looking over his or her shoulder. Testing is repeated to the opposite side. Using an inclinometer, the patient is positioned supine with the head in a neutral position and the inclinometer placed on the forehead and zeroed. The patient is instructed to roll the head into rotation, and motion is read at end range.

Segmental mobility testing of the cervical and thoracic spine

Segmental mobility testing is a useful tool for assessing restricted segmental motion and the provocation of symptoms during passive accessory intervertebral motion at each thoracic and cervical spinal segment. Mobility is typically categorized as normal, hypomobile, or hypermobile (Christensen et al., 2002; Cleland et al., 2006). In general, spinal segmental motion testing has shown poor-to-moderate kappa coefficients (Fjellner et al., 1999; Smedmark et al., 2000). Cleland et al. (2006) reported that thoracic segmental mobility testing using posterior to anterior (PA) spring testing has poor-to-fair inter-rater reliability for both pain and mobility in neck pain patients. In a study by Heiderscheit and Boissonnault (2008), reliability of segmental mobility testing of the thoracic spine in subjects without symptoms improved when considering agreement within and between raters to within +/– one thoracic vertebral level rather than one segment only. More research is required on this topic; however, one could conclude

that thoracic segmental mobility testing intrarater and inter-rater reliability is improved when assessment is based upon region (that is, upper T1–T4, middle T5–T8, and lower T9–T12) rather than one specific segment.

Despite poor-to-fair reliability of segmental mobility testing, models of examination allow the therapist to assess spinal regions and, when coupled with the history, form the basis of a movement-impairment-based diagnosis. Manually palpating tender areas and recreating pain can provide therapeutic reassurance to the patient and guide future interventions. Clinicians should avoid language that equates examination findings with spinal positional faults or malalignment as this may translate to fear–avoidance behaviors or pain catastrophizing. Given current literature, it is highly unlikely that positional faults can occur.

Atlanto-occipital segmental mobility is assessed with the patient in supine position (Figure 9.1A). The atlanto-occipital joint is responsible for upper cervical flexion and extension, allowing for a nodding motion to occur. With the occiput cradled in both hands, rotate the head approximately 30 degrees and apply an anterior glide coupled with extension and a posterior glide coupled with flexion to assess the amount and quality of motion (Figure 9.1B). The side of rotation indicates the side being tested. This is repeated on the contralateral side.

Atlantoaxial mobility is assessed with the patient in supine position. The atlantoaxial joint is primarily responsible for upper cervical rotation. To assess atlantoaxial mobility, the head is passively and maximally flexed (Figure 9.2A), followed by cervical rotation to one side (Figure 9.2B). This is repeated to the contralateral side as well. Ogince et al. (2007) coined an adaptation of this assessment as the craniocervical rotation test. This test was found to have a sensitivity of 90 per cent and a specificity of 91 per cent in differentiating individuals with cervicogenic headache involvement versus migraine with aura and

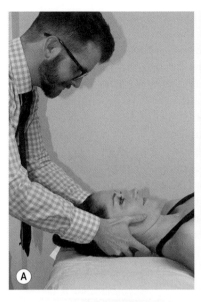

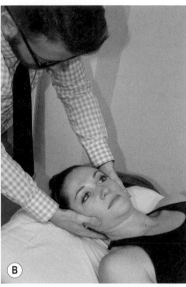

Figure 9.1
Atlanto-occipital segmental mobility assessment. The patient is in supine position while the examiner cradles the occiput as shown (A). The examiner rotates the head approximately 30 degrees and applies both an anterior glide coupled with extension and a posterior glide coupled with flexion to assess the amount and quality of motion (B).

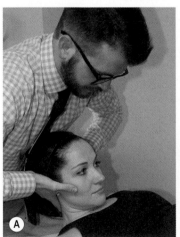

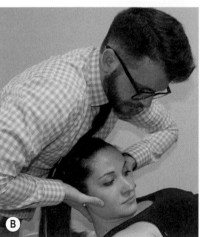

Figure 9.2
Atlantoaxial mobility assessment using the cervical flexion-rotation test. The examiner passively and maximally flexes the head of the patient (A), and then rotates the patient's head to one side (B). This is repeated for the contralateral side.

headache-free control. If craniocervical rotation was less than or equal to 32 degrees on the more restricted side, the test was considered positive. In clinical practice, range of motion is considered limited when the clinician determines a firm end feel and there is a minimum of a 10 degrees reduction from the expected range based on clinician judgment.

Segmental mobility of the lower cervical spine can be assessed in supine and using spring testing while in prone. To perform supine testing, the patient is positioned as such with the head in a neutral position. The clinician stands at the head of the table with his or her abdomen exerting a constant pressure at the top of the patient's head in order to stabilize the head, yet allow for head movement. Lateral glides are then performed from C2 to C7, assessing for available movement and symptom reproduction. Segments are determined to be hypomobile if movement in that direction is decreased compared to movement in the opposite direction and if movement in the opposite direction appears to be normal compared to other levels. Likewise, a segment can be determined to be hypermobile if it has more movement compared to other segments. A segment may also be judged to be hypermobile in a given direction if movement in that direction is increased compared to movement in the opposite direction and if movement in the opposite direction appears to be normal compared to other levels. Normal mobility is recorded as such if movement is comparable with the range of other segments. Bias into flexion and extension may also be performed.

Cervical segmental mobility may also be performed in prone via spring testing. Tissue irritability and tenderness can be assessed prior to spring testing via palpation of cervical paraspinals and adjacent musculature. With the patient prone and in a neutral cervical position, the clinician is positioned at the head of the table. Soft tissue of the posterior neck is drawn upward using the palm and digits 2–5, and the dorsal aspects of the thumbs are subsequently approximated and positioned over the articular process (Figure 9.3A) or the spinous process (Figure 9.3B) of the segment to be tested. With the elbows extended, the clinician applies a gentle, but firm, posterior-to-anterior (PA) force. This is completed from C1 to C7 segments. Mobility of each segment is determined as normal, hypomobile, or hypermobile based on the anticipation of what normal mobility would feel like and as compared to adjacent segments. Pain provocation, if present, is clarified as local or referred, and is determined as to whether this reproduces the patient's chief complaint. Kerr and Olafson (1961) demonstrated that afferents from the trigeminal nerve and the upper three cervical roots converge in the trigeminocervical nucleus in the upper cervical cord. This phenomenon may result in a reproduction of the patient's pain during upper cervical segmental mobility testing (C1–C3) that mimics symptoms of TMD. Jull et al. (1999) demonstrated a very high degree of agreement among clinicians in isolating the painful cervical segment in patients with chronic cervicogenic headaches.

Before thoracic segmental mobility is assessed, the clinician positions the patient in prone and assesses for tissue reactivity by palpating the thoracic medial gutter between the spinous processes and transverse

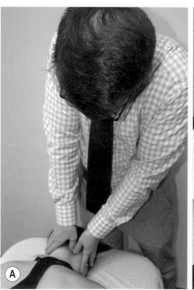
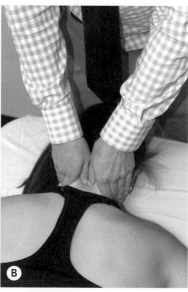

Figure 9.3
Cervical segmental mobility performed in prone using spring testing. Upper cervical segments, such as the atlanto-occipital joint (A), and lower cervical segments (B) may be assessed using this technique.

processes. With the hypothenar eminence positioned over the spinous process, the clinician performs spring testing via a posterior-to-anterior directed force to determine the presence or absence of pain and mobility. Mobility is categorized as normal, hypomobile, or hypermobile. This process can be completed unilaterally via spring testing over the transverse processes.

Deep neck flexor muscle performance

Several methods of determining deep neck flexor muscle performance have been proposed (Watson & Trott, 1993; Jull et al., 1999; Jull, 2000). Deep neck flexor strength testing has been described previously via manual resistance at the forehead while the patient simultaneously performs a chin tuck with cervical flexion (Vitti et al., 1973). However, more recent evidence supporting the deep neck flexors' role in providing postural stability motivated authors to find alternatives for endurance assessment (Silverman et al., 1991; Grimmer, 1994; Greenman, 1996; Blizzard et al., 2000). Jull et al. (1999) derived an additional testing procedure, called the craniocervical flexion test, which utilizes a progressively staged assessment of active craniocervical flexion using an air-filled stabilizer (Jull, 2000) (Figure 9.4). The techniques described above appear to have sufficient reliability (Grimmer 1994; Blizzard et al., 2000; Jull, 2000; Harris et al., 2005; Chiu et al., 2005). Deep neck flexor muscle performance testing has been shown to be diagnostic in identifying endurance deficits in patients with cervicogenic headache (Zito et al., 2006), but additional studies may be warranted regarding this relationship.

The preferred technique for assessing deep neck flexor endurance requires the patient to be positioned into a hook lying position (Figure 9.5A). The patient retracts the chin (Figure 9.5B) and lifts the head and neck until the head is approximately one inch above the table (Figure 9.5C). A line is drawn across one of the skin folds along the patient's neck and the therapist

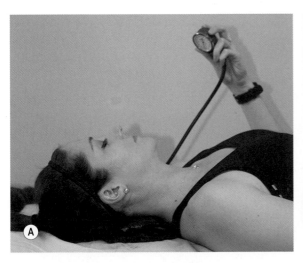
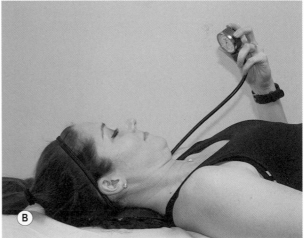

Figure 9.4

Deep neck flexor muscle performance testing using the craniocervical flexion test. Patients are positioned in supine with a pneumatic feedback device, such as a sphygmomanometer, located between the cervical spine and table (A). Active craniocervical flexion is performed in progressively staged increments (22, 24, 26, 28, and 30 mmHg), and held for 10 seconds at each stage (B).

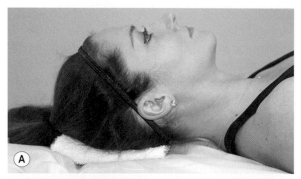

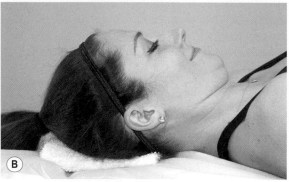

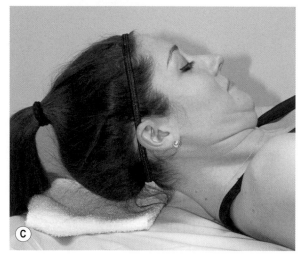

Figure 9.5
Deep neck flexor endurance testing. The patient is positioned in a hook lying position as shown (A). The patient retracts the chin (B) and lifts the head to approximately one inch above the table (C). After test completion, the time to fatigue is recorded.

supports under the occiput. When the line over the merged skin folds begin to separate or the patient's head touches the therapist's hand for more than one second, the test is complete. This technique may be preferred due to the ease of performance in a typical, busy clinical setting and because it does not require additional equipment. However, if a patient's symptom irritability threshold is considered to be low, the patient may find this test difficult to perform and it would then be of limited value.

References

Ballenberger N, von Piekartz H, Danzeisen M, Hall T. Patterns of cervical and masticatory impairment in subgroups of people with temporomandibular disorders-an explorative approach based on factor analysis. Cranio 2017; 20: 1–11. [Epub ahead of print]

Ballenberger N, von Piekartz H, Paris-Alemany A, La Touche R, Angulo-Diaz-Parreño S. Influence of different upper cervical positions on electromyography activity of the masticatory muscles. J Manipulative Physiol Ther 2012; 35: 308–318.

Blizzard L, Grimmer KA, Dwyer T. Validity of a measure of the frequency of headaches with overt neck involvement, and reliability of measurement of cervical spine anthropometric and muscle performance factors. Arch Phys Med Rehabil 2000; 1204–1210.

Bradnam L, Barry C. The role of the trigeminal sensory nuclear complex in the patho-physiology of craniocervical dystonia. J Neuroscience 2013; 33: 18358–18367.

Chiu TT, Law EYH, Chiu THS. Performance of the craniocervical flexion test in subjects with and without chronic neck pain. J Orthop Sports Phys Ther 2005; 35: 567–571.

Christensen H, Vach W, Vach K, et al. Palpation of the upper thoracic spine: an observer reliability study. J Manipulative Physiol Ther 2002; 25: 285–292.

Cleland JA, Childs JD, Fritz JM, Whitman JM. Interrater reliability of the history and physical examination in patients with mechanical neck pain. Arch Phys Med Rehabil 2006; 87: 1388–1395.

Cook C, Brown C, Isaacs R, et al. Clustered clinical findings for diagnosis of cervical spine myelopathy. J Man Manip Ther 2010; 18: 175–180.

Cook C, Roman M, Stewart KM, Leithe L, Isaacs R. Reliability and diagnostic accuracy of clinical special tests for myelopathy in patients seen for cervical dysfunction. J Orthop Sports Phys Ther 2009; 39: 172–178.

Corrêa ECR, Bérzin F. Temporomandibular disorder and dysfunctional breathing. Braz J Oral Science 2004; 10: 498–502.

Cross KM, Kuenze C, Grindstaff T, Hertel J. Thoracic spine thrust manipulation improves pain, range of motion, and self-reported function in patients with mechanical neck pain: a systematic review. J Orthop Sports Phys Ther 2011; 41: 633–642.

Fjellner A, Bexander C, Faleij R, Strender LE. Inter-examiner reliability in physical examination of the cervical spine. J Manipulative Physiol Ther 1999; 22: 511–516.

González-Iglesias J, Cleland JA, Neto F, Hall T, Fernández-de-las-Peñas C. Mobilization with movement, thoracic spine manipulation, and dry needling for the management of temporomandibular disorder: a prospective case series. Physiother Theory Pract 2013; 29: 586–595.

Greenman P. Principles of Manual Medicine. 2nd ed. Philadelphia, PA: Lippincott Williams & Wilkins; 1996.

Griegel-Morris P, Larson K, Mueller-Klaus K, Oatis CA. Incidence of common postural abnormalities in the cervical, shoulder, and thoracic regions and their association with pain in two age groups of healthy subjects. Phys Ther 1992; 72: 425–431.

Grimmer K. Measuring the endurance capacity of the cervical short flexor muscles group. Aust J Physiother 1994; 40: 251–254.

Grondin F, Hall T, von Piekartz H. Does altered mandibular position and dental occlusion influence upper cervical movement: a cross-sectional study in asymptomatic people. Musculoskelet Sci Pract 2017; 27:85–90.

Haneline MT, Rosner AL. The etiology of cervical artery dissection. J Chiroprac Med 2007; 6: 110–120.

Harris KD, Heer DM, Roy TC et al. Reliability of a measurement of neck flexor muscle endurance. Phys Ther 2005; 85: 1349–1355.

Heiderscheit B, Boissonnault W. Reliability of joint mobility and pain assessment of the thoracic spine and rib cage in asymptomatic individuals. J Man Manip Ther 2008; 16: 210–216.

Hole DE, Cook JM, Bolton JE. Reliability and concurrent validity of two instruments for measuring cervical range of motion: effects of age and gender. Man Ther 2000; 1: 36–42.

Johnson KD, Kim KM, Yu BK, Saliba SA, Grindstaff TL. Reliability of thoracic spine rotation range of motion measurements in healthy adults. J Athletic Train 2012: 47: 52–60.

Jull G. Deep cervical flexor muscle dysfunction in whiplash. J Musculoskeletal Pain 2000; 8: 143–154.

Jull G, Barrett C, Magee R, Ho P. Further clinical clarification of the muscle dysfunction in cervical headache. Cephalalgia 1999; 19: 179–185.

Kendall FP, McCreary EK, Provance PG. Muscles: Testing and Function. 4th ed. Baltimore: Williams & Wilkins, 1993.

Kerr FW, Olafson RA. Trigeminal and cervical volleys: convergence on single units in the spinal gray at C-1 and C-2. Arch Neurol 1961; 5: 171–178.

Kerry R. Examination of the upper cervical region In Petty NJ (ed.). Neuro-musculoskeletal examination and assessment: a handbook for therapists. 4th ed. Edinburgh: Churchill Livingstone, Elsevier; 2011.

La Touche R, París-Alemany A, von Piekartz H et al. The influence of cranio-cervical posture on maximal mouth opening and pressure pain threshold in patients with myofascial temporomandibular pain disorders. Clin J Pain 2011; 27: 48–55.

La Touche R, Paris-Alemany A, Mannheimer JS et al. Does mobilization of the upper cervical spine affect pain sensitivity and autonomic nervous system function in patients with cervico-craniofacial pain? A randomized-controlled trial. Clin J Pain 2013; 3: 205–215.

Lewis JS. Rotator cuff tendinopathy/sub-acromial impingement syndrome: is it time for a new method of assessment? Br J Sports Med 2009; 3: 21–24.

Molina C, Robbins D, Roberts H, et al. Reliability and validity of single inclinometer measurements for thoracic spine range of motion [abstract]. J Man Manip Ther 2000; 8: 143.

Ogince M, Hall T, Robinson K, Blackmore AM. The diagnostic validity of the cervical flexion-rotation test in C1/2-related cervicogenic headache. Man Ther 2007; 12: 256–262.

Olivo SA, Bravo J, Magee D et al. The association between head and cervical posture and temporomandibular disorders: a systematic review. J Orofacial pain 2006; 20: 9–23.

Refshauge K, Bolst L, Goodsell M. The relationship between cervico-thoracic posture and the presence of pain. J Man Manip Ther 1995; 3: 21–24.

Rushton A, Rivett D, Carlesso L, Flynn T, Hing W, Kerry R. International framework for examination of the cervical region for potential of cervical arterial dysfunction prior to orthopaedic manual therapy intervention. Man Ther 2014; 19: 222–228.

Sharp J, Purser DW. Spontaneous atlantoaxial dislocation in ankylosing spondylitis and rheumatoid arthritis. Annals Rheum Dis 1961; 20: 47–77.

Silverman JL, Rodriguez AA, Agre JC. Quantitative cervical flexor strength in healthy subjects and in subjects with mechanical neck pain. Arch Phys Med Rehabil 1991; 72: 679–681.

Smedmark V, Wallin M, Arvidsson I. Inter-examiner reliability in assessing passive inter-vertebral motion of the cervical spine. Man Ther 2000; 5: 97–101.

Thomas LC, Rivett DA, Attia JR, Parsons M, Levi C. Risk factors and clinical features of craniocervical arterial dissection. Man Ther 2011; 16: 351–356.

Uitvlugt G, Indenbaum S. Clinical assessment of atlantoaxial instability using the Sharp-Purser test. Arthr Rheum 1988; 31: 918–922.

Viikari-Juntura E. Inter-examiner reliability of observations in physical examinations of the neck. Phys Ther 1987; 67: 1526–1532.

Viikari-Juntura E, Porras M, Laasonen EM. Validity of clinical tests in the diagnosis of root compression in cervical disc disease. Spine 1989; 14: 253–257.

Vitti M, Fujiwara M, Basmanjian JM, Iida M. The integrated roles of longus colli and sternocleidomastoid muscles: an electromyographic study. Anat Rec 1973; 177: 471–484.

von Piekartz H, Hall T. Orofacial manual therapy improves cervical movement impairment associated with headache and features of temporomandibular dysfunction: a randomized controlled trial. Man Ther 2013; 4: 345–350.

von Piekartz H, Ludtke K. Effect of treatment of temporomandibular disorders (TMD) in patients with cervicogenic headache: a single-blind, randomized controlled study. Cranio 2011; 29: 43–56.

von Piekartz H, Pudelko A, Danzeisen M, Hall T, Ballenberger N. Do subjects with acute/subacute temporomandibular disorder have associated cervical impairments: a cross-sectional study. Man Ther 2016; 26: 208–215.

Walczyńska-Dragon K, Baron S, Nitecka-Buchta A, Tkacz E. Correlation between TMD and cervical spine pain and mobility: is the whole body balance TMJ related? BioMed Res Int 2014; 2014: 582414.

Watson DH, Trott PH. Cervical headache: an investigation of natural head posture and upper cervical flexor muscle performance. Cephalgia 1993; 13: 272–284.

Zito G, Jull G, Story I. Clinical tests of musculoskeletal dysfunction in the diagnosis of cervicogenic headache. Man Ther 2006; 11:118–129.

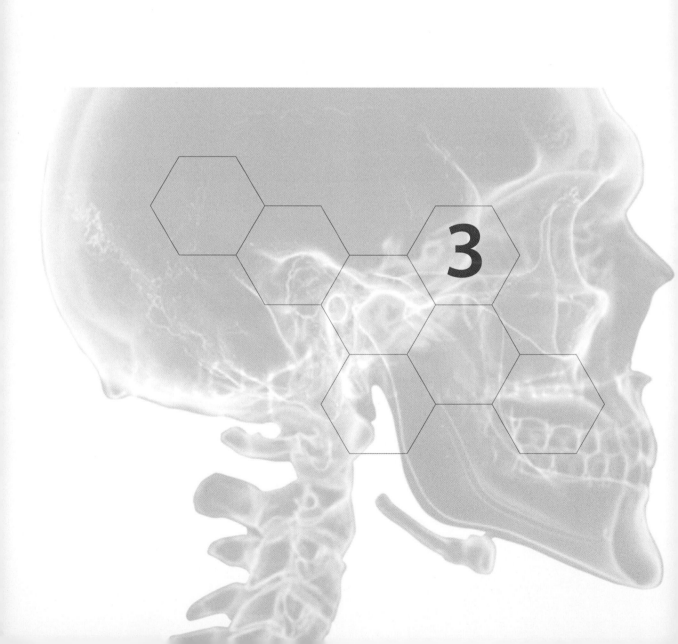

PART 3
Manual therapy for temporomandibular disorders

Chapter 10

Effectiveness of manual therapy and therapeutic exercises for temporomandibular disorders: an evidence-based approach

Susan Armijo-Olivo, Elisa Bizetti Pelai, Ambra Michelotti, Laurent Pitance,
Cristina Lozano-López, Blanca Codina García-Andrade

Introduction

The management of temporomandibular disorder (TMD) considers several types of treatments such as surgical and nonsurgical approaches (Coskun Benlidayi et al., 2016); however, the nonsurgical approach is usually the first step and is commonly preferred in managing TMD. Physical therapy interventions are one of the most common noninvasive approaches to manage TMD (Calixtre et al., 2016; Rai et al., 2016) and include many potentially effective interventions such as electrophysical agents, for example ultrasound (Rai et al., 2016), laser (Demirkol et al., 2017), and transcutaneous electrical nerve stimulation (TENS) (Awan & Patil, 2015). In addition, other physical therapy interventions such as manual therapy (Armijo-Olivo et al., 2016) and therapeutic exercises (Rocabado, 1987) are increasingly being used to manage this condition due to their favorable effects (von Piekartz & Hall, 2013; Tuncer et al., 2013b; Calixtre et al., 2016).

Manual therapy constitutes a wide variety of different techniques, which may be categorized into three major groups: manipulation, mobilization, and soft tissue (muscle energy) techniques (Clar et al., 2014). Manual therapy has been used for several years in many musculoskeletal pain conditions due to its positive effects. Specifically, for TMD, manual therapy claims to improve function by restoring the quantity and the quality of mandibular movements and reducing pain used alone or as an adjunct treatment, along with exercises, physical modalities, and splint therapy. Recent evidence suggests that manual therapy is a legitimate treatment for TMD and indeed research to date suggests that a mixed therapy involving manual therapy techniques as well as exercises improves patient's outcomes (Miller et al., 2010). Research suggests that manual therapy for TMD targeted to the orofacial region as well as to the cervical spine could be beneficial. A combination of manual therapy for the orofacial region plus therapy of the cervical spine was more effective than home exercises or treatment to the cervical spine alone in subjects with mixed TMD (Armijo-Olivo et al., 2016). Moreover, mobilization of the cervical spine was shown to decrease pain intensity and pain sensitivity (via pressure pain threshold evaluation) and to increase mandibular movements in subjects with myogenous TMD (Armijo-Olivo et al., 2016). Also, manual therapy techniques such as mobilization of the cervical spine could have an influence on orofacial pain as well as movement in the jaw through the connections of these systems in the trigeminocervical nucleus caudalis (Sessle, 1999).

Exercise therapy has been considered a cornerstone for the rehabilitation of musculoskeletal dysfunction and therapeutic exercises have been widely used in the rehabilitation and prevention of TMD, with the aim of alleviating pain and improving function (Machado et al., 2016). In general, therapeutic exercise is the prescription of muscular contraction and bodily movement to improve the overall function of the individual and to help meet the demands of daily living (Hertling & Kessler, 2006). Exercise treatment aims to restore normal function by altering sensory input, reducing potential inflammation, improving coordination and strengthening of muscles, and promoting the repair and regeneration of tissues (Taylor et al., 2007). Exercise therapy is extensively utilized for TMD, although the potential mechanisms of action are not fully understood. Therapeutic exercise interventions are prescribed to improve craniomandibular function and improve muscular coordination, relax tense muscles, increase range of motion, and increase muscular strength (Carlsson & Magnusson, 1999). Useful techniques include muscle-strengthening exercises, active joint exercises to increase oral opening and decrease pain, postural exercises, and cervical motor control exercises to optimize the functioning of the craniomandibular system (Rocabado, 1987; Armijo-Olivo & Gadotti, 2016).

Although the evidence supporting the use of manual therapy and therapeutic exercise for TMD has been historically limited, in the last few years, several systematic reviews in the area have been published. All of the systematic reviews published (McNeely et al., 2006; Medlicott & Harris, 2006; Armijo-Olivo et al., 2016) provide further evidence in support of postural exercises, and active and passive oral exercises in reducing pain and improving mouth opening in people with TMD due to disc displacement, acute arthritis, and chronic myofascial pain. In addition, evidence based on recent systematic reviews (Armijo-Olivo et al., 2016; Calixtre et al., 2016) shows that manual therapy has promising results to treat myogenous, arthrogenous, and mixed TMD, although current evidence is still limited and of low quality. After the publication of these systematic reviews, research in the area of TMD has quickly expanded and thus new randomized control trials (RCTs) investigating the effectiveness of exercises and manual therapy have been conducted. These recent studies provide new evidence in this field and their results need to be merged with the results of previous studies. Therefore, this chapter will provide an updated overview of the evidence of manual therapy and therapeutic exercise for TMD-related pain.

This chapter will focus on evidence from RCTs obtained through extensive searches of electronic databases (MEDLINE, EMBASE, Cochrane Library, ISI Web of Science, EBM reviews, and CINAHL) up to February 2017 and in consultation with experts in the field. The information gathered for this chapter was restricted to RCTs with participants meeting the following criteria:

1. diagnosis of TMD according to the research diagnostic criteria for temporomandibular disorders (RDC/TMD) (Dworkin & LeResche, 1992) or any clinical diagnosis involving signs and symptoms of TMD, (Kraus, 2007; Leeuw & Klasser, 2013);

2. adult (> 18 years of age);

3. musculoskeletal dysfunction;

4. pain impairment;

5. no previous surgery in the temporomandibular joint (TMJ) region; and,

6. no other serious comorbid conditions (for example fracture, cancer, neurological disease).

Included studies for this chapter had to compare any type of manual therapy intervention (for example, mobilization, manipulation, soft tissue mobilization) or exercise therapy alone or in combination with other therapies. Comparisons of interest were a placebo intervention, a controlled comparison intervention, or standard care (treatment that normally is offered). If the effect of any of the therapies of interest could not be determined, studies were not included.

The main outcomes of interest for this compilation of the evidence were pain, range of motion, and oral function. Oral function for this chapter focused on limitations of daily activities of TMD patients measured through different questionnaires. Pressure pain thresholds (PPTs) as well as electromyographic activity of masticatory or cervical muscles were also investigated (Armijo-Olivo et al., 2016).

It is important to highlight that we attempted to pool the results of these studies in a quantitative way where possible through a meta-analysis of the results. The studies were pooled based on TMD diagnosis (myogenous, arthrogenous or mixed), potential intervention (manual therapy and exercise), and outcome. Thus, groups of studies that were similar in terms of these characteristics were created and pooled. In the presence of clinical heterogeneity in the study population or intervention, the DerSimonian and Laird random effects model of pooling was used based on the assumption of the presence of interstudy variability to provide a more conservative estimate of the true effect (Bérard & Bravo, 1998).

For analysis of continuous outcome data, the mean difference (MD) and standardized mean difference (SMD) with 95 per cent confidence intervals to pool data were used. Heterogeneity was evaluated statistically using the I^2 statistic (Higgins & Green, 2011).

Cohen criteria (0.2, 0.5, and 0.8 as small, moderate and large effect size respectively) were used to interpret values of SMD found for our pooled estimates (Cohen, 1988). Revman 5.3 Software (RevMan 5 – Cochrane Community) was used to summarize the effects (pooled mean differences) and construct the forest plots for all comparisons. To interpret values of nonstandardized effect sizes such as mean differences, we used the clinical significance of the outcome of interest to establish the potential effectiveness of these outcomes. The following criteria were applied: the minimal clinically important difference (MCID) for pain has been reported to range from 1.5 to 3.2 points (Farrar et al., 2001; van der Roer et al., 2006; Kovacs et al., 2007; Dworkin et al., 2008; Maughan and Lewis, 2010) thus study results reporting higher values of differences between groups than these minimal values, were considered clinically relevant. The smallest detectable difference of maximal mouth opening in healthy subjects has been reported to be 5 mm, indicating that an important change of at least 5 mm can be considered clinically relevant (Kropmans et al., 1999). PPT measurements have been shown to have good or excellent inter-rater and intrarater reliability (Nussbaum & Downes, 1998; Ylinen et al., 2005; Cathcart & Pritchard, 2006). The minimal important difference (MID) for PPTs has been reported to be $\geq 1.10\,Kg/cm^2$ (Chesterton et al., 2003; Fuentes et al., 2011). Therefore, difference scores higher than this score on PPT between groups were considered clinically relevant.

Chapter 15 of this textbook describes in more detail specific exercises used to treat patients with TMDs whereas Chapter 11 describes more specifically manual therapy techniques used in these conditions.

General description of included studies

This chapter compiled data from 58 unique studies reported in 63 articles.

Diagnosis

Nineteen (n=19) unique studies examined the effectiveness of the exercise and/or manual therapy interventions in myogenous TMD (Crockett et al., 1986; Magnusson & Syrén, 1999; Komiyama et al., 1999; Wright et al., 2000; Michelotti et al., 2004; Gavish et al., 2006; Mulet et al., 2007; Kalamir et al., 2010; Craane et al., 2012a; Guarda-Nardini et al., 2012; Kalamir et al., 2012, 2013; La Touche et al., 2013; Tuncer et al., 2013a; Tuncer et al., 2013b; Gomes et al., 2014b; Kraaijenga et al., 2014; Rodriguez-Blanco et al., 2015; Espejo-Antúnez et al., 2016) 17 studies (18 articles) in patients with arthrogenous TMD (Alajbeg et al., 2015; Bae & Park, 2013; Carmeli et al., 2001; Craane et al., 2012b; Diraçoğlu et al., 2009; de Felício et al., 2008; Haketa et al., 2010; Ismail et al., 2007; Machado et al., 2016; Minakuchi et al., 2001; Nascimento et al., 2013; Schiffman et al., 2007; Stegenga et al., 1993; Yoda et al., 2003; Yoshida et al., 2005, 2011; Yuasa et al., 2001) and 22 studies (26 articles) in individuals with mixed diagnoses of TMD (including both myogenous and arthrogenous TMD) (Burgess et al., 1988; Cuccia et al., 2010; de Felício et al., 2010; Ficnar et al., 2013; Gomes et al., 2014b; Grace et al., 2002; Klobas et al., 2006; Maluf et al., 2009; Mansilla Ferragud & Boscá Gandia, 2008; Niemelä et al., 2012; Otaño & Legal, 2010; Packer et al., 2014, 2015; von Piekartz & Lüdtke, 2011; Raustia & Pohjola, 1986; Tavera et al., 2012; Tegelberg & Kopp, 1988, 1996; Truelove et al., 2006). One study looked at both myogenous and arthrogenous TMD (Maloney et al., 2002).

Twenty-eight studies (Alajbeg et al., 2015; Craane et al., 2012a, 2012b; Espejo-Antúnez et al., 2016; de Felício et al., 2008, 2010; Ficnar et al., 2013; Gavish et al., 2006; Ismail et al., 2007; Kalamir et al., 2010, 2013; Komiyama et al., 1999; La Touche et al., 2013; Machado et al., 2016; Maloney et al., 2002; Michelotti et al., 2004; Mulet et al., 2007; Nascimento et al., 2013; Niemelä et al., 2012; Packer et al., 2014, 2015; Rodriguez-Blanco et al., 2015; Truelove et al., 2006; Tuncer et al., 2013a; Tuncer et al., 2013b; Wright et al., 2000) used the RDC/TMD (Dworkin & LeResche, 1992) to make the diagnosis. The remaining studies used clinical criteria of limited range of motion and crepitus of the TMJ (Bae & Park, 2013); magnetic resonance imaging (MRI) to diagnose disc displacement (Schiffman et al., 2007); the Fonseca Patient History Index (Gomes et al., 2014b); or a general clinical diagnosis of TMD performed by a dentist or a specialist in oral and maxillofacial surgery (Gesslbauer et al., 2016).

Methodological quality assessment

Although we compiled a large amount of RCTs for this chapter, the quality of these studies reviewed is either poor or unclear. Risk of bias assessments using the risk of bias tool determined that only two studies (Gomes et al., 2014a; Rodriguez-Blanco et al., 2015) were considered low risk of bias, 53% (n=30) was considered unclear, and 44% (n=25) of them, high risk of bias.

Effectiveness of manual therapy and exercise in muscle-related pain (myogenous) temporomandibular disorder

Posture correction exercises

The effectiveness of posture correction exercises for patients with myogenous TMD was evaluated and had positive results in two studies (Komiyama et al., 1999; Wright et al., 2000). The maximum pain-free opening significantly increased in patients receiving postural training (5.54 mm, 95% CI 2.93, 8.15) (Kropmans et al., 1999) when compared with a control group. The same results were obtained for symptoms and disturbance of symptoms with daily life; the between-groups difference was SMD: 1.13 (95% CI 0.48, 1.78), indicating a large effect size, clinically significant for this outcome.

General jaw exercises alone or combined with a neck exercise program

General jaw exercises alone or combined with a neck exercise program in myogenous TMD were used in eight articles (Craane et al., 2012b; Crockett et al., 1986; Gavish et al., 2006; Kraaijenga et al., 2014; Magnusson & Syrén, 1999; Maloney et al., 2002; Michelotti et al., 2004; Mulet et al., 2007). In general, the results of these studies were inconsistent. Three articles found positive results when comparing jaw exercises with a control group in outcomes such as pain and range of motion (Gavish et al., 2006; Maloney et al., 2002; Michelotti et al., 2004); however, the remaining five articles (Craane et al., 2012b; Crockett et al., 1986; Magnusson & Syrén, 1999; Mulet et al., 2007) did not find such significant differences between groups.

The studies with similar outcomes, diagnosis, and comparing an exercise program with another type of therapy such as education (Craane et al., 2012b; Michelotti et al., 2004) or splint therapy (Magnusson & Syrén, 1999; Maloney et al., 2002) were pooled. The results from this analysis showed that there was a trend to favor exercise therapy on pain-free maximum opening and pain intensity when compared with a control group. For pain-free maximum opening, the pooled MD was 5.94 mm (95% CI −1.0, 12.87), which is considered clinically relevant favoring the exercise group (Kropmans et al., 1999). For pain intensity including data from five studies (Craane et al., 2012a; Gavish et al., 2006; Maloney et al., 2002; Michelotti et al., 2004; Mulet et al., 2007), the pooled SMD was 0.43 (95% CI −0.02, 0.87) with a moderate effect size according to Cohen guidelines (Cohen, 1988). A nonsignificant effect was found on pain-free maximum opening (1.92 mm, 95% CI −0.57, 4.41) when performing sensitivity analysis in exercise therapy versus education (Craane et al., 2012a; Michelotti et al., 2004); however, when comparing exercises versus splint therapy (Magnusson & Syrén, 1999; Maloney et al., 2002) a statistically and clinically meaningful difference was found between the groups (12.31 mm, 95% CI 7.73, 16.89) favoring jaw exercises.

Manual therapy for the orofacial region

Four RCTs looking at manual therapy targeted to the orofacial region in myogenous TMD (Kalamir et al., 2010; Guarda-Nardini et al., 2012; Kalamir et al., 2012, 2013) were found. Improvement in mouth opening and reduction in jaw pain were found in these trials when compared to a control group. Facial manipulation had similar effects to a botulinum toxin injection, although botulinum toxin injections were slightly superior in increasing range of motion at three months after treatment when compared with facial manipulation, but facial manipulation was better for reducing pain intensity. Positive results favoring manual therapy targeted to the orofacial region in myogenous TMD versus control groups were obtained on pain intensity (1.31 cm, 95% CI 0.86, 1.76). Three similar articles (Kalamir et al., 2010; Guarda-Nardini et al., 2012; Kalamir et al., 2013) with similar diagnosis, outcomes and interventions, were hence pooled and showed that manual therapy improved pain intensity (pooled MD: 1.35 cm, 95% CI 0.91, 1.78) at four to six weeks of treatment compared with a waiting list (control group) or botulinum toxin, approaching a clinically relevant value.

Manual therapy for the cervical spine

Two RCTs used manual therapy mobilization of the cervical spine in subjects with myogenous TMD (La Touche et al., 2013; Bortolazzo et al., 2015). Mobilizations targeted to the cervical spine had good results in decreasing pain intensity (visual analog scale – VAS) and pain sensitivity (PPT) in subjects with myogenous TMD when compared with a placebo treatment. The results obtained by La Touche et al. (2013) were considered clinically relevant, with an effect size for pain intensity of 28.75 points (95% CI 21.65, 35.85) and 1.12 Kg/cm^2 (95% CI 0.96, 1.29) for pain and PPT, respectively.

The other study used upper cervical manipulation compared to a placebo group in subjects with myogenous TMD (Bortolazzo et al., 2015) and found good results as well. The upper cervical manipulation results in a normalized muscular performance (surface electromyographic analysis) of the masticatory musculature and an increase in mouth opening in women with myogenic TMD. There was a between-groups difference in mouth opening of 8.20 mm (95% CI 1.56, 14.84) favoring cervical mobilizations, which is considered clinically relevant (Cohen, 1988).

Massage therapy

One study investigated the effectiveness of massage therapy alone versus splint, or massage therapy when combined with splint versus splint alone or manual therapy alone in subjects with myogenous TMD on masticatory EMG activity (Gomes et al., 2014a). The results showed that the massage therapy and occlusal splint alone did not change significantly the electromyographic activity of masseter or anterior temporal muscles. However, the combination of manual therapy plus splint therapy led to a reduction in the intensity of signs and symptoms in patients with severe TMD and sleep bruxism.

Stretching techniques targeted to the hamstring muscles

Two studies looked at stretching techniques targeted to the hamstring muscles and manual therapy techniques for masticatory and cervical muscles in myogenous TMD (Rodriguez-Blanco et al., 2015; Espejo-Antúnez et al., 2016). One study used the stretching of the hamstring muscle technique alone compared with stretching of the hamstring muscle technique plus an ischemic compression on the masseter (Espejo-Antúnez et al., 2016) and found that stretching of the hamstrings induced an improvement of all outcomes: hamstring extensibility, active mouth opening, and jaw pain. However, the addition of ischemic compression to the masseter muscle did not induce further improvements on the assessed parameters (Espejo-Antúnez et al., 2016). The reported between-groups effect sizes were small. Authors reported SMD of 0.04 for range of motion, pain (VAS) of 0.18 on the right side and 0.11 on the left side, and pain sensitivity (PPT) of 0.23 on the right side and 0.06 on the left side (Espejo-Antúnez et al., 2016).

The other study reported the effects of the neuromuscular technique over the masseter muscles, passive stretching of the hamstring musculature, and a suboccipital muscle inhibition technique when compared with neuromuscular technique over the masseter muscles, and passive stretching of the hamstring muscles (Rodriguez-Blanco et al., 2015). This study did not find differences between groups for range of motion and pain sensitivity (PPT). The authors concluded that the inclusion of a local technique at the suboccipital level did not have any impact on improving jaw mobility and orofacial sensitivity to mechanical pressure in these patients.

Effectiveness of manual therapy and exercise in arthrogenous temporomandibular disorder

Jaw and neck exercises alone

Nine studies (Bae & Park, 2013; Craane et al., 2012a; Diraçoğlu et al., 2009; de Felício et al., 2008; Maloney et al., 2002; Stegenga et al., 1993; Yoda et al., 2003; Yoshida et al., 2011; Yuasa et al., 2001) used jaw and neck exercises alone or as part of a general therapeutic regimen (medication, surgery [arthrocentesis or arthroscopy], or self-care recommendations) in subjects with arthrogenous TMD. Four studies focused on exercise therapy alone (mouth opening, lateral and anterior movement exercises, mandibular condylar exercises in different directions or exercises for recapturing the disc) comparing it to a true control group (no intervention) (Bae & Park, 2013; Yoda et al., 2003; Yoshida et al., 2011; Yuasa et al., 2001). They reported that this treatment is simple with lower costs and provides good results for patients with arthrogenous TMD in outcomes such as mouth opening, lateral movements, and pain. One study focused on exercise therapy combined with conventional treatment (education in oral habits and instructions on how to relax masticatory muscles) (Craane et al., 2012a), another study combined jaw exercises with a TheraBite® device (to increase mouth opening) (Maloney et al., 2002), and another study focused on jaw exercises with myofunctional therapy (de Felício et al., 2008). Exercise was compared with education (Craane et al., 2012a), splint therapy (Maloney et al., 2002), and waiting list (de Felício et al., 2008) respectively.

Two studies compared general exercises as part of a conventional treatment with surgery (arthrocentesis or arthroscopy) in subjects with arthrogenous TMD (Diraçoğlu et al., 2009; Stegenga et al., 1993). One of them used the arthroscopy surgery combined with conservative treatment including exercises for the jaw (Stegenga et al., 1993) comparing with the conservative treatment alone, and the other study compared the arthrocentesis surgery alone with a conventional treatment including jaw exercises (Diraçoğlu et al., 2009).

Five of these nine studies showed good results on pain intensity, range of motion, or click disappearance when analyzing the use of exercises alone or as part of a general regimen to treat subjects with arthrogenous TMD (disc displacements with or without reduction) (de Felício et al., 2008; Maloney et al., 2002; Yoda et al., 2003; Yoshida et al., 2011; Yuasa et al., 2001); however, one study found that general jaw exercises were not superior to a control group involving education (Craane et al., 2012a). In this study, the authors reported that independent of the treatment provided, all participants improved over time, which indicates that the there was no specific effect of the therapy in arthrogenous TMD, specifically in 'closed lock' patients.

The data from all the studies with similar outcomes, diagnosis, and comparing an exercise program with other forms of therapy – education (Craane et al., 2012a), splint therapy (Maloney et al., 2002), and a real control group (Bae & Park, 2013; de Felício et al., 2008; Yoshida et al., 2011; Yuasa et al., 2001) – were pooled. The meta-analysis of the studies, looking at the effectiveness of exercise alone or in combination with other conservative therapies, on pain intensity (Bae & Park, 2013; Craane et al., 2012a; de Felício et al., 2008; Maloney et al., 2002; Yuasa et al., 2001) demonstrated a statistical significance between-group difference on pain intensity favoring jaw exercises alone (Bae & Park, 2013; Yuasa et al., 2001) or combined with other therapies such as TheraBite® (Maloney et al., 2002), myofunctional therapy

(de Felício et al., 2008), or a general program approach (Craane et al., 2012a). The between-groups pooled SMD (Figure 10.1, top table) for pain intensity was −0.81 (95% CI −1.50, −0.11), which is considered a large effect size according to Cohen's guidelines (Cohen, 1988).

When the data of the studies including only a true control group as a comparison group (Bae & Park, 2013; de Felício et al., 2008; Yuasa et al., 2001) were pooled for pain intensity, similar results were found, although the SMD increased to −1.24 (95% CI −2.32, −0.16) favoring the exercise group (Figure 10.1, bottom table).

Related to mouth opening, pooling data from all of the studies including jaw exercises alone or combined with other therapies compared with different comparison groups (education, splint, true control groups) (Bae & Park, 2013; Craane et al., 2012a; Maloney

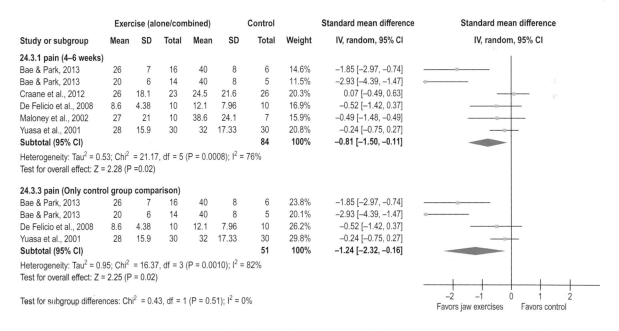

Figure 10.1

Meta-analysis pooled data of jaw exercises alone or combined with other therapies compared with other therapies (education, splint, true control groups) on pain intensity in patients with arthrogenous TMD.

et al., 2002; Yoshida et al., 2011; Yuasa et al., 2001) showed a significant mean between-group difference of 0.47 cm (95% CI 0.26, 0.68) on mouth opening favoring jaw exercises alone or combined with other therapies (Figure 10.2, top table). This difference is approaching the minimal clinically relevant cutoff of 0.5 cm indicated in the literature (Kropmans et al, 1999). Similar results were obtained when including only studies using a true control group (Figure 10.2, bottom table).

Data from the studies that used exercises plus arthrocentesis or arthroscopy versus conservative therapy (exercises alone on vertical active mouth opening at six months) were also pooled (Stegenga et al., 1993; Yoda et al., 2003). No differences between treatments were found. The pooled MD was −1.01 mm (95% CI −5.43, 3.42) implying that conservative treatment plus exercises is appropriate to treat disc displacement without reduction or when

subjects have restricted mandibular movement. In addition, these results highlight the importance of using conservative treatments as a first line of treatment in people with arthrogenous TMD.

Manual therapy plus jaw exercises

Ten articles (corresponding to eight unique studies) used manual therapy plus jaw exercises in subjects with arthrogenous TMD (Minakuchi et al., 2001; Alajbeg et al., 2015; Carmeli et al., 2001; Haketa et al., 2010; Ismail et al., 2007; Minakuchi et al., 2004; Nascimento et al., 2013; Schiffman et al., 2007; Yoshida et al., 2005). Four studies compared manual therapy and exercises for the jaw versus splint therapy and found that manual therapy plus exercises have a beneficial effect for these patients (Alajbeg et al., 2015; Carmeli et al., 2001; Haketa et al., 2010; Ismail et al., 2007). Another study (that was reported

Study or subgroup	Exercise (alone/combined) Mean	SD	Total	Control Mean	SD	Total	Weight	Mean difference IV, random, 95% CI
24.2.1 maximal active mouth opening (cm) (4–6 weeks) (all)								
Bae & Park, 2013	4.07	0.64	16	3.81	0.42	5	21.3%	0.26 [−0.20, 0.72]
Bae & Park, 2013	4.33	1.19	14	3.81	0.42	5	8.6%	0.52 [−0.20, 1.24]
Craane et al., 2012	1.6	6.56	23	3.4	6.95	26	0.3%	−1.80 [−5.58, 1.98]
Maloney et al., 2002	3.54	0.39	10	2.99	0.65	7	15.5%	0.55 [0.01, 1.09]
Yoshida et al., 2011	3.8	1.7	74	3	1.4	74	17.9%	0.80 [0.30, 1.30]
Yuasa et al., 2001	3.75	0.71	30	3.35	0.68	30	36.4%	0.40 [0.05, 0.75]
Subtotal (95% CI)			**167**			**148**	**100%**	**0.47 [0.26, 0.68]**

Heterogeneity: Tau^2 = 0.00; Chi^2 = 4.10, df = 5 (P = 0.54); I^2 = 0%
Test for overall effect: Z = 4.33 (P = 0.0001)

Study or subgroup	Mean	SD	Total	Mean	SD	Total	Weight	Mean difference IV, random, 95% CI
24.2.2 maximal active mouth opening (cm) (4–6 weeks) (only control group comparison)								
Bae & Park, 2013	4.07	0.64	16	3.81	0.42	6	25.3%	0.26 [−0.20, 0.72]
Bae & Park, 2013	4.33	1.19	14	3.81	0.42	5	10.2%	0.52 [−0.20, 1.24]
Yoshida et al., 2011	3.8	1.7	74	3	1.4	74	21.2%	0.80 [0.30, 1.30]
Yuasa et al., 2001	3.75	0.71	30	3.35	0.68	30	43.2%	0.40 [0.05, 0.75]
Subtotal (95% CI)			**134**			**115**	**100%**	**0.46 [0.23, 0.69]**

Heterogeneity: Tau^2 = 0.00; Chi^2 = 2.63, df = 3 (P = 0.450); I^2 = 0%
Test for overall effect: Z = 3.91 (P = < 0.0001)

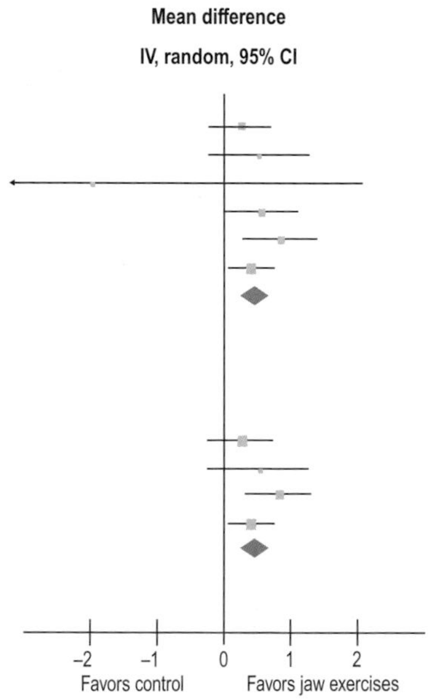

Figure 10.2

Meta-analysis pooled data of jaw exercises alone or combined with other therapies compared with other therapies (education, splint, true control groups) on mouth opening in patients with arthrogenous TMD.

in two different articles) (Minakuchi et al., 2001; 2004) compared manual therapy plus exercises with self-care and advice regarding prognosis, and three articles (two studies) compared manual therapy and exercises with nonsteroidal anti-inflammatory drugs (NSAIDs), muscle relaxants, and over-the-counter analgesics (Schiffman et al., 2007; Yoshida et al., 2005). Nascimento et al. (2013) looked at the difference between anesthetic blockage of the auriculotemporal nerve versus manual therapy and exercises plus blockage of the auriculotemporal nerve and reported that the anesthetic blockage of the auriculotemporal nerve and physical therapy were effective in the reduction of pain in subjects with arthrogenous TMD. The results showed in general that manual therapy plus jaw exercises reduced the symptoms and increased the range of motion in subjects with arthrogenous TMD, particularly for those with disc displacements without reduction ('closed lock').

Therefore, data from studies with similar interventions outcomes and diagnoses were pooled (Alajbeg et al., 2015; Carmeli et al., 2001; Haketa et al., 2010; Ismail et al., 2007; Minakuchi et al., 2001; Schiffman et al., 2007). The results showed that pain intensity was significantly reduced in subjects receiving manual therapy combined with exercises when compared with splint therapy, self-care, or medications. The pooled SMD for pain intensity at four weeks to three months was 0.44 (95% CI 0.17, 0.71) with a moderate effect size according to Cohen's guidelines (Cohen, 1988) (Figure 10.3).

Additionally, the pooled effect of the studies looking at mouth opening (Alajbeg et al., 2015; Carmeli et al., 2001; Haketa et al., 2010; Ismail et al., 2007; Minakuchi et al., 2001) found that manual therapy plus exercise significantly increased mouth opening when compared with splint therapy, self-care, or medications. The pooled MD for mouth opening at four weeks to three months was 3.60mm (95% CI 1.53, 5.66) indicating a potential clinically significant finding (Figure 10.4).

Effectiveness of manual therapy and exercise in mixed temporomandibular disorder

General jaw exercises

Twelve studies (Burgess et al., 1988; de Felício et al., 2010; Ficnar et al., 2013; Grace et al., 2002; Klobas et al., 2006; Machado et al., 2016; Maluf et al., 2009; Niemelä et al., 2012; Raustia et al., 1985;

Study or subgroup	Manual therapy plus exercise			Control (sp, sc or med)				Standard mean difference	Standard mean difference
	Mean	SD	Total	Mean	SD	Total	Weight	IV, random, 95% CI	IV, random, 95% CI
Alajbeg et al., 2015	11.5	12.25	6	−7.5	14.69	6	4.3%	1.30 [0.00, 2.59]	
Carmeli et al., 2001	1.39	1.41	18	0.17	1.71	18	15.7%	0.76 [0.08, 1.44]	
Haketa et al., 2010	30	24.1	19	15.4	27.66	25	19.6%	0.55 [−0.06, 1.16]	
Ismail et al., 2007	28	20	13	23	22	22	15.3%	0.23 [−0.46, 0.92]	
Minakuchi et al., 2001	7	15.46	25	−0.1	12.71	21	20.8%	0.49 [−0.10, 1.08]	
Schiffman et al., 2007	0.3	0.22	24	0.28	0.23	28	24.3%	0.09 [−0.46, 0.63]	
Total (95% CI)			**105**			**120**	**100%**	**0.44 [0.17, 0.71]**	

Heterogeneity: Tau^2 = 0.00; Chi^2 = 4.65, df = 5 (P = 0.46); I^2 = 0%
Test for overall effect: Z = 3.21 (P = 0.001)

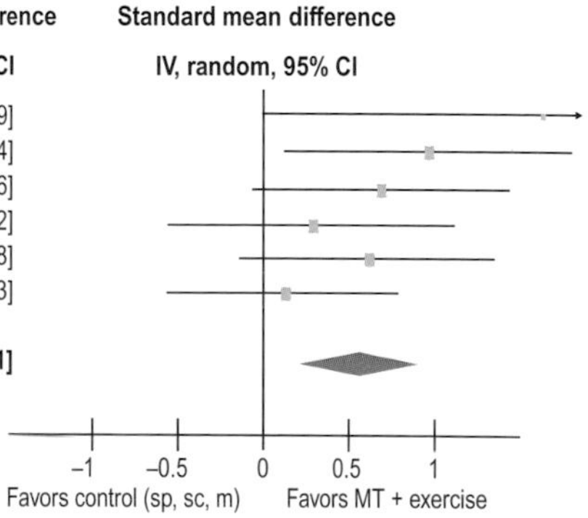

Favors control (sp, sc, m)   Favors MT + exercise

Figure 10.3

Meta-analysis pooled data of manual therapy plus exercises compared with other therapies (splint, medications) on pain intensity in patients with arthrogenous TMD. med, medications; sc, standard care; sp, splint.

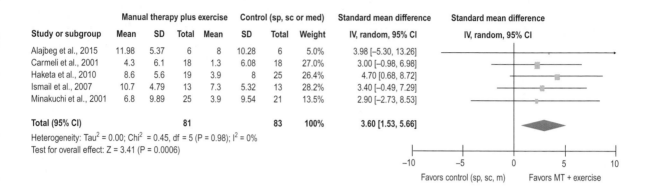

Study or subgroup	Manual therapy plus exercise			Control (sp, sc or med)			Weight	Standard mean difference	Standard mean difference
	Mean	SD	Total	Mean	SD	Total		IV, random, 95% CI	IV, random, 95% CI
Alajbeg et al., 2015	11.98	5.37	6	8	10.28	6	5.0%	3.98 [−5.30, 13.26]	
Carmeli et al., 2001	4.3	6.1	18	1.3	6.08	18	27.0%	3.00 [−0.98, 6.98]	
Haketa et al., 2010	8.6	5.6	19	3.9	8	25	26.4%	4.70 [0.68, 8.72]	
Ismail et al., 2007	10.7	4.79	13	7.3	5.32	13	28.2%	3.40 [−0.49, 7.29]	
Minakuchi et al., 2001	6.8	9.89	25	3.9	9.54	21	13.5%	2.90 [−2.73, 8.53]	
Total (95% CI)			**81**			**83**	**100%**	**3.60 [1.53, 5.66]**	

Heterogeneity: Tau^2 = 0.00; Chi^2 = 0.45, df = 5 (P = 0.98); I^2 = 0%
Test for overall effect: Z = 3.41 (P = 0.0006)

Favors control (sp, sc, m)   Favors MT + exercise

Figure 10.4

Meta-analysis pooled data of manual therapy plus exercises compared with other therapies (splint, standard care, medications) on mouth opening in patients with arthrogenous TMD. med, medications; sc, standard care; sp, splint.

Raustia & Pohjola, 1986; Tavera et al., 2012; Tegelberg & Kopp, 1996, 1988; Truelove et al., 2006) (reported in 14 articles) included a general jaw exercises program in subjects with mixed TMD. Four studies showed better results for general jaw exercises for decreasing pain intensity and pain sensitivity (PPT) and improving function of the masticatory muscles when compared with true control groups (no intervention) (Burgess et al., 1988; de Felício et al., 2010; Tegelberg & Kopp, 1996, 1988). One study found that stretching of the masticatory muscles (temporalis and masseter) when compared with a true control group or a proprioceptive neuromuscular technique (PNF) of the masticatory muscles showed better results to reduce pain; however, no statistical significant differences between groups on maximal mouth opening were found (Burgess et al., 1988). Further, it was found that a general program of mandibular exercises with and without resistance improved active mouth opening and reduced clinical symptoms of TMD (clinical dysfunction and number of tender points) when compared to a control group (Tegelberg & Kopp, 1988). Another study found positive effects of orofacial myofunctional therapy (mandible posture and mobility, symmetry and coordination of masticatory musculature) for reducing

symptoms and signs of TMD and improving masticatory muscle coordination when compared to an occlusal splint therapy group or a true control group (no intervention) (de Felício et al., 2010). Nevertheless, when general jaw exercises (and/or whiplash rehabilitation) were compared with other forms of active or passive treatments such as acupuncture (Raustia et al, 1985; Raustia & Pohjola, 1986), stabilization splints (Ficnar et al., 2013; Niemelä et al., 2012; Tavera et al., 2012; Truelove et al., 2006), global postural re-education program (Maluf et al., 2009), facial flex device (Grace et al., 2002), and/or whiplash rehabilitation alone including physical therapy, occupational therapy, and training in pain management (Klobas et al., 2006), no differences were found in terms of pain reduction between these treatments. Machado et al. (2016) found that the combination of low-level laser therapy and orofacial myofunctional therapy (exercises for tongue, lips, cheeks and jaw muscles) was more effective in promoting TMD rehabilitation than low-level laser therapy alone.

Studies with available data, similar interventions and similar outcomes (Grace et al., 2002; Maluf et al., 2009) were pooled. When determining the effectiveness of jaw general exercises on patients with mixed

TMD, on pain intensity, it was found that exercises in the form of general jaw exercises plus conventional treatment, or with the addition of an oral device (Grace et al., 2002) were not superior to other treatment modalities such as splint therapy, global postural re-education, splint plus counseling, acupuncture, or standard conservative care. The pooled SMD for pain intensity was -0.06 (95% CI −0.50; 0.38) with a very small effect size according to Cohen's guidelines (Cohen, 1988). The pooled results from these studies on mouth opening (Burgess et al., 1988; de Felício et al., 2010; Grace et al., 2002; Klobas et al., 2006; Niemelä et al., 2012; Raustia et al., 1985; Tegelberg & Kopp, 1996) also revealed a nonsignificant difference between general jaw exercises versus splint therapy, global postural re-education, splint plus counseling, or standard conservative care with an MD for mouth opening of −0.25 mm (95% CI −2.08, 1.57).

Manual therapy

Seven studies (Cuccia et al., 2010; Gesslbauer et al., 2016; Gomes et al., 2014a; Mansilla Ferragud & Boscá Gandia, 2008; O'Reilly & Pollard, 1996; Otaño & Legal, 2010; Packer et al., 2014, 2015) (with data reported in eight articles) included manual therapy (mobilization of C0–C1 [Mansilla Ferragud & Boscá Gandia, 2008; Otaño & Legal, 2010], mobilization of the cervical spine [O'Reilly & Pollard, 1996], manipulation of the upper thoracic spine [Packer et al., 2015, 2014], massage in the masticatory muscles [Gomes et al., 2014a], TMJ mobilizations [Cuccia et al., 2010], and osteopathic manipulative techniques [Gesslbauer et al., 2016]) to treat mixed TMD. The results of these studies were equivocal. Two studies (Mansilla Ferragud & Boscá Gandia, 2008; Otaño & Legal, 2010) found positive results while the remaining studies did not find differences in the outcomes of interest (Cuccia et al., 2010; Gesslbauer et al., 2016; Gomes et al., 2014a; O'Reilly & Pollard, 1996; Packer et al., 2015, 2014). No significant differences for reducing symptoms were obtained when manual therapy targeted to the jaw (manipulative procedures designed to

reduce the dysfunction of the ligaments of TMJ and to retrain the involuntary neuromuscular, reflexive control of posture and balance) was compared with conventional conservative therapy (oral appliance, physical therapy with gentle muscle stretching, and relaxing therapy, hot and/or cold pack and TENS) (Cuccia et al., 2010), or when cervical chiropractic adjustment was compared with cervical TrP therapy (O'Reilly & Pollard, 1996) or upper thoracic manipulation was compared with placebo upper thoracic technique (Packer et al., 2014) or masticatory muscles massage with splint therapy (Gomes et al., 2014a), or manipulative osteopathy versus cranial osteopathy techniques (Gesslbauer et al., 2016).

Mansilla Ferragud & Boscá Gandia (2008) and Otaño & Legal (2010) compared in their studies the effects of the mobilization or manipulation of the atlantoaxial joint (C0–C1) with a placebo group and found positive results at improving mouth range of motion and increasing PPT in the orofacial region. When pooling the results of these two studies no differences were found between mobilization of the atlantoaxial joint and the control group receiving no mobilization of the atlantoaxial joint on mouth opening. However, the pooled MD for mouth opening between the control and manual therapy groups was 17.33 mm with a wide confidence interval, and an upper bound of 45 mm approximately (95% CI −10.39, 45.06).

Manual therapy plus exercises

Four studies (Bojikian Calixtre et al., [submitted 2017]; von Piekartz & Hall, 2013; von Piekartz & Lüdtke, 2011; Tuncer et al., 2013b, 2013a) (reported in five manuscripts) used the combination of manual therapy plus exercise for subjects with mixed TMD. Tuncer et al. (2013a, 2013b) explored the specific effect of orofacial and cervical manual therapy combined with stretching techniques for the masticatory and neck muscles compared with exercises for the jaw and neck alone and education (home physical therapy) in this patient group. They found that manual therapy plus home physical therapy is more effective at decreasing pain and increasing pain-free maximum mouth opening than the jaw and neck exercise program alone. von Piekartz & Lüdtke (2011) compared the effect of orofacial physical therapy and neck exercises and manual therapy techniques targeted to both orofacial and cervical regions plus home exercises with treatment targeted to the cervical spine only in subjects with mixed TMD. The results showed that the group with manual therapy plus exercise for both regions (orofacial and cervical) was better than only treatment to the cervical region for TMD signs (mouth opening, pain intensity, and pain sensitivity). Bojikian Calixtre et al., compared the effect of a suboccipital inhibition technique, passive anterior–posterior upper cervical mobilization, sustained natural apophyseal glide (SNAG) mobilization with rotation on C1–C2 vertebrae, and neck stabilization exercises using a biofeedback with a true control group (waiting list) and found that the combination of manual therapy plus cervical motor control exercises decreased pain and headache impact in subjects with mixed TMD. Mean differences between groups in current and maximum pain scores were 2.0 cm and 1.9 cm at five weeks respectively. Those differences showed large effect sizes (d > 0.8) and were considered clinically relevant. Thus, treatment targeted to the cervical spine warrants more research in light of these promising results.

When pooling the results of three studies (von Piekartz & Hall, 2013; von Piekartz & Lüdtke, 2011; Tuncer et al., 2013b) on mouth opening, it was found that manual therapy targeted to the orofacial region or in combination with cervical treatment was better than home exercises for the jaw and neck alone or treatment to the cervical spine alone for improving mouth opening. The pooled MD for mouth opening between control and manual therapy groups was 6.10 mm (95% CI 1.11, 11.09) favoring the manual therapy group. This value of a difference could be considered clinically relevant (Kropmans et al., 1999).

Conclusion

Manual therapy techniques and jaw exercises aim to reduce pain, increase joint mobility, improve relaxation, and optimize jaw function. The mechanism behind manual therapy techniques is still not clearly understood and different hypotheses have been proposed. Nevertheless, the current literature suggests that manual therapy initiates a cascade of neurophysiological responses from the peripheral and the central nervous systems, which can be responsible for the clinical outcomes (Bialosky et al., 2009). Other psychological and nonspecific factors related to the patient could also explain why manual therapy may be effective (Bishop et al., 2015). A large and heterogeneous amount of different manual therapy techniques has been reported in this chapter. Some of them were directly focused on the TMJ and others were targeted to the cervical or thoracic spine such as mobilization or manipulation.

The effects of jaw exercises are considered to be a result of reciprocal muscle inhibition, proprioceptive neuromuscular facilitation, increased awareness, improved motor control, muscular endurance, strength, and improved muscular length through stretching. It has been reported that the most useful techniques for re-education and rehabilitation of the masticatory musculature are strengthening exercises and stretching (Hertling & Kessler, 2006). The exercise programs can be executed in a number of different ways. Usually exercise programs contain relaxation exercises, free movement of the mandible, as well as resistive movements with a small resistance, combined with stretching of the jaw muscles.

Although the quality of the evidence is mostly uncertain, the evidence gathered in this chapter supports the use of active and passive oral exercises to reduce pain intensity, improve relaxation, and optimize jaw mobility or function in myogenous, arthrogenous, and mixed TMD. Also, postural exercises targeted to the head and neck, as well as neck exercises and manual therapies targeted to the neck are also effective interventions for the management of TMD pain and dysfunction.

Most of these exercise programs were part of a general conservative treatment approach including other therapies such as counseling and splint. Exercise programs should be considered as the first-choice treatment for TMD pain because of their low risk of side effects. However, the execution of exercise programs has been diverse and clear information regarding their dosage, frequency, duration, number of repetitions or compliance has not been yet provided and thus, the optimal treatment regimen for treating TMD is uncertain. Therefore, more research on exercise therapy and manual therapy regarding dosages is necessary to allow for clinical replication. Furthermore, most of the studies did not investigate the isolated effect of exercises or manual therapy, which made it difficult to determine the sole contribution of these therapies to treat TMD. In addition, no trial investigated the use of other forms of exercise therapy, such as aerobic exercises to manage TMD. Aerobic exercise has been shown to improve muscle strength, flexibility, and functional capacity and could induce analgesia in people with chronic pain (Sharma et al., 2010). Further research is required to investigate the usefulness of aerobic exercise and other forms of exercise not used in the analyzed studies such as exercises modifying visual feedback (Sanneke et al., 2017) in subjects with TMD.

One of the highlights of this evidence compilation was that there is emerging evidence supporting the use of cervical spine treatment through neck exercises plus cervical mobilizations to improve pain.

A few new RCTs have tested the combination of cervical exercises with manipulation or mobilization of neck structures to manage TMD symptoms. These studies have obtained promising results in reducing pain with large effect sizes. However, there is still a need for investigating the isolated effect of exercises targeted to cervical muscles to improve jaw symptoms. None of the studies looked at this type of treatment. Thus, there is a clear need for well-designed RCTs examining manual therapy interventions for TMD and ideally in isolation. Given the positive effects of active and passive exercise, postural exercises, and manual therapy for TMD, high-quality trials with larger samples are required.

Finally, the results of this chapter have some limitations. First, the findings of this chapter compilation are specific to TMD (nonsurgical) and to exercise and manual therapy. Second, as with any systematic approach to synthesize the literature, there is the potential for selection bias yet our group used a comprehensive search strategy and included databases as well as manual searches. Third, there was great heterogeneity in the analyzed studies in terms of diagnoses, treatment description, comparison groups used, outcomes, and their quality. This hindered the possibility to quantitatively pool study results. Although only 28 studies used a diagnostic tool that has been demonstrated as being valid, reliable, and reproducible to diagnose TMD, we feel that study populations included in all trials appeared to be representative of patients seen in clinical practice. We encourage clinicians and researchers to use the new diagnostic criteria for TMD (DC/TMD) (Schiffman et al., 2014) in future studies to allow consistent diagnoses according to the same criteria and allow compilation of data across studies.

Chapter 10

References

Alajbeg I, Gikić M, Valentić Peruzović M. Mandibular range of movement and pain intensity in patients with anterior disc displacement without reduction. Acta Stomatol Croat 2015; 49: 119–127.

Armijo-Olivo S, Gadotti, I. Temporomandibular disorders. In Magee DJ, Zachazewski JE, Quillen WS, Manske RC. Pathology and Intervention in Musculoskeletal Rehabilitation. 2nd ed. 2016, pp. 119–156.

Armijo-Olivo S, Pitance L, Singh V et al. Effectiveness of manual therapy and therapeutic exercise for temporomandibular disorders: Systematic review and meta-analysis. Phys Ther 2016; 96: 9–25.

Awan KH, Patil S. The role of transcutaneous electrical nerve stimulation in the management of temporomandibular joint disorder. J Contemp Dent Pract 2015; 16: 9846.

Bae Y, Park Y. The effect of relaxation exercises for the masticatory muscles on temporomandibular joint dysfunction (TMD). J Phys Ther Sci 2013; 25: 583–586.

Bérard A, Bravo G. Combining studies using effect sizes and quality scores: application to bone loss in postmenopausal women. J Clin Epidemiol 1998; 51: 801–807.

Bialosky JE, Bishop MD, Price DD, Robinson ME, George SZ. The mechanisms of manual therapy in the treatment of musculoskeletal pain: a comprehensive model. Man Ther 2009; 14: 531–538.

Bishop MD, Torres-Cueco R, Gay CW, Lluch-Girbés E, Beneciuk JM, Bialosky JE. What effect can manual therapy have on a patient's pain experience? Pain Manag 2015; 5: 455–464.

Bojikian Calixtre L, Oliveira AB, Ramalho de Sena Rosa L et al. Effects of upper cervical mobilizations and neck exercises on pain, mandibular function, and headache impact in women with TMD. A single-blinded randomized controlled trial [submitted to Physical Therapy, 2017].

Bortolazzo GL, Pires PF, Dibai-Filho AV et al. Effects of upper cervical manipulation on the electromyographic activity of the masticatory muscles and the opening range of motion of the mouth in women with temporomandibular disorder: randomized and blind clinical trial. Fisioter E Pesqui 2015; 22: 426–434.

Burgess JA, Sommers EE, Truelove EL, Dworkin SF. Short-term effect of two therapeutic methods on myofascial pain and dysfunction of the masticatory system. J Prosthet Dent 1988; 60: 606–610.

Calixtre LB, Grüninger BL da Silva, Haik MN, Alburquerque-Sendín F, Oliveira AB. Effects of cervical mobilization and exercise on pain, movement and function in subjects with temporomandibular disorders: a single group pre-post-test. J Appl Oral Sci 2016; 24: 188.

Carlsson G, Magnusson T. Treatment modalities. In Carlsson G, Magnusson T (eds). Management of Temporomandibular Disorders in the General Dental Practice. Berlin: Quintessence Publishing Company, Inc. 1999, pp. 93–122.

Carmeli E, Sheklow SL, Bloomenfeld I. Comparative study of repositioning splint therapy and passive manual range of motion techniques for anterior displaced temporomandibular discs with unstable excursive reduction. Physiotherapy 2001; 87: 26–36.

Cathcart S, Pritchard D. Reliability of pain threshold measurement in young adults. J Headache Pain 2006; 7: 21–26.

Chesterton LS, Foster NE, Wright CC, Baxter GD, Barlas P. Effects of TENS frequency, intensity and stimulation site parameter manipulation on pressure pain thresholds in healthy human subjects. Pain 2003; 106: 73–80.

Clar C, Tsertsvadze A, Court R, Hundt GL, Clarke A, Sutcliffe P. Clinical effectiveness of manual therapy for the management of musculoskeletal and non-musculoskeletal conditions: systematic review and update of UK evidence report. Chiropr Man Ther 2014; 22: 12.

Cohen J. Statistical Power Analysis for the Behavioral Sciences, 2nd ed. Routledge; 1988.

Coskun Benlidayi I, Salimov F, Kurkcu M, Guzel R. Kinesio-taping for temporo-mandibular disorders: Single-blind, randomized, controlled trial of effectiveness. J Back Musculoskelet Rehabil 2016; 29: 373–380.

Craane B, Dijkstra PU, Stappaerts K, De Laat A. Randomized controlled trial on physical therapy for TMJ closed lock. J Dent Res 2012a; 91: 364–369.

Craane B, Dijkstra PU, Stappaerts K, De Laat A. One-year evaluation of the effect of physical therapy for masticatory muscle pain: a randomized controlled trial. Eur J Pain Lond Engl 2012b; 16: 737–747.

Crockett DJ, Foreman ME, Alden L, Blasberg B. A comparison of treatment modes in the management of myofascial pain dysfunction syndrome. Biofeedback Self-Regul 1986; 11: 279–291.

Cuccia AM, Caradonna C, Annunziata V, Caradonna D. Osteopathic manual therapy versus conventional conservative therapy in the treatment of temporomandibular disorders: a randomized controlled trial. J Bodyw Mov Ther 2010; 14: 179–184.

Demirkol N, Usumez A, Demirkol M, Sari F, Akcaboy C. Efficacy of low-level laser therapy in subjective tinnitus patients with temporomandibular disorders. Photomed Laser Surg 2017; 35: 427–431.

Diraçoğlu D, Saral IB, Keklik B et al. Arthrocentesis versus nonsurgical methods in the treatment of temporomandibular disc displacement without reduction. Oral Surg Oral Med Oral Pathol Oral Radiol Endod 2009; 108: 3–8.

Dworkin SF, LeResche L. Research diagnostic criteria for temporomandibular disorders: review, criteria, examinations and specifications, critique. J Craniomandib Disord 1992; 6: 301–355.

Dworkin RH, Turk DC, Wyrwich KW et al. Interpreting the clinical importance of treatment outcomes in chronic pain clinical trials: IMMPACT recommendations. J Pain 2008; 9: 105–121.

Espejo-Antúnez L, Castro-Valenzuela E, Ribeiro F, Albornoz-Cabello M, Silva A, Rodríguez-Mansilla J. Immediate effects of hamstring stretching alone or combined with ischemic compression of the masseter muscle on hamstrings extensibility, active mouth opening and pain in athletes with temporomandibular dysfunction. J Bodyw Mov Ther 2016; 20: 579–587.

Farrar JT, Young JP, LaMoreaux L, Werth JL, Poole RM. Clinical importance of changes in chronic pain intensity measured on an 11-point numerical pain rating scale. Pain 2001; 94: 149–158.

de Felício CM, Melchior M de O, Ferreira CLP, Da Silva MA. Otologic symptoms of temporomandibular disorder and effect of orofacial myofunctional therapy. Cranio2008; 26: 118–125.

de Felício CM, de Oliveira MM, da Silva MA. Effects of orofacial myofunctional therapy on temporomandibular disorders. Cranio 2010; 28: 249–259.

Ficnar T, Middelberg C, Rademacher B, Hessling S, Koch R, Figgener L. Evaluation of the effectiveness of a semi-finished occlusal appliance: a randomized, controlled clinical trial. Head Face Med 2013; 9: 5.

Fuentes C J, Armijo-Olivos S, Magee DJ, Gross DP. A preliminary investigation into the effects of active interferential current therapy and placebo on pressure pain sensitivity: a random crossover placebo controlled study. Physiotherapy 2011; 97: 291–301.

Gavish A, Winocur E, Astandzelov-Nachmias T, Gazit E. Effect of controlled masticatory exercise on pain and muscle performance in myofascial pain patients: A pilot study. Cranio 2006; 24: 184–190.

Gesslbauer C, Vavti N, Keilani M, Mickel M, Crevenna R. Effectiveness of osteopathic manipulative treatment versus osteopathy in the cranial field in temporomandibular disorders: a pilot study. Disabil Rehabil 2016: 1–6.

Gomes CAF de P, El Hage Y, Amaral AP, Politti F, Biasotto-Gonzalez DA. Effects of massage therapy and occlusal splint therapy on electromyographic activity and the intensity of signs and symptoms in individuals with temporomandibular disorder and sleep bruxism: a randomized clinical trial. Chiropr Man Ther 2014a; 22: 43.

Gomes CAF de P, Politti F, Andrade DV et al. Effects of massage therapy and occlusal splint therapy on mandibular range of motion in individuals with temporomandibular disorder: a randomized clinical trial. J Manipulative Physiol Ther 2014b; 37: 164–169.

Grace EG, Sarlani E, Reid B, Read B. The use of an oral exercise device in the treatment of muscular TMD. Cranio 2002; 20: 204–208.

Guarda-Nardini L, Stecco A, Stecco C, Masiero S, Manfredini D. Myofascial pain of the jaw muscles: comparison of short-term effectiveness of botulinum toxin injections and fascial manipulation technique. Cranio 2012; 30: 95–102.

Haketa T, Kino K, Sugisaki M, Takaoka M, Ohta T. Randomized clinical trial of treatment for TMJ disc displacement. J Dent Res 2010; 89: 1259–1263.

Hertling D, Kessler RM. Management of Common Musculoskeletal Disorders: Physical Therapy Principles and Methods. 4th ed. 2006.

Higgins JPT, Green S (eds). Cochrane Handbook for Systematic Reviews of Interventions Version 5.1.0 [updated March 2011]. The Cochrane Collaboration, 2011. Available: http://handbook.cochrane.org [Nov 23, 2017].

Ismail F, Demling A, Hessling K, Fink M, Stiesch-Scholz M. Short-term efficacy of physical therapy compared to splint therapy in treatment of arthrogenous TMD. J Oral Rehabil 2007; 34: 807–813.

Kalamir A, Bonello R, Graham P, Vitiello AL, Pollard H. Intraoral myofascial therapy for chronic myogenous temporomandibular disorder: a randomized controlled trial. J Manipulative Physiol Ther 2012; 35: 26–37.

Kalamir A, Graham PL, Vitiello AL, Bonello R, Pollard H. Intra-oral myofascial therapy versus education and self-care in the treatment of chronic, myogenous temporomandibular disorder: a randomised, clinical trial. Chiropr Man Ther 2013; 21: 17.

Kalamir A, Pollard H, Vitiello A, Bonello R. Intra-oral myofascial therapy for chronic myogenous temporomandibular disorders: a randomized, controlled pilot study. J Man Manip Ther 2010; 18: 139–146.

Klobas L, Axelsson S, Tegelberg A. Effect of therapeutic jaw exercise on temporomandibular disorders in individuals with chronic whiplash-associated disorders. Acta Odontol Scand 2006; 64: 341–347.

Komiyama O, Kawara M, Arai M, Asano T, Kobayashi K. Posture correction as part of behavioural therapy in treatment of myofascial pain with limited opening. J Oral Rehabil 1999; 26: 428–435.

Kovacs FM, Abraira V, Royuela A et al. Minimal clinically important change for pain intensity and disability in patients with nonspecific low back pain. Spine 2007; 32: 2915–2920.

Kraaijenga S, van der Molen L, van Tinteren H, Hilgers F, Smeele L. Treatment of myogenic temporomandibular disorder: a prospective randomized clinical trial, comparing a mechanical stretching device (TheraBite®) with standard physical therapy exercise. Cranio 2014; 32: 208–216.

Kraus S. Temporomandibular disorders, head and orofacial pain: cervical spine considerations. Dent Clin North Am 2007; 51: 161–193.

Kropmans TJ, Dijkstra PU, Stegenga B, Stewart R, de Bont LG. Smallest detectable difference in outcome variables related to painful restriction of the temporomandibular joint. J Dent Res 1999; 78: 784–789.

La Touche R, París-Alemany A, Mannheimer JS et al. Does mobilization of the upper cervical spine affect pain sensitivity and autonomic nervous system function in patients with cervico-craniofacial pain? A randomized-controlled trial. Clin J Pain 2013; 29: 205–215.

Leeuw R de, Klasser GD (eds). Orofacial pain: guidelines for assessment, diagnosis, and management. Fifth ed. Chicago: Quintessence Publishing Company, Inc. 2013.

Machado BC, Mazzetto MO, Da Silva MA, de Felício CM. Effects of oral motor exercises and laser therapy on chronic temporomandibular disorders: a randomized study with follow-up. Lasers Med Sci 2016; 31: 945–954.

Magnusson T, Syrén M. Therapeutic jaw exercises and interocclusal appliance therapy. A comparison between two common treatments of temporomandibular disorders. Swed Dent J 1999; 23: 27–37.

Maloney GE, Mehta N, Forgione AG et al. Effect of a passive jaw motion device on pain and range of motion in TMD patients not responding to flat plane intraoral appliances. Cranio 2002; 20: 55–66.

Maluf S, Moreno BGD, Osvaldo C, Marques AP. A Comparison of two muscular stretching modalities on pain in women with myogenous temporomandibular disorders. Pain Pract 2009; 9.

Mansilla Ferragud P, Boscá Gandia JJ. Efecto de la manipulación de la charnela occipito-atlo-axoidea en la apertura de la boca. Osteopat Científica 2008; 3: 45–51.

Maughan EF, Lewis JS. Outcome measures in chronic low back pain. Eur Spine J 2010; 19: 1484–1494.

McNeely ML, Armijo Olivo S, Magee DJ. A systematic review of the effectiveness of physical therapy interventions for temporomandibular disorders. Phys Ther 2006; 86: 710–725.

Medlicott MS, Harris SR. A systematic review of the effectiveness of exercise, manual therapy, electrotherapy, relaxation training, and biofeedback in the management of temporomandibular disorder. Phys Ther 2006; 86: 955–973.

Michelotti A, Steenks MH, Farella M, Parisini F, Cimino R, Martina R. The

additional value of a home physical therapy regimen versus patient education only for the treatment of myofascial pain of the jaw muscles: short-term results of a randomized clinical trial. J Orofac Pain 2004; 18: 114–125.

Miller J, Gross A, D'Sylva J, Burnie SJ, Goldsmith CH, Graham N, et al. Manual therapy and exercise for neck pain: a systematic review. Man Ther 2010; 15: 334–354.

Minakuchi H, Kuboki T, Matsuka Y, Maekawa K, Yatani H, Yamashita A. Randomized controlled evaluation of non-surgical treatments for temporomandibular joint anterior disk displacement without reduction. J Dent Res 2001; 80: 924–928.

Minakuchi H, Kuboki T, Maekawa K, Matsuka Y, Yatani H. Self-reported remission, difficulty, and satisfaction with nonsurgical therapy used to treat anterior disc displacement without reduction. Oral Surg Oral Med Oral Pathol Oral Radiol Endod 2004; 98: 435–440.

Mulet M, Decker KL, Look JO, Lenton PA, Schiffman EL. A randomized clinical trial assessing the efficacy of adding 6 × 6 exercises to self-care for the treatment of masticatory myofascial pain. J Orofac Pain 2007; 21: 318–328.

Nascimento MM, Vasconcelos BC, Porto GG, Ferdinanda G, Nogueira CM, Raimundo RC. Physical therapy and anesthetic blockage for treating temporomandibular disorders: a clinical trial. Med Oral Patol Oral Cirugia Bucal 2013; 18:e81–85.

Niemelä K, Korpela M, Raustia A, Ylöstalo P, Sipilä K. Efficacy of stabilisation splint treatment on temporomandibular disorders. J Oral Rehabil 2012; 39: 799–804.

Nussbaum E, Downes L. Reliability of clinical pressure-pain algometric measurements obtained on consecutive days. Phys Ther 1998; 78: 160–169.

O'Reilly A, Pollard H. TMJ pain and chiropractic adjustment: a pilot study. Chiropr J Aust 1996; 26: 125–129.

Otaño L, Legal L. Modificaciones radiológicas del espacio entre el occipucio y el cuerpo del atlas tras una manipulación global (OAA) de Fryette. Osteopat Científica 2010; 5: 38–46.

Packer AC, Pires PF, Dibai-Filho AV, Rodrigues-Bigaton D. Effects of upper thoracic manipulation on pressure pain sensitivity in women with temporomandibular disorder: a randomized, double-blind, clinical trial. Am J Phys Med Rehabil 2014; 93: 160–168.

Packer AC, Pires PF, Dibai-Filho AV, Rodrigues-Bigaton D. Effect of upper thoracic manipulation on mouth opening and electromyographic activity of masticatory muscles in women with temporomandibular disorder: a randomized clinical trial. J Manipulative Physiol Ther 2015; 38: 253–261.

Rai S, Ranjan V, Misra D, Panjwani S. Management of myofascial pain by therapeutic ultrasound and transcutaneous electrical nerve stimulation: A comparative study. Eur J Dent 2016; 10: 46.

Raustia AM, Pohjola RT. Acupuncture compared with stomatognathic treatment for TMJ dysfunction. Part III: Effect of treatment on mobility. J Prosthet Dent 1986; 56: 616–623.

Raustia AM, Pohjola RT, Virtanen KK. Acupuncture compared with stomatognathic treatment for TMJ dysfunction. Part I: A randomized study. J Prosthet Dent 1985; 54: 581–585.

RevMan 5 – Cochrane Community [n.d.]. Available: http://community.cochrane.org/tools/review-production-tools/revman-5/revman-5-download [14 Nov, 2017].

Rocabado M. The importance of soft tissue mechanics in stability and instability of the cervical spine: a functional diagnosis for treatment planning. Cranio 1987; 5: 130–138.

Rodriguez-Blanco C, Cocera-Morata FM, Heredia-Rizo AM et al. Immediate effects of combining local techniques in the craniomandibular area and hamstring muscle stretching in subjects with temporomandibular disorders: a randomized controlled study. J Altern Complement Med 2015; 21: 451–459.

van der Roer N, Ostelo RWJG, Bekkering GE, van Tulder MW, de Vet HCW. Minimal clinically important change for pain intensity, functional status, and general health status in patients with nonspecific low back pain. Spine 2006; 31: 578–582.

Sanneke D, De Kooning, Voogt L, Ickmans K, Daenen L, Nijs J. The effect of visual feedback of the neck during movement in people with chronic whiplash-associated disorders: an experimental study. J Orthop Sports Phys Ther 2017; 47: 190–199.

Schiffman EL, Look JO, Hodges JS et al. Randomized effectiveness study of four therapeutic strategies for TMJ closed lock. J Dent Res 2007; 86: 58–63.

Schiffman E, Ohrbach R, Truelove E et al. Diagnostic Criteria for Temporomandibular Disorders (DC/TMD) for Clinical and Research Applications: Recommendations of the International RDC/TMD Consortium Network and Orofacial Pain Special Interest Group. J Oral Facial Pain Headache 2014; 28: 6–27.

Sessle BJ. Neural mechanisms and pathways in craniofacial pain. Can J Neurol Sci 1999; 26: S7-S11.

Sharma NK, Ryals JM, Gajewski BJ, Wright DE. Aerobic exercise alters analgesia and neurotrophin-3 synthesis in an animal model of chronic widespread pain. Phys Ther 2010; 90: 714–725.

Stegenga B, de Bont LG, Dijkstra PU, Boering G. Short-term outcome of arthroscopic surgery of temporomandibular joint osteoarthrosis and internal derangement: a randomized controlled clinical trial. Br J Oral Maxillofac Surg 1993; 31: 3–14.

Tavera AT, Montoya MCP, Calderón EFGG, Gorodezky G, Wixtrom RN. Approaching temporomandibular disorders from a new direction: a randomized controlled clinical trial of the TMDes ear system.

Cranio J Craniomandib Pract 2012; 30: 172–182.

Taylor NF, Dodd KJ, Shields N, Bruder A. Therapeutic exercise in physiotherapy practice is beneficial: a summary of systematic reviews 2002–2005. Aust J Physiother 2007; 53: 7–16.

Tegelberg A, Kopp S. Short-term effect of physical training on temporomandibular joint disorder in individuals with rheumatoid arthritis and ankylosing spondylitis. Acta Odontol Scand 1988; 46: 49–56.

Tegelberg A, Kopp S. A 3-year follow-up of temporomandibular disorders in rheumatoid arthritis and ankylosing spondylitis. Acta Odontol Scand 1996; 54: 14–18.

Truelove E, Huggins KH, Mancl L, Dworkin SF. The efficacy of traditional, low-cost and nonsplint therapies for temporomandibular disorder: a randomized controlled trial. J Am Dent Assoc 1939 2006; 137: 1099–1107.

Tuncer AB, Ergun N, Karahan S. Temporomandibular disorders treatment: Comparison of home exercise and manual therapy. Fiz Rehabil 2013a; 24: 9–16.

Tuncer AB, Ergun N, Tuncer AH, Karahan S. Effectiveness of manual therapy and home physical therapy in patients with temporomandibular disorders: a randomized controlled trial. J Bodyw Mov Ther 2013b; 17: 302–308.

von Piekartz H, Hall T. Orofacial manual therapy improves cervical movement impairment associated with headache and features of temporomandibular dysfunction: a randomized controlled trial. Man Ther 2013; 18: 345–350.

von Piekartz H, Lüdtke K. Effect of treatment of temporomandibular disorders (TMD) in patients with cervicogenic headache: a single-blind, randomized controlled study. Cranio 2011; 29: 43–56.

Wright EF, Domenech MA, Fischer JR. Usefulness of posture training for patients with temporomandibular disorders. J Am Dent Assoc 2000; 131: 202–210.

Ylinen J, Takala E-P, Kautiainen H et al. Effect of long-term neck muscle training on pressure pain threshold: a randomized controlled trial. Eur J Pain 2005; 9: 673–681.

Yoda T, Sakamoto I, Imai H et al. A randomized controlled trial of therapeutic exercise for clicking due to disk anterior displacement with reduction in the temporomandibular joint. Cranio 2003; 21: 10–16.

Yoshida H, Fukumura Y, Suzuki S et al. Simple manipulation therapy for temporo-mandibular joint internal derangement with closed lock. Asian J Oral Maxillofac Surg 2005; 17: 256–260.

Yoshida H, Sakata T, Hayashi T, Shirao K, Oshiro N, Morita S. Evaluation of mandibular condylar movement exercise for patients with internal derangement of the temporomandibular joint on initial presentation. Br J Oral Maxillofac Surg 2011; 49: 310–313.

Yuasa H, Kurita K, Treatment Group on Temporomandibular Disorders. Randomized clinical trial of primary treatment for temporomandibular joint disk displacement without reduction and without osseous changes: a combination of NSAIDs and mouth-opening exercise versus no treatment. Oral Surg Oral Med Oral Pathol Oral Radiol Endod 2001; 91: 671–675.

Chapter 11

Joint mobilization and manipulation interventions for the cervical spine and temporomandibular joint

César Fernández-de-las-Peñas, Juan Mesa-Jiménez, Joshua A. Cleland

The evidence for joint manipulation and mobilization

Joint mobilization is usually defined as low-velocity, high-amplitude passive motion inducing intra-capsular movement at different amplitudes, whereas joint manipulation is defined as a high-velocity, low-amplitude motion facilitating joint gliding (Hengeveld et al., 2005; Maitland, 1986). Due to inconsistencies in terminology, use of standardized manipulation terminology in physical therapy practice has been proposed (Mintken et al., 2008).

Maitland (1986) originally described five different grades of mobilization according to the amplitude of motion and resistance offered by the surrounding tissues (Hengeveld et al., 2005). Grades I and IV refer to small amplitude oscillations at the beginning and end of tissue resistance, while Grades II and III indicate large amplitude oscillations in the mid-resistance range. Clinically Grades I–II are typically used for individuals where pain is the dominant symptom and a patient's disorder is considered irritable in nature (pain dominant); whereas Grades III–IV are usually applied to individuals where the main symptom relates to limitation of range of motion and this restriction is associated with some pain provocation (resistance dominant). Finally, Grade V refers to high-velocity low-amplitude thrust manipulation (Hengeveld et al., 2005; Maitland, 1986).

Joint mobilization is provided in the limits of range, and the therapist expects a pain response, which should settle immediately or within seconds of the mobilization being completed. In current clinical practice, a Grade I mobilization is rarely used since large-amplitude mobilizations with short pain provocation (Grade II or III) offer the patient the advantage of increasing range and reducing pain.

It is clinically important to consider that the temporomandibular joint (TMJ) has dense ligaments (Cuccia et al., 2011) and several muscles supporting the joint; therefore, clinicians will experience significant tissue resistance during manual joint mobilizations. In fact, the treatment dose (how many, for how long) is crucial for the TMJ and is decided based on the clinical presentation of the patient. In our clinical experience, in individuals with temporomandibular disorder (TMD), two to three repetitions for 120–180 seconds are usually required since the TMJ is generally extremely stiff. It has recently been suggested that mobilization of the TMJ is able to improve the extensibility of noncontractile tissue and increase range of motion while decreasing pain and related disability via peripheral, spinal, and supraspinal mechanisms (Butts et al., 2017).

As has been discussed in Chapter 10 of this textbook, there is enough evidence supporting the use of manual therapy for the management of TMD. Most of the studies using manual therapy for the management of TMD have included both joint and soft tissue approaches. Briefly and in relation to joint-biased interventions, Calixtre et al. (2015) reported moderate evidence supporting upper cervical spine manipulation and/or mobilization techniques for patients with TMD. Armijo-Olivo et al. (2016) found that manual therapy, including manipulation and/or mobilization to the TMJ and/or the cervical spine, was effective when administered alone or in combination with exercise for TMD, although effect sizes were low to moderate and related to the type of TMD. The meta-analysis conducted by Martins et al. (2016) found moderate evidence and large clinical effects supporting TMJ mobilization, particularly when combined with multimodal therapy, for improving pain and active mouth opening in patients with TMD. However, other reviews did not find evidence supporting the effectiveness of TMJ mobilization for individuals with disc displacement without reduction, although this was based on just two trials (Alves et al., 2013). It is probable that joint-biased interventions would not be indicated in all types of TMD, being more effective in arthrogenous TMD.

Additionally, since TMD pain is a multidimensional disorder, a multimodal treatment approach including manual therapy (applied to the joint and soft tissues), exercise, medication, splint therapy, and neuroscience pain education is required (Shaffer et al., 2014; Miernik & Więckiewicz, 2015). In fact, manual therapy interventions should combine mobilization and/or manipulation of the cervical and thoracic spine with techniques that target the TMJ (Jayaseelan & Tow, 2016; Sault et al., 2016). This is important since an isolated application of thoracic spine manipulation does not have a direct effect on pressure pain sensitivity (Packer et al., 2014) or active mouth opening (Packer et al., 2015) in women with TMD; however, the inclusion of cervicothoracic

manipulation in a multimodal treatment approach can be crucial (Jayaseelan & Tow, 2016). Furthermore, each treatment session should be personalized using an impairment-based model of care where the clinician prioritizes identified physical impairments related to the patient's symptomatology. In fact, a clinical pragmatic approach including manual therapies directed at identified impairments has been found to be effective for TMD (Nicolakis et al., 2001; Furto et al., 2006). This chapter describes the most common mobilization and manipulation interventions for the cervical spine and the TMJ in clinical practice.

Mobilization and manipulation of the cervical spine

Upper cervical spine posterior-to-anterior mobilization (C1–C2)

The application of posterior-to-anterior (PA) upper cervical nonthrust mobilization has been shown to be effective for decreasing pain intensity and

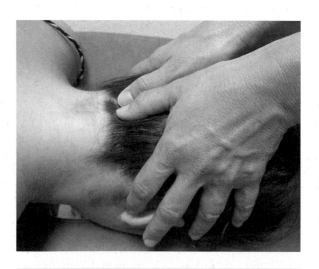

Figure 11.1
Central upper cervical spine posterior-to-anterior mobilization (C1-C2).

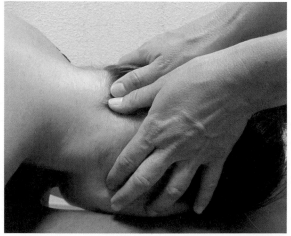

Figure 11.2
Unilateral upper cervical spine posterior-to-anterior mobilization (C1-C2).

pressure pain sensitivity in subjects with myogenous TMD when compared with a placebo treatment (La Touche et al., 2013).

For this technique, the patient lies in prone. The clinician stands at the head of the table and leans forward over the patient with arms straight and sternum over thumbs. For a central PA technique the clinician contacts with the pads of both thumbs over the spinous process of C2 (Figure 11.1), whereas for an unilateral PA, the contact is over the zygapophyseal joint of the C1–C2 joint (Figure 11.2). A gradual PA mobilization force is applied based on the reproduction of pain during the intervention.

Upper cervical spine flexion mobilization (C0–C2)

A case series found that application of a multimodal manual therapy approach including flexion and PA nonthrust mobilizations of the upper cervical spine reduced pain and increased mouth opening in patients with myogenous TMD (La Touche et al., 2009).

For this technique, the patient lies in supine. The cervical spine of the patient is in neutral and the clinician introduces occipital traction and head flexion until a palpated sense of resistance is perceived. The clinician mobilizes the upper cervical spine into a craniocervical flexion motion (Figure 11.3).

Upper cervical spine lateral flexion mobilization (C0–C1)

The patient lies in supine. The cervical spine is in neutral. With one hand, the clinician contacts the mastoid process of the temporal bone with the proximal phalanx of the index finger. The clinician's other hand cradles the patient's head. The clinician performs a slight displacement of the head at the same time inducing a side-bending motion of the occiput on the atlas (Figure 11.4).

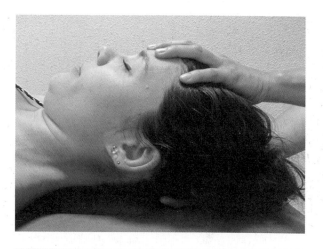

Figure 11.3
Upper cervical spine flexion mobilization (C0–C2).

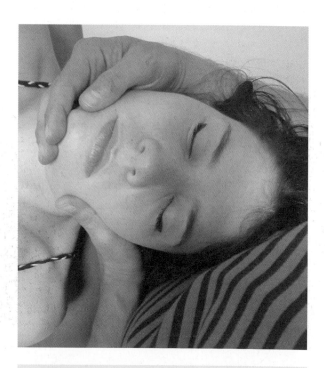

Figure 11.4
Upper cervical spine lateral flexion mobilization (C0-C1).

Chapter 11

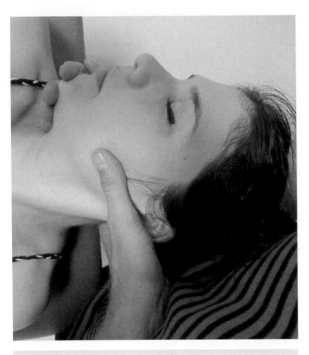

Figure 11.5
Upper cervical spine thrust manipulation (C1–C2).

Upper cervical spine thrust manipulation (C1–C2)

Mansilla-Ferragut et al. (2009) found that the application of an upper cervical spine thrust manipulation resulted in an increase in active mouth opening and a decrease in pressure pain sensitivity over a trigeminal nerve distribution area (sphenoid bone) in women with mechanical neck pain. Oliveira-Campelo et al. (2010) also reported that the application of an upper cervical spine thrust manipulation led to an immediate increase in pressure pain thresholds over latent TrPs in the masseter and temporalis muscles and an increase in maximum active mouth opening. Bortolazzo et al. (2015) showed that upper cervical spine manipulation was more effective than placebo for normalization of performance of the masticatory muscles and for increasing mouth opening in women with muscular TMD. Nielsen et al. (2017), in a review of systematic reviews, concluded that all reviews with higher standard quality had a higher chance of expressing that spinal manipulative therapy of the upper cervical spine seems to be

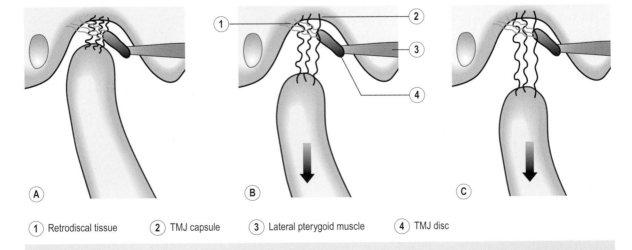

① Retrodiscal tissue　② TMJ capsule　③ Lateral pterygoid muscle　④ TMJ disc

Figure 11.6
Inferior gliding during the mandibular distraction mobilization technique in a neutral position (A), Grades I–II (B), and Grades III–IV (C).

safe; nevertheless, good clinical reasoning is highly imperative (Puentedura et al., 2012). It is also important to recognize that no clear patient profile, related to the risk of adverse events after upper cervical spine manipulation, could be identified (Kranenburg et al., 2017).

For this technique, the patient lies in supine. With one hand, the clinician contacts the posterior–lateral aspect of the articular process of the atlantoaxial (C1–C2) joint on the targeted side. The clinician cups the patient's chin and cradles the side of the head with the other hand. The upper cervical spine is flexed. The clinician performs contralateral cervical rotation and minimal side-bending until slight tension is perceived in the tissues at the contact point. A lateral glide of the C1–C2 joint is gradually introduced to increase the tension. A high-velocity low-amplitude upper cervical spine thrust manipulation is performed horizontally in the direction of the patient's contralateral eye (Figure 11.5).

Mobilization and manipulation of the temporomandibular joint

Mandibular distraction mobilization technique

The normal movement of the TMJ disc requires a low friction coefficient. In patients with TMD a compression or stiffness of the joint is usually observed. Therefore, the objective of this technique is to obtain a distraction (inferior glide) of the TMJ (Figure 11.6). Taylor et al. (1994) reported that an oscillatory Grade IV mandibular distraction mobilization technique was effective in increasing jaw range of motion and decreasing bilateral masseter muscle EMG activity in a symptomatic population compared to sham treatment. Carmeli et al. (2001) found that TMJ mobilizations progressively applied from Grade I to Grade IV combined with active jaw exercise were more effective than soft repositioning splint therapy in patients with anterior displaced disc. Ismail et al. (2007) also observed that application of mandibular translation

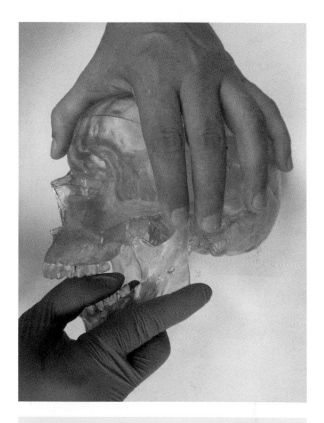

Figure 11.7
Intraoral contact for mobilization techniques of the temporomandibular joint.

mobilization combined with a Michigan splint was more effective than the use alone of the Michigan splint for improving active mouth opening and pain intensity in individuals with arthrogenous TMD. Some authors have proposed that this intervention can also be applied for reduction of TMJ disc, but there is no evidence for this hypothesis (Yabe et al., 2014).

For this technique, the patient lies supine. The clinician places the thumb of one hand on top of the back upper mandibular molars and the index finger on the inferior portion of the mandible. The clinician's other hand stabilizes the patient's head and the index and middle fingers palpate the TMJ (Figure 11.7). The clinician applies an inferior (distraction) force through the thumb and the

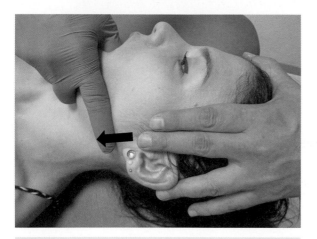

Figure 11.8
Mandibular distraction mobilization technique.

mobilization is performed using elbow extension or ulnar deviation (Figure 11.8). The patient's mouth should be relaxed during the technique; opening the mouth will decrease the effectiveness of the technique since an increase in stiffness of the TMJ can be perceived.

Anterior-to-posterior translation mobilization technique

Once the TMJ has been distracted and has less friction coefficient, an anterior-to-posterior translation mobilization can be performed to improve the gliding of the TMJ (Figure 11.9). This technique can be conducted with compression and/or distraction force with the aim of focusing on the upper or lower TMJ compartment. Additionally, given the more intimate relationship of the superior and inferior heads of the lateral pterygoid to the TMJ capsule, this mobilization may have an even stronger impact on this muscle, particularly the posterior translation of the mandible.

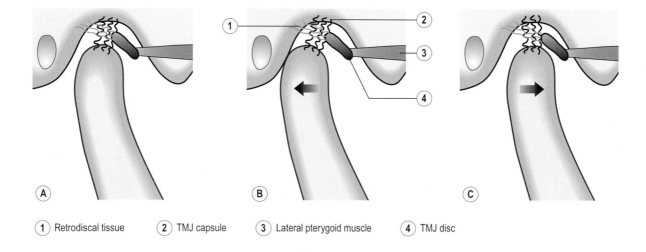

1 Retrodiscal tissue   2 TMJ capsule   3 Lateral pterygoid muscle   4 TMJ disc

Figure 11.9
Anterior-to-posterior gliding during the translation mobilization technique in a neutral position (A); posterior (B); and anterior (C) translation.

For this technique, the patient lies in supine. The contact is the same as for the distraction technique (see Figure 11.7). The clinician applies an anterior-to-posterior translation mobilization through the thumb contact (Figure 11.10).

Transverse medial accessory temporomandibular joint mobilization

A recent case series reported that the application of transverse medial accessory TMJ mobilization combined with education and advice was effective for reducing head and neck symptoms in patients with arthrogenous TMD (Grondin & Hall, 2017).

For this technique, the patient lies in supine. With one hand, the clinician contacts the lateral part of the mandibular condyle and mandibular ramus, and with the other hand provides a stabilizing force either through the contralateral zygomatic arch of the temporal bone and/or the contralateral mandibular condyle (Figure 11.11). A lateral-to-medial force is applied with the hand on the mandibular condyle.

This technique can be conducted with the patient's mouth open or closed.

A recapture technique for a displaced disc

The final objective of the TMJ mobilization is to recapture the displaced disc. The common technique to recapture the disc consists of pulling the condyle of the affected side downward and forward to locate the condyle on the anteriorly displaced disc (Miernik & Więckiewicz, 2015). It is difficult to predict the therapeutic effect of this mobilization since it depends not on the duration of locking, but rather on the stage of internal derangement. According to Pihut et al. (2013) the unlocking of the TMJ disc could be achieved in 71.8 per cent of patients who performed the active recapturing exercises. After successful unlocking of the disc, it is recommended that the subject be provided with an anterior repositioning splint to eliminate acoustic symptoms in the TMJ (Pihut et al., 2013).

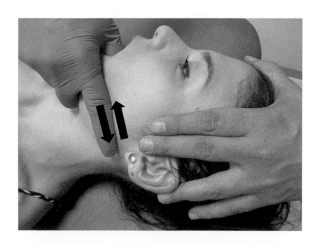

Figure 11.10
Anterior-to-posterior translation mobilization technique.

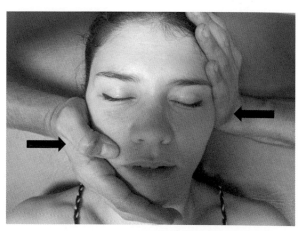

Figure 11.11
Transverse medial accessory temporomandibular joint mobilization.

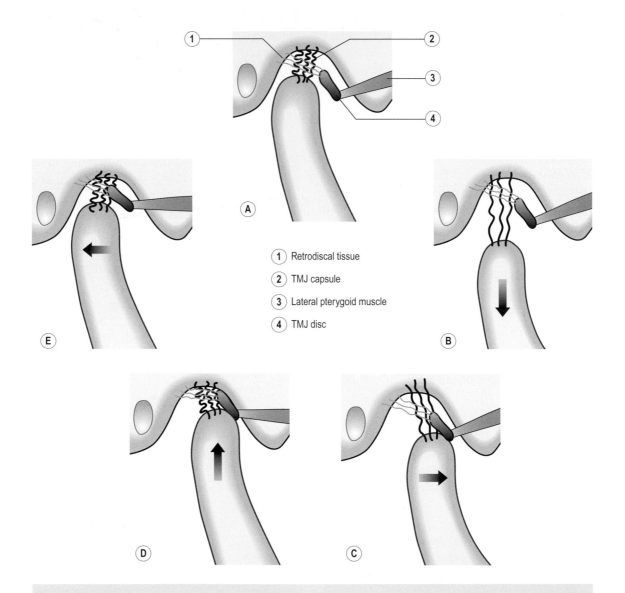

1. Retrodiscal tissue
2. TMJ capsule
3. Lateral pterygoid muscle
4. TMJ disc

Figure 11.12
Sequence of step for the recapture of a displaced disc. (A) Initial position. (B) Inferior gliding. (C) Anterior translation. (D) Compression. (E) Posterior translation.

For this technique, the patient lies in supine. The contact is the same as for the distraction technique (see Figure 11.7). First, the clinician applies an inferior force through the thumb; secondly, an anterior translation of the mandibular condyle is applied; thirdly, a compression force against the temporal fossa is applied; and, finally, maintaining the compression force, a posterior translation of the mandibular condyle is applied (Figures 11.12 and 11.13).

The disc recapturing may be also achieved not just by mandibular manipulation performed by the clinician as described, but also by active repositioning of the disc performed by the patient. In such a scenario, the anterior translation is actively performed by the patient, and not passively performed by the clinician.

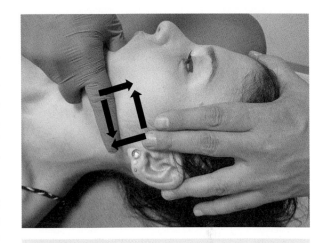

Figure 11.13
Recapture technique for a displaced disc.

References

Alves BM, Macedo CR, Januzzi E, Grossmann E, Atallah ÁN, Peccin S. Mandibular manipulation for the treatment of temporomandibular disorder. J Craniofac Surg 2013; 24: 488–493.

Armijo-Olivo S, Pitance L, Singh V, Neto F, Thie N, Michelotti A. Effectiveness of manual therapy and therapeutic exercise for temporomandibular disorder: Systematic review and meta-analysis. Phys Ther 2016; 96: 9–25.

Bortolazzo GL, Pires PF, Dibai-Filho AV, dos Santos Berni KC, Rodrigues BM, Rodrigues-Bigaton D. Effects of upper cervical manipulation on the electromyographic activity of the masticatory muscles and the opening range of motion of the mouth in women with temporomandibular disorder: randomized and blind clinical trial. Fisioter Pesqui 2015; 22: 426–434.

Butts R, Dunning J, Pavkovich R, Mettille J, Mourad F. Conservative management of temporomandibular dysfunction: a literature review with implications for clinical practice guidelines. J Bodyw Mov Ther 2017; 21: 541–548.

Calixtre LB, Moreira RF, Franchini GH, Alburquerque-Sendín F, Oliveria AB. Manual therapy for the management of pain and limited range of motion in subjects with signs and symptoms of temporomandibular disorder: a systematic review of randomized controlled trials. J Oral Rehabil 2015; 42: 847–861.

Carmeli E, Sheklow S, Bloomenfeld I. Comparative study of repositioning splint therapy and passive manual range of motion techniques for anterior displaced temporomandibular discs with unstable excursive reduction. Physiother 2001; 87, 26–36.

Cuccia AM, Caradonna C, Caradonna D. Manual therapy of the mandibular accessory ligaments for the management of temporomandibular joint disorders. J Am Osteopath Assoc 2011; 111: 102–112.

Furto ES, Cleland JA, Whitman JM, Olson KA. Manual physical therapy interventions and exercise for patients with temporomandibular disorders. Cranio 2006; 24: 283–291.

Grondin F, Hall T. Changes in cervical movement impairment and pain following orofacial treatment in patients with chronic arthralgic temporomandibular disorder with pain: a prospective case series. Physiother Theory Pract 2017; 33: 52–61.

Hengeveld E, Banks K, Wells P. Maitland's Peripheral Manipulation, 4th ed. Elsevier Health Sciences: London; 2005.

Ismail F, Demling A, Hessling K, Fink M, Stiesch-Scholz M. Short-term efficacy of physical therapy compared to splint therapy in treatment of arthrogenous TMD. J Oral Rehabil 2007; 34: 807–813.

Jayaseelan DJ, Tow NS. Cervicothoracic junction thrust manipulation in the multimodal management of a patient with temporomandibular disorder. J Man Manip Ther 2016; 24: 90–97.

Kranenburg HA, Schmitt MA, Puentedura EJ, Luijckx GJ, van der Schans CP. Adverse events associated with the use of cervical spine manipulation or mobilization and patient characteristics: a systematic review. Musculoskelet Sci Pract 2017; 28: 32–38.

La Touche R, Fernández-de-las-Peñas C, Fernández-Carnero J et al. The effects of manual therapy and exercise directed at the cervical spine on pain and pressure pain sensitivity in patients with myofascial temporomandibular disorders. J Oral Rehabil 2009; 36: 644–652.

La Touche R, París-Alemany A, Mannheimer JS et al. Does mobilization of the upper cervical spine affect pain sensitivity and autonomic nervous system function in patients with cervico-craniofacial pain? A randomized-controlled trial. Clin J Pain 2013; 29: 205–215.

Maitland GD. Vertebral Manipulation, 5th ed. Butterworth-Heinemann Medical; 1986.

Mansilla-Ferragut P, Fernández-de-las-Peñas C, Alburquerque-Sendín F, Cleland JA, Boscá-Gancía JJ. Immediate effects of atlanto-occipital joint manipulation on active mouth opening and pressure pain sensitivity in women with mechanical neck pain. J Manipulative Physiol Ther 2009; 32: 101–106.

Martins W, Blasczyk JC, Aparecida Furlan de Oliveira M et al. Efficacy of musculoskeletal manual approach in the treatment of temporomandibular joint disorder: a systematic review with meta-analysis. Man Ther 2016; 21: 10–17.

Miernik M, Więckiewicz W. The basic conservative treatment of temporomandibular joint anterior disc displacement without reduction – review. Adv Clin Exp Med 2015; 24: 731–735.

Mintken PE, DeRosa C, Little T, Smith B. AAOMPT clinical guidelines: a model for standardizing manipulation terminology in physical therapy practice. J Orthop Sports Phys Ther 2008; 38: A1-6.

Nicolakis P, Burak EC, Kollmitzer J, Kopf A, Piehslinger E, Wiesinger GF, Fialka-Moser V: An investigation of the effectiveness of exercise and manual therapy in treating symptoms of TMJ osteoarthritis. J Craniomandib Pract 2001; 19: 26–32.

Nielsen SM, Tarp S, Christensen R, Bliddal H, Klokker L, Henriksen M. The risk associated with spinal manipulation: an overview of reviews. Syst Rev 2017; 6: 64.

Oliveira-Campelo NM, Rubens-Rebelatto J, Martí N-Vallejo FJ, Alburquerque-Sendín F, Fernández-de-las-Peñas C. The immediate effects of atlanto-occipital joint manipulation and suboccipital muscle inhibition technique on active mouth opening and pressure pain sensitivity over latent myofascial trigger points in the masticatory muscles. J Orthop Sports Phys Ther 2010; 40: 310–317.

Packer AC, Pires PF, Dibai-Filho AV, Rodrigues-Bigaton D. Effects of upper thoracic manipulation on pressure pain sensitivity in women with temporomandibular disorder: a randomized, double-blind, clinical trial. Am J Phys Med Rehabil 2014; 93: 160–168.

Packer AC, Pires PF, Dibai-Filho AV, Rodrigues-Bigaton D. Effect of upper thoracic manipulation on mouth opening and electromyographic activity of masticatory muscles in women with temporomandibular disorder: a randomized clinical trial. J Manipulative Physiol Ther 2015; 38: 253–261.

Pihut M, Wiśniewska G, Majewski S. Active repositioning of temporomandibular disc displacement without reduction. J Stoma 2013; 66: 650–662.

Puentedura EJ, March J, Anders J, Perez A, Landers MR, Wallmann HW, Cleland JA. Safety of cervical spine manipulation: are adverse events preventable and are manipulations being performed appropriately? A review of 134 case reports. J Man Manip Ther 2012; 20: 66–74.

Sault JD, Emerson Kavchak AJ, Tow N, Courtney CA. Regional effects of orthopedic manual physical therapy in the successful management of chronic jaw pain. Cranio 2016; 34: 124–132.

Shaffer SM, Brismée JM, Sizer PS, Courtney CA. Temporomandibular disorders. Part 2: conservative management. J Man Manip Ther 2014; 22: 13–23.

Taylor M, Suvinen T, Reade P. The effect of Grade IV distraction mobilization on patients with temporomandibular pain-dysfunction disorder. Physiother Theory Pract 1994; 10: 129–136.

Yabe T, Tsuda T, Hirose S, Ozawa T, Kawai K. Treatment of acute temporomandibular joint dislocation using manipulation technique for disk displacement. J Craniofac Surg 2014; 25: 596–597.

Chapter 12

Manual therapy for myofascial trigger points in temporomandibular disorders

César Fernández-de-las-Peñas, María Palacios-Ceña

Evidence for the effectiveness of manual therapy in the treatment of trigger points

There are several interventions proposed for the management of trigger points (TrPs): dry needling, ultrasound, laser therapy, electrotherapy or manual therapies (Desai et al., 2013; Dommerholt & Fernández-de las-Peñas, 2013). Of these interventions, manual therapies are the most commonly used in the management of TMD (Wieckiewicz et al., 2015).

As explained in the previous chapters of this textbook, muscle tissue plays an important role in the genesis of TMD symptoms. Therefore, this chapter will focus on the different manual approaches that may be used to inactivate myofascial TrPs within the masticatory musculature. Several manual therapies are suggested in the literature for the treatment of muscle TrPs: ischemic compression, TrP pressure release, massage, passive stretching, myofascial induction (see Chapter 13), spray and stretch, muscle energy techniques, and neuromuscular approaches (Simons et al., 1999, Dommerholt & McEvoy, 2011; Shah et al., 2015).

Several systematic reviews investigating the effectiveness of manual therapies have concluded that there is moderate to strong evidence supporting the use of manual pressure interventions for immediate pain relief of TrPs, but limited evidence exists for long-term pain relief (Fernández-de-las-Peñas et al., 2005; Rickards, 2006; Vernon & Schneider, 2009). These results were confirmed in a meta-analysis concluding that muscle manual therapies had a favorable effect on pressure-pain sensitivity when compared with no-treatment and sham groups and comparable effects when compared with other active treatments (Gay et al., 2013). This conclusion was further supported by another meta-analysis showing that the pain relief obtained with ischemic compression was greater than that obtained through active range of motion exercises and placebo interventions, but similar to other therapeutic approaches (Cagnie et al., 2015). A recent meta-analysis also reported a moderate effect size improvement in mouth opening following soft tissue interventions; however, this effect was based on two studies conducted on subjects diagnosed with latent TrPs in the masseter, which does not represent patients commonly seen in clinical practice (Webb & Rajendran, 2016). In fact, it is interesting to note that TrP manual therapy does not exhibit tolerance to repetitive applications since single and multiple applications decreased the sensitivity to pressure at the TrP area (Moraska et al., 2017).

As discussed in Chapter 10, there is enough evidence to support the use of manual therapy in the management of TMD. Briefly and in relation to soft tissue interventions, Calixtre et al. (2015) found low to moderate evidence supporting that myofascial release and massage over the masticatory muscles were more effective than placebo for the management of patients with TMD. Armijo-Olivo et al. (2016) concluded that manual therapy alone or combined with exercises showed promising benefits for TMD, although effect sizes were low to moderate and related to the type of TMD. Finally, the meta-analysis conducted by Martins et al. (2016) also showed significant differences and large clinical effects on active mouth opening and on pain during mouth opening favoring musculoskeletal manual techniques compared to other conservative treatments for TMD. Nevertheless, it is difficult to draw firm clinical conclusions from current evidence since most studies had investigated single modalities for TMD, whereas multimodal approaches are commonly used in clinical practice.

There are clinical studies demonstrating the effectiveness of the inclusion of TrP techniques in multimodal manual therapy protocols for the management of some chronic pain conditions. Kim et al. (2013) demonstrated that the application of ischemic compression after TrP injection was more effective than TrP injection alone for TrPs in the upper trapezius muscle. This assumption is also supported by a recent meta-analysis concluding that exercise has small to moderate effects on pain intensity in the short term in people with myofascial pain and that a combination of different types of exercise seems to achieve greater benefits (Mata Díz et al., 2017). It is becoming clear that manual TrP techniques should be combined with other manual therapy interventions, including neuroscience education and exercises.

Manual therapy in the management of trigger points

There are several types of soft tissue intervention that can be used in the management of TrPs in the masticatory musculature (Miernik et al., 2012). Clinicians should select the appropriate technique based on the clinical presentation of the patient and the patient's preferences.

Compression interventions

Different compression techniques have been described with variations on the amount of pressure, duration of application, position of the muscle (shortened or lengthened), or presence or absence of pain during the intervention. In clinical practice, the pressure level, duration of application, and position of the muscle are determined based on the sensitization mechanisms of the patient and the degree of irritability of the tissue. In a patient with a low degree of sensitization, more intense and/or painful techniques

may be applied. Simons (2002) proposed that compressing the sarcomeres by direct pressure in a vertical or perpendicular manner combined with active contraction of the affected muscle may equalize the length of the sarcomeres in the TrP and consequently decrease the pain; however, this notion has not been scientifically investigated (Dommerholt & Shah, 2010). Other hypotheses suggest that pain relief from direct pressure may result from reactive hyperemia within the TrP or a spinal reflex mechanism for the relief of muscle tension (Hou et al., 2002).

One of the compression techniques applied over TrPs that has been most expanded on is known as 'ischemic compression' (Simons et al., 1999). With the muscle in a lengthened position, the clinician applies pressure to the TrP until the sensation of pressure becomes painful. At the moment of pain occurrence, the pressure is maintained until the pain level is eased by around 50–75 per cent, as perceived by the patient under treatment, at which moment the pressure is increased until discomfort or pain appears again. This process is usually repeated for 90 seconds (Simons et al., 1999). There is no consensus as to how much pressure should be applied or for how long for this technique. Hou et al. (2002) found that low pressure below the pain threshold for a prolonged period (90 seconds) and high pressure over the pain threshold (pain tolerance) for a shorter period (30 seconds) were equally effective for decreasing pressure pain sensitivity over TrPs. Gay et al. (2013) found that the perceived intensity of pressure applied during muscle-biased techniques may be an important parameter for a positive effect. This positive effect may be related to the fact that inducing a tolerable amount of pain during treatment may activate the conditioned pain modulation, also known as diffuse noxious inhibitory control (Gay et al., 2013). In clinical practice, the pressure level used is dependent on the sensitization mechanisms of the patient, the degree of irritability of the TrP, and the patient's preferences and expectations.

Some clinicians have proposed the use of the 'TrP pressure release technique' instead of ischemic compression (Lewit, 1999). This technique consists of an application of pressure over the TrP until an increase in muscle resistance (tissue barrier) is perceived by the clinician (Lewit, 1999). The pressure is maintained until the clinician perceives a release of the taut band. At this stage the pressure is increased to return to the previous level of muscle tension and the process is repeated for 90 seconds. In most subjects, the muscle tension is usually perceived by the clinician before painful perception, thereby resulting in a pain-free technique (Lewit, 1999).

Massage therapy

Massage is performed along the taut band (longitudinal strokes) or across the taut band (transverse strokes) (Miernik et al., 2012). Hong et al. (1993) reported that deep tissue massage was more effective for decreasing pressure pain sensitivity than spray and stretch and other manual therapies. It has been hypothesized that massage may exert a lengthening effect similar to compression techniques when applied over a TrP (Hong et al., 1993; Simons, 2002). For instance, transverse friction massage offers a transverse mobilization to the taut band, whereas stroking may offer a longitudinal mobilization of the taut band. In muscles where pincer palpation is being applied, the therapist's fingers should grasp the taut band from both sides of the TrP area, stroking centrifugally and elongating away from the TrP (Simons, 2002).

Stretching interventions

There are many methods of applying a stretching procedure: passive stretching (where the clinician passively stretches the muscle without participation of the patient), active stretching (where the patient actively stretches the muscle without participation of the clinician), spray and stretch, or postisometric relaxation (Hong et al., 1993; Simons et al., 1999;

Lewit, 1999). In the orofacial region, it is important to keep in mind that patients with benign hypermobility should not perform any stretching exercises, as stretching will most likely contribute to increased laxity in connective tissue and ligaments without any positive effect on muscles, taut bands, and TrPs.

Hong et al. (1993) demonstrated that spray and stretch showed immediate positive effects on pressure pain sensitivity and was more effective when combined with deep pressure massage. Hou et al. (2002) found that the application of spray and stretch in combination with other modalities was more effective for inactivating TrPs. Emad et al. (2012) showed that TrP injections combined with stretching was more effective than TrP injections alone for reducing pain. Again, stretching interventions should be used as a part of multimodal therapeutic approaches, and not just as isolated treatment.

Dynamic interventions

As TrPs are located in active muscle tissues, dynamic interventions, which involve contraction or stretching of the affected muscle at the same time as clinicians apply the manual technique, may be extremely helpful. For instance, during TrP manual compression, the patient is asked to actively contract the affected muscle (Gröbli & Dejung, 2003). During longitudinal stroking, the patient may also be asked to actively move the area (Gröbli & Dejung, 2003). An active contraction may increase the stretching over the shortened sarcomeres (Simons, 2002). The mechanisms of dynamic techniques are still unknown, but may be related to activation of intrafascial mechanoreceptors.

Clinical application of manual therapy over trigger points

In this section, different TrP manual therapies are described in relation to the various masticatory muscles. The featured techniques are not exclusive and

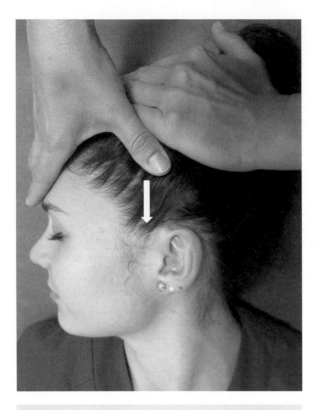

Figure 12.1
Longitudinal strokes applied to the taut band of the temporalis. The arrow shows the direction of the strokes.

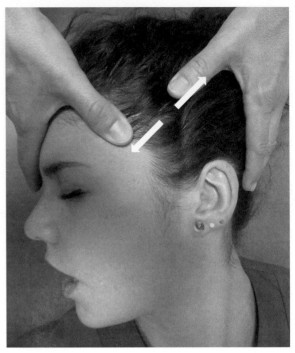

Figure 12.2
Dynamic longitudinal strokes applied to the taut band of the temporalis. The arrow shows the direction of the strokes.

are not the only possibilities. Clinicians are encouraged to develop other techniques based on established principles. The selection of techniques will depend on the irritability of TrPs, the sensitization of the patient's central nervous system and the patient's preferences.

Manual therapy for the temporal muscle

TrPs in the temporal muscle or temporalis refer pain to the head and/or the teeth in individuals with tension-type headache (Fernández-de-las-Peñas et al., 2007) or TMD (Fernández-de-las-Peñas et al., 2010). This is an important muscle responsible for dynamic control of the TMJ. In the authors' clinical practice, the application of longitudinal strokes to the temporalis is extremely useful for relaxing TrP taut bands without increasing tension in the TMJ. Longitudinal strokes are usually performed with the thumb from a cranial to caudal direction (Figure 12.1). The degree of pressure applied is determined by the feedback reported by the patient or the tension felt within the patient's tissue. If the patient has an exquisitely tender TrP or a tender taut band, a dynamic longitudinal stroke may be applied. In such a scenario, the clinician's thumbs are placed at both sides of the TrP and a divergent longitudinal stroke is be applied at the same time as the patient slowly opens the mouth (Figure 12.2).

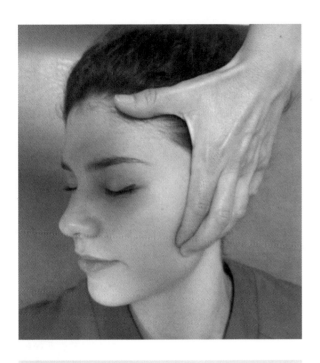

Figure 12.3
Transverse friction applied to the taut band of
the masseter.

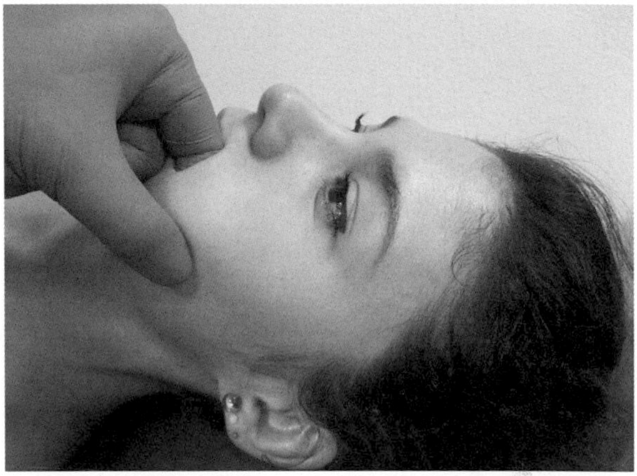

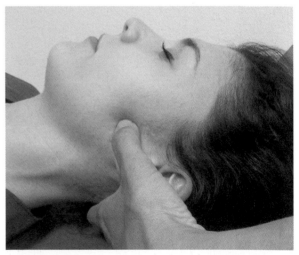

Figure 12.4
Intraoral pincer compession applied to the taut
band of the masseter.

Figure 12.5
Compression applied to the taut band of the
deep masseter.

Manual therapy for the masseter muscle

The masseter muscle refers pain to the teeth or deep into the TMJ in patients with TMD (Fernández-de-las-Peñas et al., 2010). It can also refer pain to the eyebrow in patients with tension-type headache (Simons et al., 1999).

The masseter has high-density connective tissue architecture, and it is divided into deep and superficial parts. Therefore, direct techniques, such as transverse friction massage, can be applied to the superficial part of the muscle (Figure 12.3). In addition, intraoral compression of superficial masseter TrPs may also be applied; this technique is performed with a pincer palpation (Figure 12.4). The deep part of the masseter is located at the most posterior part of the zygomatic bone, just in front of the TMJ. At this point, a manual compression technique may be applied (Figure 12.5).

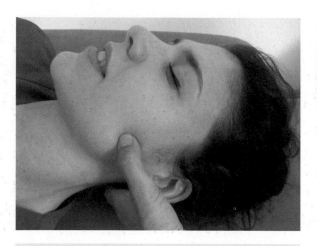

Figure 12.6
Compression and contraction applied to the taut band of the masseter.

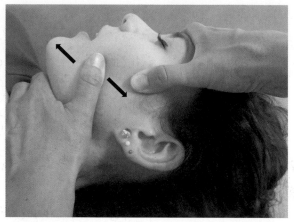

Figure 12.7
Dynamic longitudinal strokes applied to the taut band of the masseter. The arrows show the direction of the strokes.

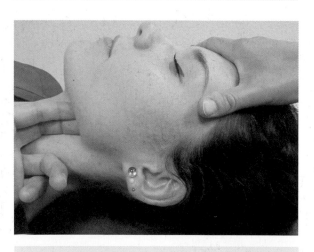

Figure 12.8
Compression applied to the lower part of the medial pterygoid.

Dynamic techniques, such as compression and contraction, may also be applied to the masseter. This technique combines a manual compression with an active contraction of the compressed muscle

(Gröbli & Dejung, 2003). For the masseter, manual compression is applied over the TrP and the patient is asked to clench the teeth (Figure 12.6). A dynamic longitudinal or transverse stroke is also applied. For this technique, the clinician applies longitudinal or transverse strokes over the TrP taut band with both thumbs from a cranial (zygomatic) to caudal (mandible) direction and at the same time the patient opens the mouth (Figure 12.7).

Manual therapy for the medial pterygoid muscle

The medial pterygoid is the main agonist of the masseter during mouth closing with the temporalis. The referred pain elicited by TrPs in this muscle is perceived inside the TMJ, ear, and some parts of the mouth (Simons et al., 1999). This muscle is difficult to access with manual palpation, but the lower part can be reached at the inferior border of the mandible angle. In this anatomical area, a static compression is applied with two fingers (Figure 12.8). For the middle part, intraoral contact is needed. The patient opens the mouth and the clinician's index finger contacts

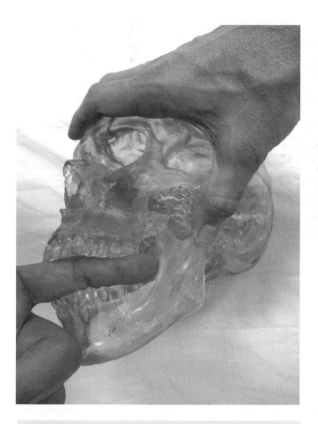

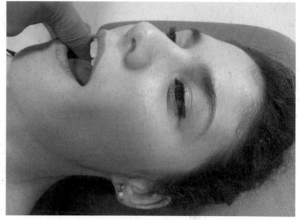

Figure 12.10

Intraoral compression of the middle part of the medial pterygoid.

Figure 12.9

Intraoral contact for compression applied to the middle part of the medial pterygoid.

the middle part of the medial pterygoid between the dental arcades (Figure 12.9). In this position, a static compression is applied (Figure 12.10).

Manual therapy for the lateral pterygoid muscle

The lateral pterygoid is an important muscle for movement and control of the jaw since it is anatomically attached to the TMJ disc, particularly the superior head (Usui et al., 2008). TrPs in the lateral pterygoid may refer pain in and around the maxillary sinus and deep into the TMJ (Simons et al., 1999). Manual palpation of the lateral pterygoid is

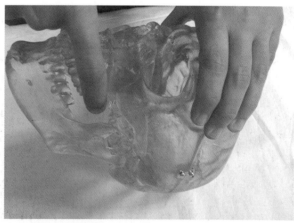

Figure 12.11

Intraoral contact for compression applied to the lateral pterygoid.

a controversial issue due to its anatomical location (Turp & Minagi, 2001). A recent study has confirmed that palpation of the anterior area of the muscle is feasible (Stelzenmueller et al., 2016). The lateral pterygoid can be palpated using intraoral contact in the cheek. The index finger of the clinician palpates along the oral vestibule parallel to the upper section of the alveolar process of the maxilla, onto the maxillary tuberosity, until the lateral plate of the pterygoid process is reached (Figure 12.11). In this position, a manual compression is applied (Figure 12.12). A stretching compression technique combining compression with an active stretching of the muscle can also be applied. From the same palpation position, the patient can be asked to perform active mandible retraction, which will stretch the lateral pterygoid.

Manual therapy for the suprahyoid muscles

The anterior neck muscles, particularly the suprahyoid musculature, participate in the overall stability of the cervical spine, provide support for swallowing, and are involved in mastication. In general, TrPs in the suprahyoid muscle contribute to pain in multiple areas including the anterior neck, larynx, tongue, and lower facial area. The digastric muscle is probably the muscle most accessible for

palpation and is therefore the main target of our techniques. A direct compression technique may be applied to the anterior (Figure 12.13) or posterior (Figure 12.14) belly of the muscle. Care should be taken when palpating the posterior belly as it is a highly sensitive anatomical area. When the sensitivity has decreased, dynamic transverse strokes may be applied to the suprahyoid musculature. For this technique, the clinician contacts bilaterally with both digastric muscles and applies strokes over the inferior border of the mandible (transverse strokes in relation to the anatomical attachments of the suprahyoid muscles) (Figure 12.15).

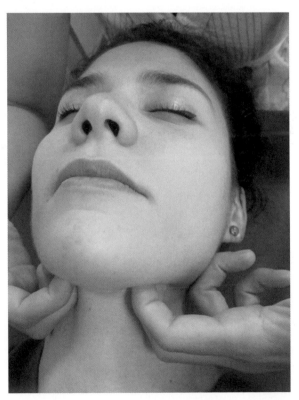

Figure 12.13
Compression applied to the taut band of the anterior part of the digastric muscle.

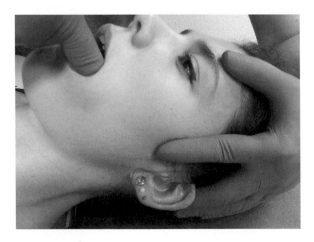

Figure 12.12
Intraoral compression applied to the lateral pterygoid.

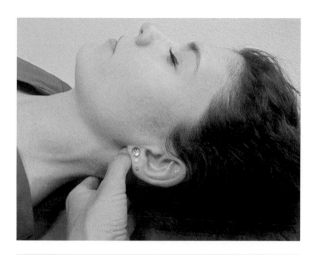

Figure 12.14
Compression applied to the taut band of the posterior part of the digastric muscle.

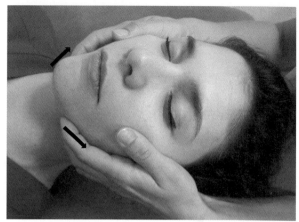

Figure 12.15
Dynamic longitudinal strokes applied to the suprahyoid musculature. The arrows show the direction of the strokes.

Conclusion

There are several manual therapies that can be used to inactivate myofascial TrPs in the masticatory muscles. Current evidence supports the use of a single application of manual therapy; however, manual therapy is usually part of a multimodal approach to pain relief. Some trials have reported the effectiveness of the inclusion of TrP manual therapy in different multimodal approaches for treating chronic pain. Clinicians should choose the appropriate manual therapy technique according to the characteristics of the patient.

References

Armijo-Olivo S, Pitance L, Singh V, Neto F, Thie N, Michelotti A. Effectiveness of manual therapy and therapeutic exercise for temporomandibular disorder: Systematic review and meta-analysis. Phys Ther 2016; 96: 9–25.

Cagnie B, Castelein B, Pollie F, Steelant L, Verhoeyen H, Cools A. Evidence for the use of ischemic compression and dry needling in the management of trigger points of the upper trapezius in patients with neck pain: a systematic review. Am J Phys Med Rehabil 2015; 94: 573–583.

Calixtre LB, Moreira RF, Franchini GH, Alburquerque-Sendín F, Oliveria AB. Manual therapy for the management of pain and limited range of motion in subjects with signs and symptoms of temporomandibular disorder: a systematic review of randomized controlled trials. J Oral Rehabil 2015; 42: 847–861.

Desai MJ, Saini V, Saini S. Myofascial pain syndrome: a treatment review. Pain Ther 2013; 2: 21–36.

Dommerholt J, Fernández-de-las-Peñas C. Trigger Point Dry Needling: An Evidence and Clinical-Based Approach. 1st ed. London: Churchill Livingstone: Elsevier; 2013.

Dommerholt J, McEvoy J. Myofascial trigger point release approach. In: Wise CH (ed.). Orthopaedic Manual Physical Therapy: From Art to Evidence. Philadelphia: FA Davis; 2011.

Dommerholt J, Shah J Myofascial pain syndrome. In Ballantyne JC, Rathmell JP, Fishman SM (eds). Bonica's Management of Pain. Baltimore: Lippincott, Williams & Williams; 2010, pp. 450–471.

Emad MR, Roshanzamir S, Ghasempoor MZ, Sedghat SMP. Effectiveness of stretching after trigger point injections. J Musculoskel Res 2012; 14: 1250002.

Fernández-de-las-Peñas C, Sohrbeck-Campo M, Fernández J, Miangolarra-Page JC.

Manual therapies in myofascial trigger point treatment: a systematic review. J Bodyw Mov Ther 2005; 9: 27–34.

Fernández-de-las-Peñas C, Ge H, Arendt-Nielsen L, Cuadrado ML, Pareja JA. The local and referred pain from myofascial trigger points in the temporalis muscle contributes to pain profile in chronic tension-type headache. Clin J Pain 2007; 23: 786–792.

Fernández-de-las-Peñas C, Galán-Del-Río F, Alonso-Blanco C et al. Referred pain from muscle trigger points in the masticatory and neck-shoulder musculature in women with temporomandibular disorders. J Pain 2010; 11: 1295–1304.

Gay CW, Alappattu MJ, Coronado RA, Horn ME, Bishop MD. Effect of a single session of muscle-biased therapy on pain sensitivity: a systematic review and meta-analysis of randomized controlled trials. J Pain Res 2013; 6: 7–22.

Gröbli C, Dejung B. Nichtmedikamentöse Therapie myofaszialer Schmerze. Schmerz 2003; 17: 475–480.

Hong CZ, Chen YC, Pon CH, Yu J. Immediate effects of various physical medicine modalities on pain threshold of an active myofascial trigger point. Journal of Musculoskeletal Pain 1993; 1 (1): 37–53.

Hou CR, Tsai LC, Cheng KF et al. Immediate effects of various physical therapeutic modalities on cervical myofascial pain and trigger-point sensitivity. Arch Phys Med Rehabil 2002; 83: 1406–1414.

Kim SA, Oh KY, Choi WH, Kim IK. Ischemic compression after trigger point injection affects the treatment of myofascial trigger points. Ann Rehabil Med 2013; 37: 541–546.

Lewit K. Manipulative therapy in rehabilitation of the locomotor system. 3rd ed. Oxford: Butterworth Heinemann; 1999.

Martins W, Blasczyk JC, Aparecida Furlan de Oliveira M et al. Efficacy of musculoskeletal manual approach in the treatment of temporomandibular joint disorder: a systematic review with meta-analysis. Man Ther 2016; 21: 10–17.

Mata Díz JB, de Souza J, Leopoldino A, Oliveira V. Exercise, especially combined stretching and strengthening exercise, reduces myofascial pain: a systematic review. J Physiother 2017; 63: 17–22.

Miernik M, Wieckiewicz M, Paradowska A, Wieckiewicz W. Massage therapy in myofascial TMD pain management. Adv Clin Exp Med 2012; 21: 681–685.

Moraska AF, Schmiege SJ, Mann JD, Butryn N, Krutsch JP. Responsiveness of myofascial trigger points to single and multiple trigger point release massages: a randomized, placebo-controlled trial. Am J Phys Med Rehabil 2017; 96: 639–645.

Rickards LD. The effectiveness of non-invasive treatments for active myofascial trigger point pain: a systematic review of the literature. Int J Osteopathic Med 2006; 9: 120–136.

Shah JP, Thaker N, Heimur J, Aredo JV, Sikdar S, Gerbet L. Myofascial trigger points then and now: a historical and scientific perspective. PM R 2015; 7: 746–761.

Simons DG. Understanding effective treatments of myofascial trigger points. J Bodyw Mov Ther 2002; 6: 81–88.

Simons DG, Travell JG, Simons LS. Travell & Simons' Myofascial Pain & Dysfunction: The Trigger Point Manual. Vol. 1: Upper Half of Body. Baltimore: Williams & Wilkins; 1999.

Stelzenmueller W, Umstadt H, Weber D, Goenner-Oezkan V, Kopp S, Lisson J. Evidence - the intraoral palpability of the lateral pterygoid muscle - a prospective study. Ann Anat 2016; 206: 89–95.

Turp JC, Minagi S. Palpation of the lateral pterygoid region in TMD: where is the evidence? J Dent 2001; 29: 475–483.

Usui A, Akita K, Yamaguchi K. An anatomic study of the divisions of the lateral pterygoid muscle based on the findings of the origins and insertions. Surg Radiol Anat 2008; 30: 327–333.

Vernon H, Schneider M. Chiropractic management of myofascial trigger points and myofascial pain syndrome: a systematic review of the literature. J Manipul Physiol Ther 2009; 32: 14–24.

Webb TR, Rajendran D. Myofascial techniques: what are their effects on joint range of motion and pain? - A systematic review and meta-analysis of randomised controlled trials. J Bodyw Mov Ther 2016; 20: 682–699.

Wieckiewicz M, Boening K, Wiland P, Shiau YY, Paradowska-Stolarz A. Reported concepts for the treatment modalities and pain management of temporomandibular disorders. J Headache Pain 2015; 16: 106.

Chapter 13

Myofascial induction approaches in temporomandibular disorders

Andrzej Pilat, Eduardo Castro-Martín

Introduction

Definition

The American Association of Orofacial Pain (AAOP) defines temporomandibular disorder (TMD) as 'a collective term embracing a number of clinical problems that involve the masticatory musculature, TMJ and associated structures, or both' (McNeill, 1990). The AAOP classification divides TMD broadly into 2 syndromes: 1, muscle-related TMD (myogenous TMD), sometimes called TMD secondary to myofascial pain and dysfunction; and 2, joint-related (arthrogenous) TMD, or TMD secondary to 'true' articular disease (Schiffman & Ohrbach, 2016); however, it is difficult to draw a line between both syndromes and generally both coexist in a majority of patients. Readers are referred to Chapter 2 of the current textbook for further data on TMD classification.

Relevant anatomical aspects

The difficulties in an accurate classification are related to the specific anatomical characteristics of the TMJ:

1. It is the only joint of the human body that, being bilateral and symmetrical, involves a *single bone* (the mandible) which in turn is articulated with the two temporal bones.

2. It is located in front of the ear canal on both sides of the head, which will determine its design, related to the protection of the auditory system. In fact, the axis of TMJ movement during opening/closing of the mouth, is not performed within the joint. It is separated approximately 4-6 cm from the posterior condyle of the mandible.

3. It is a synovial joint; however, its dynamics are not usually analyzed, as in other synovial joints, in the assessment from global body movement.

4. The articular surfaces of the mandibular fossa and the maxilla head are incongruent, which requires the presence of a disc for proper functioning of the joint. This disc fills the space between two articular surfaces and through its continuous *deformation*, adapts to the needs of the joint movement.

5. The TMJ and its related structures receive their innervation from the first three cervical roots (C1-C3) and up to five cranial nerves (V, VII, IX, X and XII). Few anatomical locations receive this much attention of the nervous system to perform their function.

Based on these findings, it can be concluded that dysfunction of one TMJ will affect the contralateral one triggering potential bilateral symptoms. Thus, even a small dysfunction in either joint will generate the need for extensive adjustments in all components of the masticatory system, in order to maintain optimum functionality.

It is often difficult to determine the precise cause of TMD, as well as establish the diagnosis, and clinical behavior is challenging. Even so, TMD is a common diagnosis and affects a large part of the population (Proffit et al., 1980). The symptoms are varied and include pain, tenderness, spasm of the masticatory muscles and changes in the resting jaw position. It is considered that the most common causes of TMD are muscle dysfunctions, due to para-functional activities, hyperactivity or malocclusion of varying degrees. Therefore, considering the singularity of the masticatory system, it is interesting to investigate how the central nervous system coordinates the sophisticated complex. In recent years, research on the fascia has provided interesting information on this issue and will be discussed in this chapter.

Chapter 13

Controversies in definition

In the last ten years, the research related to the temporomandibular area has been increasing, gathering almost 8000 scientific publications (PubMed, US National Library of Medicine National Institutes of Health). Generally, the analysis focuses on the unit of the mandibula–cervical spine–skull 'comprised of the head, neck and jaw, considering the dynamic interaction and the close relationship that exists between its components' (Rocabado, 1983). Thus, proper understanding of the prevalence, potential etiologies, natural progression and treatment of TMD focuses both on the position of the head and the orthostatic stability of the skull on the cervical spine, as a whole.

However, despite the availability of extensive research related to the TMJ, there is no clear advance in the understanding of the TMJ's dynamics, such as in biting, biting, chewing, swallowing, talking, facial expression and breathing. The complexity of TMJ performance and its ability to adapt to a changing biomechanical environment is manifested, for example, in occlusion. In this task, which involves six axes of movement, co-activated by sixteen groups of muscles, the forces generated between the teeth, depending on the functional demands, range from small precise to large crushing dental contacts. Further, there could even be infinite patterns of muscle co-activation to produce an accurate occlusion (Peck, 2016). Nevertheless, certain aspects of the TMJ complex remain controversial:

1. Although the TMJ is widely known to function under compression (Kang & Yi, 2000; Okeson, 2013; Isberg, 2001), the two bone components of this joint are deformed in different ways during the same movements. Compression is present in the mandibular condyle (with fine trabeculae oriented vertically), and traction within the temporal eminence (with transversely oriented trabeculae) (Herring & Liu, 2001).

2. The amount of optimal compression during mastication is not clearly defined (Scarr & Harrison, 2016), despite the systematization of the electromyographic studies of the masticatory muscles (Chaves et al., 2017; Matsuda et al., 2016). The approach is usually analytical without an integrated functional conclusion.

3. There are discrepancies on the function of the ligaments and other periarticular structures (Bag et al., 2014; Lobbezoo et al., 2004; Koolstra, 2002). It is assumed that they are passive limiting devices to restrict joint movement (Okeson, 2013). On the contrary, other authors suggest their dynamic attitude (van der Wal, 2009). One of the examples of this controversy is represented by the behavior of the retrodiscal tissue (Coombs et al., 2017). It is described as a structure of loose connective tissue with long elastic fibers, richly innervated and vascularized, that acts as an anchor against the excessive forward slip of the disc (Westesson et al., 1989; Langendoen et al., 1997); it means just having a passive action. However, the ligament also participates in repositioning of the disc during mouth closing to return the mandible to its starting position, a potential key action to prevent dislocation. The kinetic discharge, due its previous stretching, is frequently performed by the connective tissue in coordination with the contractile elements (Pilat, 2015).

4. The influence of hyperlaxity in relation to TMJ dysfunctions is unclear. It has been suggested that this laxity facilitates the formation of dysfunctions (Khan & Pedlar, 1996; Ögren et al., 2012); however, others showed that this association was not clear (Dijkstra et al., 2002; Pasinato et al., 2011).

5. Manfredini et al. (2017) suggest discarding the occlusion paradigm as a hypothesis in the pathophysiology of TMD, while others maintain this relationship (Bilgiç & Gelgör, 2017; Michelotti et al., 2016).

Temporomandibular disorders and central sensitization

The main reason for the consultation and the primary concern for individuals with TMD is pain. An erroneous processing of nociceptive sensory input is an essential factor in central nervous system dysfunctions associated with chronic TMD (readers are referred to Chapter 6 of this textbook for further information on this topic). In recent years, research on chronic pain has focused on central sensitization mechanisms (La Touche et al., 2017). It is considered that the neuropeptides and other inflammatory mediators such as tumor necrosis factor, interleukins, or cytokines, in the joint environment, can stimulate a peripheral response accompanied by a neurogenic inflammation that causes hyperexcitability of the nervous system and hypersensitivity.

This situation may lead to hyperactivity and synaptic changes at the spinal and central level, including the decrease in gray matter volume in the anterior and posterior cingulate cortex, in the insula, in the anterior frontal and in the superior temporal gyrus. Likewise, functional and structural changes in the thalamus, basal ganglia and primary somatosensory cortex can, in consequence, cause central sensitization. In this way, the central processes of pain, cognitive-behavioral and emotional aspects, would be altered. The presence of spinal and central hyperexcitability in patients with TMD has been documented in previous papers (Milam et al., 1998; Fernández-de-las-Peñas et al., 2009; Gerstner et al., 2011; Ichesco et al., 2012; Lin, 2014; La Touche et al., 2017).

The issues raised so far, as well as the neurological implications, including the latest findings in relation to central sensitization, force clinicians to locate TMDs beyond the TMJ itself and to extend the concept to the perception of a system.

Temporomandibular disorders and the systemic approach

It seems that the craniomandibular region represents an extremely precise system in which all parts and processes are perfectly coordinated. We define a system as 'an ordered set of elements in interaction, to achieve a certain objective'. The objectives are the intrinsic reasons of the system and constitute the aspect that integrates all its parts. The alteration of one part of the system will affect the others and, therefore, will change the behavior of the whole system. A body system assembles different types of elements with diverse activities (subsystems) that are associated with other subsystems, through an uninterrupted and innervated structure of functional stability, that is, the three-dimensional collagenous matrix that is the fascia.

The TMJ as the biological entity manifests itself as a complex biological system, in which the total is not equal to the sum of its parts. The communication capacities of subunits (subsystems) are essential for the evolution of the system, since without such capacities this paradigm of systemic functioning cannot be implemented. It is suggested that the model that fulfills the proposed objectives is the biotensegrity model.

Biotensegrity from the temporomandibular disorder perspective

Biotensegrity concept

Biotensegrity is a concept previously adopted in the analysis of human body structures such as the shoulder (Levin, 1997), spine (Levin, 2002), pelvis (Levin, 2007; Pardehshenas et al., 2014), skull (Scarr, 2008), elbow (Scarr, 2012), knee (Hakkak et al., 2015), foot (Wilson & Kiely, 2016) and the TMJ itself (Scarr & Harrison, 2017). The term 'tensegrity' defines a structural organization, in the form of 'tensional integrity.' The architect and philosopher Richard

Buckminster Fuller defined the pattern in the early 1950s, with the collaboration of the sculptor Kenneth Snelson.

An example of tensegrity is an assemblage of 'wires' (extensible elements subject to tensile forces) and 'bars' (rigid elements subject to compression), in which the wires form an uninterrupted external network linking the ends of the bars, internally located (Motro, 2003). The tensegrity structures are characterized by a remarkable stability either in static or dynamic behavior; a force applied at any one vertex is transmitted to all the others, and equally with deformations (Scarr, 2014; Gordon, 1978) (Figure 13.1).

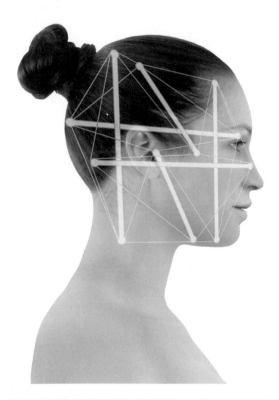

Figure 13.1
The biotensegrity model.

Emphasized by Fuller, as a universal principle of organization, tensegrity attracted the attention of biologist Donald Ingber (1998). According to Ingber, the structure of the cell follows the tensegrity principles, allowing the cell to assume different forms according to its position, function, destiny, and proper adaptation to the environment. When applying the tensegrity concept to living organisms, for example the human body, the term biotensegrity is frequently used.

Thus, rising to a higher level in the body hierarchy, it is evident that a model inspired on tensegrity can describe the anatomy of a joint, reproducing the conditions which allow the bones to 'float', one relative to the other without touching, while the surrounding tissues are integrated into the 'fascia', the functional unit that also involves the organs and the whole organism (Scarr, 2014; Levin, 2006).

It is proposed that the fascia can be considered as the tensegritic organism of the human body with the aim of guaranteeing and maintaining structural and functional integrity; therefore, it should be the focus of the primary objective of therapeutic attention (Huijing & Baan, 2003). The craniomandibular region represents a deformable structure that receives continuous charges and discharges, acting in favor of and against gravitational force. The movements of the TMJ are carried out in different axes, they require stability and, at the same time, a great adaptive capacity. This emphasizes the prompt response coordinated by the central nervous system during mastication or phonation, in the continuous search for stability.

In the TMJ biotensegrity model, the tensile reactivity is provided by ligaments, musculature, connective tissue matrix, blood vessels, and articular discs, which ensure strength, integrity and pre-stress; whereas compression is secured by the bones and fluids enclosed in the compartments. Therefore, advantages of the concept of the TMJ biotensegrity system includes:

1. Stability: Associated with the whole system and not just with a single element, which allows an efficient process of adjustments.

2. Dynamic coherence: the joint's dynamic components (ligaments, joint capsules, aponeurosis) are under continuous tension (required to maintain movements' independence).

3. Selectivity: the continuous adjustment process allows bone dynamics to be independent (demands due to musculotendinous and fascial tensions) of the intra-articular disc dynamics. In this way, it can act selectively (for example phonation) or with a related overall task (for example cervico-cranial-mandibular concomitance).

4. Multifunctionality: functional optimization and inherent stability.

Synergism in TMJ biomechanics

The biotensegrity model moves away from the structural one. In fact, studies focusing on the dynamic stability between the neck and TMJ open new perspectives (Solow & Tallgren, 1976; Higbie et al., 1999; Visscher et al., 2000; Ohmure et al., 2008; La Touche et al., 2011; Moon & Lee, 2011). The systemic approach based on biotensegrity focuses on a three-dimensional global movement model, based on synergisms of the whole system, rather than just on the 'head-neck-jaw' structure of muscular balance. For instance:

1. In cervical extension, the mouth tends to open, the hyoid rises (modifying its behavior), the occlusal plane rises and the dental contacts are posteriorized (occlusal disorder that responds to the central nervous system requesting the masticatory muscles). If a cervical flexion posture is adopted (when looking at the ground), the opposite occurs. With cervical lateroflexion the occlusal plane is tilted, following the craniocervical and atlas plane tilt.

2. Cephalic protrusion involves mouth opening and mandibular retraction while the disc is positioned anteriorly. Consequently, it facilitates disc luxation, and the excessive elongation of the retrodiscal tissue. On the other hand, if an open-mouth behavior is adopted (for example mouth breather), the cervical spine is positioned in extension. This phenomenon is present when using intraoral splints, which increase the vertical mouth dimension (opening the mouth) and cause cervical lordosis; the phenomenon is observed in patients with bruxism.

3. Craniocervical extension/flexion movements are associated with phonation and chewing. This association is modified depending on the sort of words articulated or the size of the food bolus. In particular, mouth opening is accompanied by cervical extension (occuring when we want to bite a large volume of food). Cervical movements recruit the craniomandibular muscles (Funakoshi et al., 1976; Forsberg et al., 1985; Ballenberger et al., 2012) into latero-flexion, rotation, and flexion-extension. The temporal and masseter musculature get into tension as an antigravitational strategy of the mandible.

4. A forward head posture (Milidonis et al., 1993; McLean, 2005; Ohmure et al., 2008) recruits the masseter, temporal, digastric and genioglossus muscles generating an anterior lingual resting position, which may lead to lingual and also chewing and swallowing action disorders.

5. The dynamics of the mandible recruit cervical muscles (Davies, 1979; Clark et al., 1993; Hochberg et al., 1995; Armijo-Olivo & Magee, 2007; Rodriguez et al., 2011; Hellmann et al., 2012; Häggman-Henrikson et al., 2013). Chewing, opening the mouth against resistance and clenching the teeth (that is, bruxism) activate the sternocledomastoid, splenius, semispinalis, multifidus and levator scapulae muscles.

6. The TMJ region absorbs extensive attention from the central nervous system in activities such as

phonation, breathing, swallowing and chewing. In order to achieve these goals, it is necessary to coordinate the chewing muscles with the tongue (Carlson et al., 1997; Takahashi et al., 2005; Kakizaki et al., 2002). Messina (2017) mentions a lingual-mandibular-hyoid system, which connects the skull, buccal and nasal cavity, pharynx, hyoid and mandible in a complex biomechanical relationship involving a multitude of ligaments, thirty-four muscles, five cranial pairs (V, VII, IX, X and XII) and the nerve root that emerges from C2. These activities also mobilize muscles from the cranial, TMJ, scapular, paravertebral, prevertebral, and infrahyoid levels, as well as the tongue.

Fascia as a system

Definition of fascia and characteristics of the fascial system

It is suggested that fascia represents the fundamental structure that ensures structural and functional continuity between components of the craniomandibular region. The fascial system supports all components of the body: bones, muscle fibers, nerves, lipids, liquids, blood vessels and diverse groups of receptors. Fascia also manages biochemical signals, repels pathogen aggressions, acts dynamically in scar formation, and supports the extracellular matrix allowing communication between cells throughout the body. Fascia acts as a synergistic whole, absorbing and distributing local stimuli to all parts of the system. Its sensor network registers thermal, chemical, pressure, vibration and movement stimuli, influencing the experience of pain, and also participating in corrective actions generated at the periphery or ordered from higher neurological levels.

There is a great discrepancy in opinions of how to define fascia (Langevin & Huijing 2009; Kumka & Bonar 2012; Schleip et al., 2012; Swanson, 2013). It has been suggested that 'fascial system' is the most appropriate term to use, considering that the terms

'cardiovascular system' or 'nervous system' describe structures formed by different types of cells with different activities.

'The fascial system consists of the three-dimensional continuum of soft, collagen-containing, loose and dense fibrous connective tissues that permeate the human body. It incorporates elements such as adipose tissue, adventitia and neurovascular sheaths, aponeuroses, deep and superficial fasciae, epineurium, joint capsules, ligaments, membranes, meninges, myofascial expansions, periostea, retinacula, septa, tendons, visceral fasciae, and all intramuscular and inter-muscular connective tissues including endo-/peri-/epi-mysium'.

—Adstrum et al., 2017

This system represents a complex communication architecture, receiving a wide range of mechanoreceptive information, not only through its topographic body distribution, but mainly by patterns of interaction with other structures of the body, particularly the muscles. From its fibrous construction, it is characterized by its property to align and accommodate to intrinsic and extrinsic tensional requests. Tensional alterations, created outside the physiological biomechanical patterns of movement, can reorient body dynamics. The density, distribution and organoleptic characteristics of the fascial system differ along its paths; however, its continuity is fundamental and allows the fascia to act as a synergistic whole, absorbing and distributing a local stimulus to the remaining elements of the body. The intrinsic structural synergy of the fascial system assures the body the relative independence from gravitational force and also enjoys a high adaptability, according to requirements coming from outside and inside the system. All these activities are related to the availability of energy and nutrients in the surrounding environment. In addition to its structural function, the fascia assumes and distributes the stimuli that the body receives: its network of receptors registers thermal, chemical, pressure, vibration

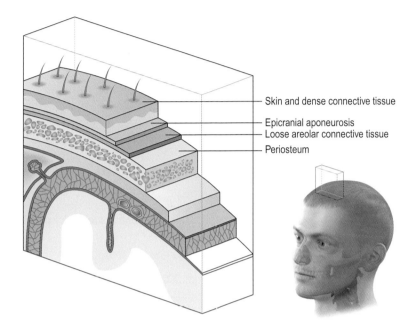

Figure 13.2
Fascial distribution in the
cranium.

Skin and dense connective tissue
Epicranial aponeurosis
Loose areolar connective tissue
Periosteum

and motion impulses. It sends these impulses to the central nervous system, which generates the necessary corrective actions. Thus, the amount of information is linked by the system for a specific purpose (Pilat, 2014).

Fascial anatomy related to the craniomandibular region

The fascial system extends throughout the human body with numerous variants; however, its continuity is always present. From the cranial vertex, the fascial system expands like a 'cap' in the form of a triple layer (Norton, 2007) (Figures 13.2 and 13.3):

1. A dense connective tissue, located under the skin, related to fat and strongly vascularized with free anastomoses derived from internal and external carotid arteries and the occipital artery. The emissary veins connect this layer with the venous sinuses of the dura mater. This fascial layer is innervated by the trigeminal nerve branches, the cervical plexus branches and posterior cervical branches (C2-C3) (Figure 13.2).

2. Epicranial aponeurosis or aponeurotic 'galea' is in tension due to the presence of two muscles that are inserted at its anterior (frontal) and posterior (occipital) ends. This fascial relationship allows us to focus to a single muscle called occipitofrontal. On both sides, the epicranial aponeurosis gives origin to the anterior, superior and posterior auricular muscles (Figure 13.3).

3. Loose areolar connective tissue, the deepest, thinnest and most mobile, extends from the eyebrows to the upper nuchal line and the outer occipital protuberance. The next stratum would be the pericranium or periosteum.

This fascial 'cap' expands:

- Backward: becoming the posterior cervical fascia.

- Forward: it continues with the myofascia of the frontal muscle and then continues to cover the nasal, palpebral and orbital structures. From here, it is transformed into a single myofascial layer (the superficial fascia is transformed into a deep fascia) connecting the muscles of the mimic and the skin,

Chapter 13

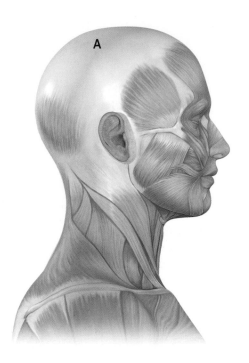

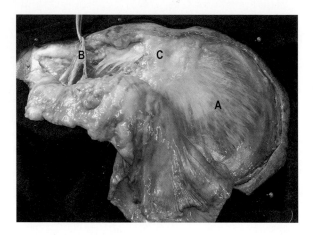

Figure 13.4
Temporalis fascia.
A. Temporalis fascia.
B. Masseter fascia.
C. Zygomatic arch.

Figure 13.3
Epicranial aponeurosis (A). From the cranial vertex the fascial system expands like a 'cap'.

reaching the buccal and mandibular region denominated facial fascia or facial musculoaponeurotic system, where it will continue with the superficial cervical fascia and platysma. Platysma and cervical fascia expand towards the deltoid, pectoral and sternal fascia on the anterior region of the thorax.

- Laterally: it transforms into the temporoparietal fascia (Demirdover et al., 2011). Here we find the fascia of the temporalis muscle, a double leaf (superficial and deep) of a fibrous, flexible character. The surface leaf of the temporal (also called temporoparietal) muscle originates in the temporal line, up to the zygomatic arch, from where it expands to become the parotideomasseteric fascia. The deep leaf is related to the temporalis muscle. Between

the two leaves, just above the zygomatic arch is the temporal fat pad that can be extended to become the oral fat (Lam & Carlson, 2014) (Figure 13.4).

The superficial temporalis fascia progresses inferiorly to the face and joins the masseteric, parotid, and tympanic regions. A complex fascial connection is built in front of the external auditory canal. In the depth, the system contains the masseter muscle (masseter fascia), which envelops the parotid (parotid fascia) and expands to the tympanomastoid fissure forming the tympanoparotid fascia (Hwang et al., 2008). Interestingly, the risorius muscle originates within the parotid fascia. The masseter fascia is continued with the platysma and cervical fascia until it joins the thorax.

An interesting point is the relations between different units of the chewing system. For example, the medial pterygoid aponeurosis is continuous with the periosteum of the mandible angle to become that of the masseter muscle, so the fascial system involves

Table 13.1
Organization of deep cervical fascial tissue.

Sheet	Location	Insertion	Comments
SUPERFICIAL SHEET OF DEEP CERVICAL FASCIA			
Superficial sheet of the deep cervical fascia, also known as cervical fascia	Around the neck Deep to superficial fascia and platysma	Anterior: chin, hyoid and sternum Posterior: cervical spinosus, nuchal-ligament, scapular spine Upper: occiput, mastoid, zygomatic arch, angle and horizontal mandibular branch Lower: sternum, clavicles and acromion	Involves sternocleidomastoid and trapezius Transforms into the parotideomasseteric fascia
MEDIUM SHEET OF DEEP CERVICAL FASCIA			
Infrahyoid fascia	Around the infrahyoid space	Upper: thyroid cartilage and hyoid Lower: sternum	Involves the infrahyoid muscles
Visceral fascia and pretracheal fascia	Deep to the infrahyoid fascia Posterior to the pharynx	Upper: base of the skull Lower: mediastinum	Contains thyroid, esophagus and trachea
DEEP SHEET OF DEEP CERVICAL FASCIA			
Alar fascia	Deep to visceral and pretracheal fascia	Upper: base of the skull Lower: up to T2	Separates the retropharyngeal space
Prevertebral fascia	Deep to the fascia alar Around the prevertebral and paravertebral muscles	Upper: base of the skull Lower: coccyx	Involves the prevertebral and paravertebral musculature

T2: Second thoracic vertebra.

both muscles in relation to the mandibular bone, allowing them to work as a stirrup, suspending the lower jaw to the depressing forces (Pilat, 2003). Another connection is the interlobed fascia that connects the aponeurotic envelope of the lateral and medial pterygoids in the pterygoid fossa, which in turn contains the sphenomandibular ligament (Perlemuter & Waligora, 1971).

The ligaments form the integral part of the fascial system (Pilat, 2003; van der Wal, 2009). An example is the stylomandibular ligament arising as a result of increased density of the deep cervical fascia (Norton, 2007).

Returning to the face, the aponeurosis of the buccinator muscle originates posteriorly, in the pterygomandibular raphe where it constitutes the buccinator pharyngeal fascia when it is related to the constrictor muscle of the pharynx. In this fascial location, the pharyngobasilar fascia that emerges from the basilar occipital portion (Sobotta, 2000) is integrated; an encounter between the region of the mimic, the pharynx and the skull.

In relation to the supra- and infrahyoid muscles, the craniocervical fascia forms a series of spaces (with a mainly longitudinal orientation), which compartmentalize, envelop, support and connect muscles, bones, viscera, blood vessels and the peripheral nervous system. They are tubes allowing the passage of the structures, but they also manage the quantity and quality of their movement. The fascial system of the neck represents a dynamic link between the head and the trunk (Pilat, 2009) (Table 13.1; Figures 13.5–13.9).

Myofascial force transmission

The discovery of the ultrastructure and the mechanobiology of the sarcomeral unit, gave shape to a new model of myofibrils, embedded inside the extracellular matrix, which, at the same time, participates (from its own dynamic) in the contractile phenomenon (Yucesoy, 2010). The shortening of the myofibril

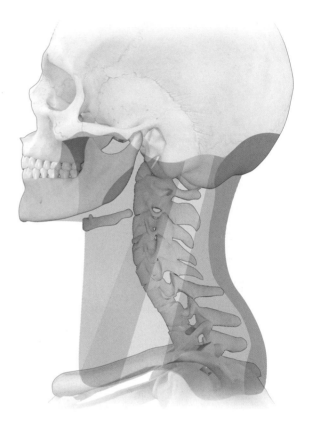

Figure 13.5
Cervical fascia distribution.

exerts a force from within the myofascial structure (endomysium, perimysium and epimysium) and resembles more the principles of the tensegrity model (Gillies & Lieber, 2011) rather than a simple linear analysis (movements arranged in series). The new, 'epimysmal' transmission paths, are parallel to tendinous ones (Huijing, 2007). In this model, the muscle does not act as an isolated and independent entity. Instead, those collagenous linkages between epimysia of adjacent muscles, such as the neurovascular tracts, provide indirect intermuscular connections.

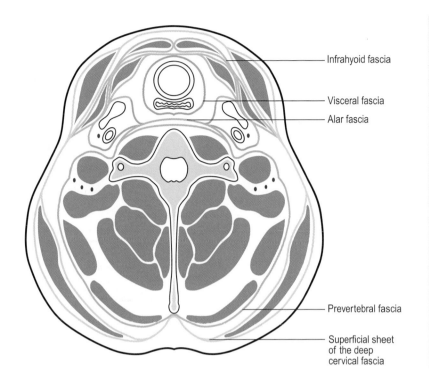

Infrahyoid fascia

Visceral fascia

Alar fascia

Prevertebral fascia

Superficial sheet of the deep cervical fascia

Figure 13.6
Cervical fascia distribution.

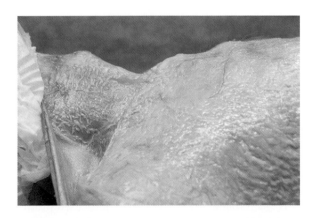

Figure 13.7
The superficial fascia in the cervical, pectoral and brachial areas. Note the continuity of its structure and the high fat content.

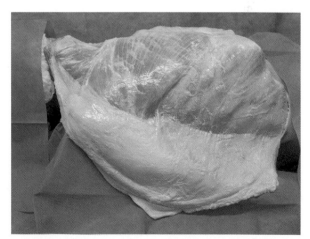

Figure 13.8
The deep fascia in the cervical, pectoral and brachial areas. Note the continuity of its structure and fibrous appearance.

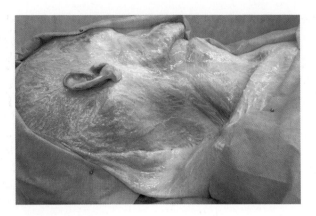

Figure 13.9
The continuity of the superficial fascia in the head, cervical and clavicular areas. Note the continuity of the structure.

Fascia as a sensitive organ

Fascia appears as the mechanosensitive structure (Vaticón 2009; Langevin, 2011). Usually the neuroanatomical studies focus mainly on discs, facet joints, muscle fibers, tendons or ligaments and there is limited information related to the innervation of the fascia. Our interest focuses on the functional connection, which involves mainly the communication throughout the loose connective tissue structures through its unique network of mechanoreceptors, particularly the so-called interstitial mechanoreceptors (type III and IV free nerve endings) (Taguchi et al., 2008; Corey et al, 2011). The main findings related to fascial innervation include:

- Fascia manifests itself as a structure that extends throughout the body with numerous muscular expansions maintaining its basal tension.

- During muscle contraction, fascial expansions transmit the effect to a specific area of the fascia, stimulating proprioceptors in that area (Tesarz et al., 2011).

- The presence of mechanoreceptors suggests active involvement of the fascia in proprioception, transmission of force, and motor control (Mense & Hoheisel, 2016).

- The proprioceptive role of the fascial network means that it can update the central nervous system in mechanical stress to operate the motor units at the time, rate and appropriate force level.

- Tissue microtrauma, inflammation and fibrosis cannot only change the intrinsic biomechanics of the soft tissues (for example increasing their stiffness), but it can also alter the sensory input derived from the affected tissues.

- Continuous activation of the nociceptors can worsen fibrosis and inflammation, causing tissue stiffness and consequent alteration of movement (Schidler et al., 2014).

- Microtrauma and resulting repetitive irritation of the free nerve terminals could create a continuous alert response. The deformation of the tissue due to an injury, hypomobility or excessive load can model the proprioceptive response and through it increase the alertness response (Chou & Shekelle, 2010).

- Irritation of other tissues, which share with fascia the innervation by the same spinal segment, can modify the threshold of sensitivity, with a painful response.

Myofascial Induction Therapy (MIT®) applied to temporomandibular disorders

MIT® definition

MIT® is a manual therapy approach focused on the functional restoration of the fascial system. It consists of the process of evaluation and treatment, where the clinician applies gentle manual mechanical stress transfer (traction or compression) to a targeted dysfunctional tissue. The outcome is a reciprocal reaction from the body that involves biochemical, signaling, metabolic, and finally physiological responses. This process aims to remodel the tissue matrix responsiveness to facilitate and optimize information transfer to, and throughout, the fascial system. The term 'induction' relates to the recovery of movement facilitation, rather than a passive stretching of the fascial system. This is primarily a learning process, in the search for a restored homeostatic level, recovering range of motion, normalization of appropriate tension, strength and,

mainly, movement coordination. The main MIT® application's goal is to restore the internal balance of the fascial system and improve the body's movement ability in musculoskeletal, neural, vascular, cranial and visceral components. It is a focused process, controlled by the central nervous system, in which the clinician acts as a facilitator. The therapeutic action focuses on the provision of resources for homeostatic balance adjustment. The final objective of the therapeutic process is not settlement of stable hierarchies, rather facilitation of optimal adaptation to

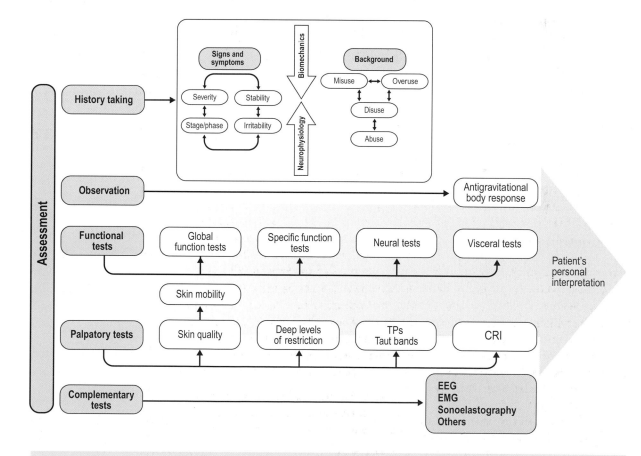

Figure 13.10

Schematic of the assessment process suggested in MIT®. CRI, cranial rhythmic impulse; EEG, electroencephalogram; EMG, electromyogram; TPs, trigger points.

environmental and personal demands (Pilat, 2014). The outcome (body image change, improvement in functional skills) should be assessed not only by the therapist but also the patient. MIT® aspires to be an individualized patient-focused treatment (Pilat, 2017).

The applications of MIT® suggested below are based on the clinical experience of the author (Pilat, 2003), and are based on the theoretical framework discussed above. The MIT® process may be combined with other therapies, or as an isolated intervention.

Myofascial dysfunction definition

Fascial system dysfunction is defined as an alteration of the highly organized assortment of specialized movements and as incorrect transfer of information through the matrix (Pilat, 2003). If proper fascial dynamics (gliding between endofascial fibers and interfascial planes) are impaired, optimal body behavior may be affected. This is also related to the proper exchange of fluids.

Assessment process

The suggested clinical evaluation proposal is summarized in Figure 13.10 and Tables 13.2 and 13.3. Special attention should be given to global functional tests when the patient performs integrated movements, often similar to everyday activities. MIT® method is a patient-oriented therapy, so her/his personal interpretation of assessment is significant. The signs and symptoms related to TMD are summarized in Figure 13.11.

Treatment objectives

The objectives of MIT® are to:

- Mobilize superficial fascial entrapments.
- Change the 'stationary attitude' of collagen structures.

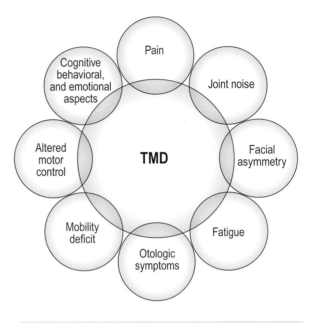

Figure 13.11
Signs and symptoms related to temporomandibular disorder (TMD).

- Facilitate the recovery of the sliding properties of the extracellular matrix.
- Stimulate physiological orientation in the mechanics of fibroblasts.
- Avoid the formation of tissue adhesions.
- Acquire a more efficient circulation of antibodies in the matrix.
- Improve blood supply (histamine release) in the restriction region.
- Improve blood supply to the nervous system.

Contraindications to MIT®

The main contraindications for MIT® include aneurysms, systemic diseases, an inflammatory process in the acute phase, acute circulatory deficiency, advanced diabetes, anticoagulant therapy, and general contraindications to any manual therapy procedure.

Table 13.2
Suggested clinical evaluation.

Postural and facial observation	Sensitivity scan	Intraoral observation	Passive joint analysis	Active mobility	Joint sounds
■ Parallelism between facial lines ■ Middle vertical face line ■ Asymmetries between facial distances ■ Head position	■ Pain ■ Touch ■ Temperature ■ Vibration	■ Tooth wear ■ Lingual indentations ■ Indentations in the oral cavity	■ Mandibular sliding and traction ■ Ligamentous and capsular test ■ Test for bilaminar zone ■ End-feel sensation	■ Depression ■ Elevation ■ Grinding movement ■ Protraction ■ Retraction	■ Auscultation ■ Palpation ■ Click ■ Crepitations ■ Pop

Table 13.3
Suggested clinical evaluation.

Muscle status	Motor control	Fascial Asymmetry	Neural mechano-sensitivity	Cervical exploration	Thoracic exploration
■ Palpation ■ Hypertrophy ■ Pain ■ Evaluation of length and strength	■ Mandibular deviation ■ Mandibular deflection ■ Facial synkinesis during grinding movement ■ Cephalic protrusion during oral opening ■ Craniocervical extension during mouth opening ■ Hyolingual dynamics during swallowing ■ Masticatory dynamics ■ Fatigue	■ Observation and palpation of the fascial system at local and regional level	■ Slump test ■ Cervicocranial flexion test ■ Mandibular nerve test	■ Posture ■ Passive mobility ■ Active mobility ■ Motor control ■ Muscle status	■ Posture ■ Passive mobility ■ Active mobility ■ Respiratory pattern ■ Muscle status

Chapter 13

Basis of clinical applications (Pilat 2003, 2009, 2014, 2015, 2017)

In the MIT® approach, the therapist applies a manual low-intensity/long-time load to the fascial system. Through it, recovery of the quality of fascial tissue (extracellular matrix) is facilitated. This process is mediated by molecular mechanisms associated with cellular mechanotransduction, piezoelectricity, and viscoelasticity, and regulated by the central nervous system. It is mainly a 'didactic' process, in the search for new, homeostatic levels through recovery of range of movement, adequate tension, strength and coordination. The final result is transmitted in a better functionality with lower energy spending. Figure 13.12 summarizes the details of this process.

Clinical procedure principles (Pilat 2003, 2009, 2014, 2015, 2017)

1. All procedures must be individualized according to the treated dysfunction and patient's individual needs regarding their age, physical and emotional conditions, cultural aspects and gender. The election of the specific technique also depends on the therapist's skills.

2. Biomechanically, the myofascial system responds to compression and traction forces. These are two mechanical strategies used when applying MIT®.

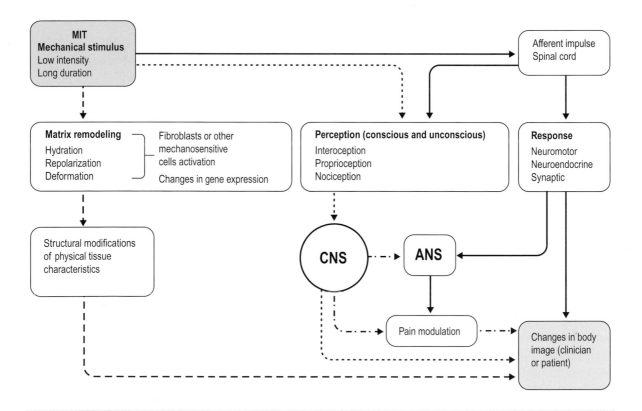

Figure 13.12
The MIT® process mechanism. ANS, autonomic nervous system; CNS, central nervous system.

3. The direction of the releasing movement is towards facilitation. The clinician should refrain from performing movements in an arbitrary direction.

4. The clinician chooses the body region affected by the myofascial dysfunction that may be associated with pain and/or dysfunction (hypo-/hypermobility, incoordination, lack of force, etc.). This region should be identified during the initial assessment process discussed above.

5. Each region affected by dysfunction requires the application of a specific procedure (Pilat, 2003).

6. The clinician tenses the tissue referred to as the first restriction barrier, by applying a three-dimensional, slow and gradual compression and/or traction. The pressure is constant for at least 60–90 seconds, the time required for releasing the first restriction barrier (beginning of the viscoelastic response).

7. During the first phase of the application the therapist barely induces the tissue to move.

8. Upon overcoming the first restriction barrier, the therapist accompanies the movement in the direction of the facilitation, pausing at each additional barrier.

9. For each technique, one must overcome at least three to six consecutive barriers and the minimum time of application is 3 to 5 minutes.

10. The tension on the tissue must be constant, but the pressure applied by the therapist may be modified after overcoming the first barrier. Pressure should be reduced when abundant activity and/or pain is perceived.

Examples of MIT® application

The following techniques are examples of the therapeutic strategies used to treat myofascial restrictions and are related to the most common clinical dysfunctions and pain symptoms associated to TMD.

Myofascial induction of the suboccipital region

The aim of this technique is to release restrictions located in the connective tissue bridges between the rectus capitis posterior minor and major musculature, and the dura mater (Hack et al., 1995; Kahkeshani & Ward, 2012). In a recent systematic review, Palomeque-del-Cerro et al. (2017) stated there is 'a continuity of soft tissue between the cervical muscles and the cervical dura mater; this might have physiological, pathophysiological, and therapeutic implications, and going some way to explaining the effect of some therapies in craniocervical disorders'.

The patient is supine and the clinician is seated at the head of the table with the forearms firmly over its surface. The clinician places both hands under the patient's head. Then, the clinician touches the suboccipital space with the second to fourth fingers, attempting to place the fingers vertically. Subsequently the clinician, with the tips of the aforementioned fingers, applies a sustained force in a direction towards the ceiling (Figure 13.13).

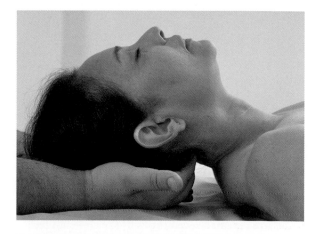

Figure 13.13
Myofascial induction of the suboccipital region.

The pressure should be painless and be maintained for at least a minimum of 4 minutes until the fascia is released.

Myofascial induction of the hyoid area

The aim of these techniques is to release fascial restriction of the suprahyoid and infrahyoid areas (Pilat, 2003). The hyoid bone is fixed to both the pre-vertebral and superficial fascia. Also, the anatomical relationships of hyoids are unique, due to the lack of the cartilaginous correlation with nearby bones. Nevertheless, the hyoid plays an important role in the biomechanical equilibrium of the fascial system of the cervical and orofacial structures. Also relevant is the fact that the hyoid bone supports the tongue muscles such as genioglossus, hyoglossus, and chondroglossus, which control the tongue's movements through reciprocal contraction. There are 14 pairs of muscles and other connective structures related to the hyoid (Figure 13.14). The hyoid participates in activities such as swallowing, speaking, chewing, and blowing. The positional balance of the hyoid controls three myofascial systems composed of:

- Suprahyoid muscles: move the hyoid cranially.

- Infrahyoid muscles: move the hyoid caudally.

- Retrohyoid muscles: move the hyoid dorsally.

A. Myofascial induction of the digastric fascia (suprahyoid procedure)

The patient is supine and the clinician is seated at the head of the table. With the unilateral hand the clinician makes contact under the mandible bone, using the middle and ring fingers. The other hand stabilizes the patient head. From this position, the fingertips of the clinician (sliding on the skin) move to the angle of the mandible (Figure 13.15). These slides are repeated seven times. If the clinician feels a restricted point, a slight and smooth pressure should be applied for 7 seconds to release the fascial restriction (Figure 13.16). If the fascial restriction is deep, the clinician should use the hand placed on the head

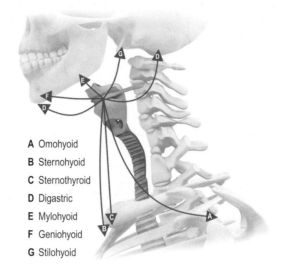

A Omohyoid
B Sternohyoid
C Sternothyroid
D Digastric
E Mylohyoid
F Geniohyoid
G Stilohyoid

Figure 13.14
The dynamics of the hyoid region. The myofascial relationships between the bones and muscles (A-G) are shown.

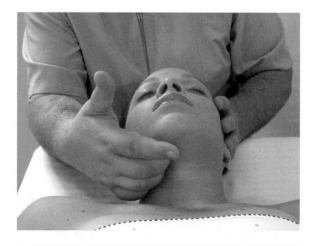

Figure 13.15
Myofascial induction on the digastric fascia.

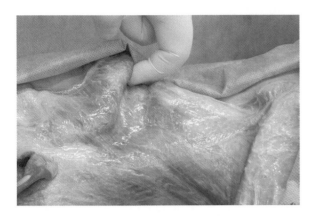

Figure 13.16
The finger position in the digastric induction process. Note: The image shows contact with a single finger so as not to cover the anatomical components.

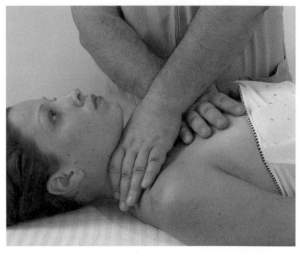

Figure 13.17
Cross-hand technique on the infrahyoid fascia.

of the patient to follow the involuntary movement of the head. Note: It is very important to avoid the application of pressure over the submandible glands.

B. Myofascial induction of the infrahyoid area (cross-hand technique)

The patient is supine and the clinician stands at one side of the table at the patient's shoulder level. The clinician applies a cross-hand position contact as follows: the cranial hand embraces the hyoid bone, whereas the caudal hand is placed in the space between the clavicles and the hyoid bone. In this position, the cranial hand applies a soft caudal traction, whereas the hyoid hand pulls in the cranial direction (Figure 13.17). The clinician waits 60 to 90 seconds until the first response is elicited by the tissue. The pressure should be constant during the entire technique.

Myofascial induction of masticatory musculature

The following procedures address the three most important masticatory muscles. The temporalis muscle acts on the parietal, temporal, frontal, sphenoid and mandible bones. With a complete occlusion, a prolonged and excessive tension of the temporalis muscle can negatively affect the dynamics of the articular disc. The masseter muscle (outside) acts together with the medial pterygoid (inside) to suspend the jaw. The lateral pterygoid runs between two bellies of the medial pterygoid, and its path is practically horizontal. It moves the coronoid process forward during mouth opening. The posterior fibers of the temporalis muscle perform the antagonistic movement leading the apophysis back when closing the mouth.

A. Temporalis fascia induction (Figure 13.18)

The patient is supine and the clinician is seated at the head of the table. The clinician, with the fingertips of both hands, contacts the temporalis muscle bilaterally (Figures 13.19 and 13.20). Subsequently, he glides his hands gently (moving the hands together along with the skin of the head), transversely to the fascial fibers' orientation (Figure 13.18) in intervals of 2 to 2.5 cm. In the clinic, it is common to perform 15 sliding cycles at each contact site. The technique should be pain-free.

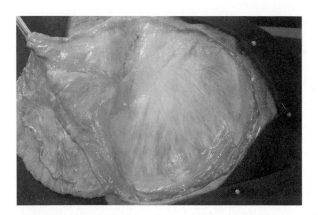

Figure 13.18
Temporalis fascia.

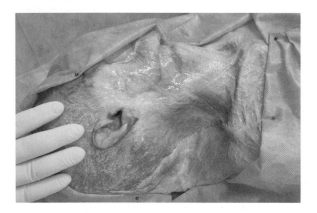

Figure 13.19
Hand positioning for the temporalis fascia induction.

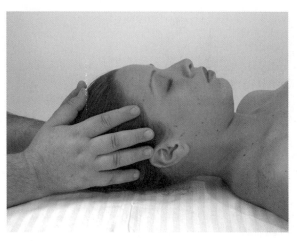

Figure 13.20
Temporalis fascia induction.

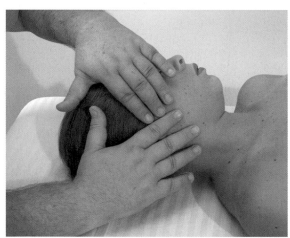

Figure 13.21
Pterygoid fascia induction.

B. Pterygoid fascia induction

The clinician places the index finger (of his dominant hand) above the third molar in the pterygoid fossa. The index, middle and ring fingers of the other hand contact the temporomaxillary region (Figure 13.21). The pressure must be exerted in all directions in a consecutive manner until relaxation is perceived. Special care must be taken because this area is usually extremely sensitive.

C. Masseter fascia induction

The clinician places the tips of the middle and ring fingers of both hands symmetrically over the insertion point of the masseter in the zygomatic arch on each side (Figure 13.22). Subsequently, he

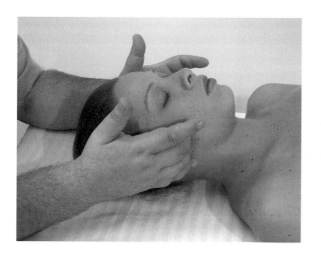

Figure 13.22
Masseter fascia induction.

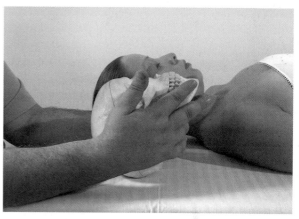

Figure 13.23
TMJ decompression procedure (hand position on the skull).

exerts a sustained pressure towards the midline of the patient's body. The principles of induction are followed.

TMJ decompression procedure
(Figures 13.23–13.25)

The use of this procedure is suggested as the final phase of the application, in the search for optimum dynamic stability. The patient is supine and the clinician is seated at the head of the table. The clinician places his middle finger just below the TMJ along the vertical ramus of the jaw; the hand fits the patient's head. Subsequently, the clinician applies a gentle caudal tension (at the fascial level) and waits until relaxation is perceived. At the end of the treatment, the patient should open and close the mouth several times.

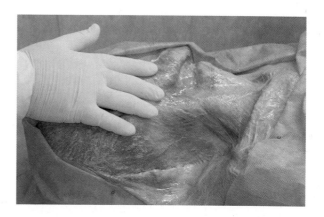

Figure 13.24
TMJ decompression procedure (hand position on the cadaver).

Conclusion

The applications of MIT® may be of benefit in the treatment of TMDs. We suggest the inclusion of MIT® into the multimodal therapeutic process. Despite the fact that research related to the scientific basis of MIT® is lacking but growing, clinical evidence remains limited, requiring unified research criteria including more objective evaluation processes, classification of strategies (local vs. global approach), unification of parameters as to force, timing, intensity and frequency of application,

Chapter 13

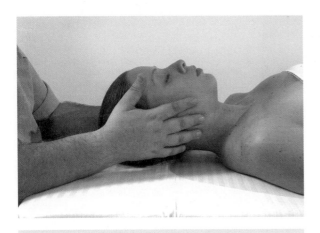

Figure 13.25
TMJ decompression procedure (hand position on a patient).

identification and analysis of responses in different body systems, identification and classification of responders versus non-responders, and analysis of long-term results (Pilat, 2017). In fact, one factor is the difficulty of quantifying proper outcomes. The development of new assessment methods (for example sonoelastography) will help in this challenge.

Clinicians familiar with other myofascial therapy approaches, (for example Myofascial Release, according to Robert Ward (2003), originated by Andrew Taylor Still, and also widely described by Carol Manheim (2008) and John F. Barnes (1990) and others) will find similarities with MIT®, each with different details, based on a similar clinical reasoning concept that allows them to complement one another.

References

Adstrum S, Hedley G, Schleip R, Stecco C, Yucesoy CA. Defining the fascial system. J Bodywork Mov Ther 2017; 21: 173–177.

Armijo-Olivo S, Magee DJ. Electromyographic activity of the masticatory and cervicalmuscles during resisted jaw opening movement. J Oral Rehabil 2007; 34: 184–194.

Bag AK, Gaddikeri S, Singhal A, Hardin S, Tran BD, Medina JA, Curé JK. Imaging of the temporomandibular joint: An update. World J Radiol 2014; 6; 567–582.

Ballenberger N, von Piekartz H, Paris-Alemany A, La Touche R, Angulo-Diaz-Parreño S. Influence of different upper cervical positions electromyography activity of the masticatory muscles. J Manipulative Physiol Ther 2012; 35:308–318.

Barnes J. Myofascial Release MFR. Seminars: Paoli. Eastern Myofascial Release Treatment Center, Malvern. 1990.

Bilgiç F, Gelgör E. Prevalence of temporomandibular dysfunction and its association with malocclusion in children: An epidemiologic study. J Clin Pediatr Dent 2017; 41:161–165.

Carlson CR, Sherman JJ, Studts JL, Bertrand PM. The effects of tongue position on mandibular muscle activity. J Orofacial Pain 1997; 11: 291–297.

Chaves TC, Dos Santos Aguiar A, Felicio LR, Greghi SM, Hallak Regalo SC, Bevilaqua-Grossi D. Electromyographic ratio of masseter and anterior temporalis muscles in children with and without temporomandibular disorders. Int J Pediatr Otorhinolaryngol 2017; 97: 35–41.

Chou R, Shekelle P. Will this patient develop persistent disabling low back pain? JAMA 2010; 303: 1295–1302.

Clark GT, Browne PA, Nakano M, Yang Q. Co-activation of sternocleidomastoid muscles during maximum clenching. J Dental Res 1993; 72: 1499–1502.

Coombs MC, Petersen JM, Wright GJ, Lu SH, Damon BJ, Yao H. Structure-function relationships of temporomandibular retrodiscal tissue. J Dental Res 2017; 96: 647–653.

Corey SM, Vizzard MA, Badger GJ, Langevin HM. Sensory innervation of the non-specialized connective tissues in the low back of the rat. Cells Tissues Organs 2011; 194: 521–530.

Davies PL. Electromyographic study of superficial neck muscles in mandibular function. J Dental Res 1979; 58: 537–538.

Demirdover C, Sahin B, Vayvada H, Oztan HY. The versatile use of temporoparietal fascial flap. Int J Medical Sci 2011; 8: 362–368.

Dijkstra PU, Kropmans TJ, Stegenga B. The association between generalized joint hypermobility and temporomandibular joint disorders: a systematic review. J Dent Res 2002; 81: 158–163.

Fernández-de-las-Peñas C, Galán-del-Río F, Fernández-Carnero J, Pesquera J, Arendt-Nielsen L, Svensson P. Bilateral widespread mechanical pain sensitivity in women with myofascial temporomandibular disorder: evidence of impairment in central nociceptive processing. J Pain 2009; 10:1170–1178.

Forsberg CM, Hellsing E, Linder-Aronson S, Sheikholeslam A. EMG activity in neck and masticatory muscles in relation to extension and flexion of the head. Eur J Orthodont 1985; 7:177–184.

Funakoshi M, Fujita N, Takehana S. Relations between occlusal interference and jaw muscle activities in response to changes in head position. J Dental Res 1976; 55: 684–690.

Gerstner G, Ichesco E, Quintero A, Schmidt-Wilcke T. Changes in regional gray and white matter volume in patients with myofascial-type temporomandibular disorders: a voxel-based morphometry study. J Orofacial Pain 2011; 25: 99–106.

Gillies A, Lieber R. Structure and function of the skeletal muscle extracellular matrix. Muscle Nerve 2011; 44:318–331.

Gordon J E. Structures, or why things don't fall down. London: Penguin Books Ltd. 1978.

Hack GD, Koritzer RT, Robinson WL, Hallgren RC, Greenman PE. Anatomic relation between the rectus capitis posterior minor muscle and the dura mater. Spine 1995; 20: 2484–2486.

Häggman-Henrikson B, Nordh E, Eriksson PO. Increased sternocleidomastoid, but not trapezius, muscle activity in response to increased chewing load. Eur J Oral Sci 2013; 121: 443–449.

Hakkak F, Jabalameli M, Rostami M, Parnianpour M. The tibiofemoral joint gaps: an arthroscopic study. SDRP Journal of Biomedical Engineering. 2015 [online] Available at: http://www.openaccessjournals.siftdesk.org/articles/pdf/The-Tibiofemoral-Joint-Gaps20151112000118.pdf [Accessed 03/6/2017].

Hellmann D, Giannakopoulos NN, Schmitter M, Lenz J, Schindler HJ. Anterior and posterior neck muscle activation during a variety of biting tasks. Eur J Oral Sci 2012; 120: 326–334.

Herring SW, Liu ZJ. Loading of the temporo-mandibular joint: anatomical and in vivo evidence from the bones. Cells Tissue Organs 2001; 169: 193–200.

Higbie EJ, Seidel-Cobb D, Taylor LF, Cummings GS. Effect of head position on vertical mandibular opening. J Orthop Sports Phys Ther 1999; 29: 127–130.

Hochberg MC, Altman RD, Brandt KD et al. Guidelines for the medical management of osteoarthritis. Part I. Osteoarthritis of the hip. American College of Rheumatology. Arthr Rheumatol 1995; 38:1535–1540.

Huijing PA. Epimuscular myofascial force transmission between antagonistic and synergistic muscles can explain movement limitation in spastic paresis. J Electromyogr Kinesiol 2007; 17: 708–724.

Huijing PA, Baan GC. Myofascial force transmission: muscle relative position and length determine agonist and synergist muscle force. J Appl Physiol 2003; 94: 1092–1107.

Hwang K, Nam YS, Kim DJ, Han SH. Anatomy of tympanoparotid fascia relating to neck lift. J Craniofacial Surg 2008; 19:648–651.

Ichesco E, Quintero A, Clauw DJ, Peltier S, Sundgren PM, Gerstner GE, Schmidt-Wilcke T. Altered functional connectivity between the insula and the cingulate cortex in patients with temporomandibular disorder: a pilot study. Headache 2012; 52: 441–454.

Ingber DE. The architecture of life. Scientific American 1998; 278: 48–57.

Isberg A. Temporomandibular joint dysfunction: a practitioner's guide. London: Isis Medical Media Ltd; 2001.

Kahkeshani K, Ward PJ. Connection between the spinal dura mater and suboccipital musculature: evidence for the myodural bridge and a route for its dissection: a review. Clin Anat 2012; 25: 415–422.

Kakizaki Y, Uchida K, Yamamura K, Yamada Y. Coordination between the masticatory and tongue muscles as seen with different foods in consistency and in reflex activities during natural chewing. Brain Res 2002; 929: 210–217.

Kang H, Yi X. Biomechanics of temporomandibular joint. Sheng Wu Yi Xue Gong Cheng Xue Za Zhi 2000; 17:324–327.

Khan FA, Pedlar J. Generalized joint hypermobility as a factor in clicking of the temporomandibular joint. Int J Oral Maxillofacial Surg 1996; 25: 101–104.

Koolstra JH. Dynamics of the human masticatory system. Crit Rev Oral Biol Med 2002; 13: 366–376.

Kumka M, Bonar J. Fascia: a morphological description and classification system based on a literature review. J Can Chiropr Assoc 2012; 56: 179–191.

Lam D, Carlson ER. The temporalis muscle flap and temporoparietal fascial flap. Oral Maxillofac Surg Clin North Am 2014; 26: 359–369.

Langendoen J, Müller J, Jull GA. Retrodiscal tissue of the temporomandibular joint: clinical anatomy and its role in diagnosis and treatment of arthropathies. Man Ther 1997; 2: 191–198.

Langevin HM. Fibroblast cytoskeletal remodeling contributes to connective tissue tension. J Cell Physiol 2011; 226: 1166–1175.

Langevin HM, Huijing PA. Communicating about fascia: history, pitfalls, and recommendations. Int J Ther Massage Bodywork 2009; 2: 3–8.

La Touche R, París-Alemany A, von Piekartz H et al. The influence of cranio-cervical posture on maximal mouth opening and pressure pain threshold in patients with myofascial temporomandibular pain disorders. Clin J Pain 2011; 27: 48–55.

La Touche R, Paris-Alemany A, Hidalgo-Pérez A et al. Evidence for central sensitization in patients with temporomandibular disorders: a systematic review and meta-analysis of observational studies. Pain Practice 2017; May 29. [Epub ahead of print]

Levin SM. Putting the shoulder to the wheel: a new biomechanical model for the shoulder girdle. Biomed Sci Instrument 1997; 33: 412–417.

Levin SM. The tensegrity truss as a model for spine mechanics: biotensegrity. J Mecha Med Biol 2002; 2: 375–388.

Levin SM. Tensegrity: the new biomechanics. In: Hutson M, Ellis R (eds). Texbook of musculoskeletal medicine. Oxford: Oxford University Press. 2006.

Levin SM. A suspensory system for the sacrum in pelvic mechanics: biotensegrity. In: Vleeming A, Mooney V, Stoeckart R (eds). Movement, Stability and Lumbopelvic Pain. Edinburgh: Churchill Livingstone, Elsevier. 2007. Pp. 229–237.

Lin CS. Brain signature of chronic orofacial pain: a systematic review and meta-analysis on neuroimaging research of trigeminal neuropathic pain and temporo-mandibular joint disorders. PLoS One 2014; 9: e94300.

Lobbezoo F, Drangsholt M, Peck C, Sato H, Kopp S, Svensson P. Topical review: new insights into the pathology and diagnosis of disorders of the temporomandibular joint. J Orofacial Pain 2004; 18: 181–191.

Manfredini D, Lombardo L, Siciliani G. Dental angle class asymmetry and temporo-mandibular disorders. J Orofacial Orthop 2017; 78: 253–258.

Manheim C. The Myofascial Release Manual. Thorofare: Slack Incorporation. 2008.

Matsuda S, Yamaguchi T, Mikami S, Okada K, Gotouda A, Sano K. Rhythm and amplitude of rhythmic masticatory muscle activity during sleep in bruxers - comparison with gum chewing. Cranio 2016; 34: 234–241.

McLean L. The effect of postural correction on muscle activation amplitudes recorded from the cervicobrachial region. J Electromyogr Kinesiol 2005; 15: 527–535.

McNeill C. Temporomandibular Disorders. Guidelines for Classification, Assessment and Management. Chicago, IL: Quintessence. 1990.

Mense S, Hoheisel U. Evidence for the existence of nociceptors in rat thoracolumbar fascia. J Bodywork Mov Ther 2016; 20: 623–628.

Messina G. The tongue, mandible, hyoid system. Eur J Translational Myol 2017; 27: 6363.

Michelotti A, Iodice G, Piergentili M, Farella M, Martina R. Incidence of temporo-mandibular joint clicking in adolescents with and without unilateral posterior cross-bite: a 10-year follow-up study. J Oral Rehabil 2016; 43:16–22.

Milam SB, Zardeneta G, Schmitz JP. Oxidative stress and degenerative temporo-mandibular joint disease: a proposed hypothesis. J Oral Maxillofacial Surg 1998; 56: 214–223.

Milidonis MK, Kraus SL, Segal RL, Widmer CG. Genioglossi muscle activity in response to

changes in anterior/neutral head posture. Am J Orthodo Dentofacial Orthop 1993; 103: 39–44.

Moon HJ, Lee YK. The relationship between dental occlusion/temporomandibular joint status and general body health: part 1. Dental occlusion and TMJ status exert an influence on general body health. J Altern Complem Med 2011; 17: 995–1000.

Motro R. Tensegrity, Structural Systems for the future. London: Kogan Page Limited. 2003.

Norton NS. Netter. Anatomía de cabeza y cuello para odontólogos. Barcelona: Elsevier Masson. 2007.

Ögren M, Fältmars C, Lund B, Holmlund A. Hypermobility and trauma as etiologic factors in patients with disc derangements of the temporomandibular joint. Int J Oral Maxillofacial Surg 2012; 41: 1046–1050.

Ohmure H, Miyawaki S, Nagata J, Ikeda K, Yamasaki K, Al-Kalaly A. Influence of forward head posture on condylar position. J Oral Rehabil 2008; 35: 795–800.

Okeson JP. Tratamiento de oclusión y afecciones temporoman-dibulares. 7th ed. Barcelona: Elsevier. 2013.

Palomeque-del-Cerro L, Arráez-Aybar LA, Rodríguez-Blanco C, Guzmán-García R, Menendez-Aparicio M, Oliva-Pascual-Vaca A. A systematic review of the soft-tissue connections between neck muscles and dura mater: The myodural bridge. Spine 2017; 42: 49–54.

Pardehshenas H, Maroufi N, Sanjari MA, Parnianpour M, Levin SM. Lumbopelvic muscle activation patterns in three stances under graded loading conditions: Proposing a tensegrity model for load transfer through the sacroiliac joints. J Bodywork Mov Ther 2014; 18: 633–642.

Pasinato F, Souza JA, Corrêa EC, Silva AM. Temporomandibular disorder and generalized joint hypermobility: application of diagnostic criteria. Braz J Otorhinolaryngol 2011; 77: 418–425.

Peck C. Biomechanics of occlusion-implications for oral rehabilitation. Review. J Oral Rehabil 2016; 43: 205–214.

Perlemuter L, Waligora J. Cahiers d´anatomie. Préparation aux concours. Tête et cou. Paris: Masson & Cie. 1971.

Pilat A. Inducción Miofascial. Madrid: MacGraw-Hill. 2003.

Pilat A. Myofascial induction approaches for patients with headache. In: Fernández-de-las-Peñas C, Arendt-Nielsen L, Gerwin RD (eds). Tension type and cervicogenic headache: patho-physiology, diagnosis and treatment. Baltimore: Jones and Bartlett, Sudbury, MA. 2009.

Pilat A. Myofascial Induction Approach. In: Chaitow L (ed). Fascial Dysfunction. Manual Therapy Approaches. Edinburgh: Handspring Publishing. 2014.

Pilat A. Myofascial induction approaches. In: Fernández-de-las-Peñas C, Cleland J, Dommerholt J (eds). Manual therapy for musculoskeletal pain syndromes of the upper and lower quadrants: An evidence and clinical informed approach. London: Elsevier; 2015.

Pilat A. Myofascial Induction Therapy. In: Liem T, Tozzi P, Chila A (eds). Fascia in Orthopaedic Field. Edinburgh: Handspring Publishing. 2017.

Proffit WR, Epker BN, Ackerman JL. Systematic description of dentofacial deformities: the database. In: Bell WH, Proffit WR, White RP (eds). Surgical correction of dentofacial deformities. Philadelphia: W.B. Saunders. 1980. Pp.105–154.

PubMed. US National Library of Medicine National Institutes of Health. [online] Available at: < https://www.ncbi.nlm.nih.gov/pubmed> [Accessed 10 June 2017].

Rocabado M. Biomechanical relationship of the cranial, cervical and hyoid regions. J Cranio-Mandibular Pract 1983; 1: 61–66.

Rodríguez K, Miralles R, Gutiérrez MF et al. Influence of jaw clenching and tooth grinding on bilateral sternocleidomastoid EMG activity. Cranio 2011; 29: 14–22.

Scarr G. A model of the cranial vault as a tensegrity structure and its significance to normal and abnormal cranial development. Int J Osteop Med 2008; 11: 80–89.

Scarr G. A consideration of the elbow as a tensegrity structure. Int J Osteop Med 2012; 16: 114–120.

Scarr G. Biotensegrity, the structural basis of life. Edinburgh: Handspring Publishing. 2014.

Scarr G, Harrison H. Resolving the problems and controversies surrounding temporo-mandibular mechanics. J Appl Biomed 2016; 14: 177–185.

Scarr G, Harrison H. Examining the temporomandibular joint from a biotensegrity perspective: A change in thinking. J Appl Biomed 2017; 15: 55–62.

Schiffman E, Ohrbach R. Executive summary of the diagnostic criteria for temporo-mandibular disorders for clinical and research applications. J Am Dental Assoc 2016; 147: 438–445.

Schilder A, Hoheisel U, Magerl W, Benrath J, Klein T, Treede RD. Sensory findings after stimulation of the thoracolumbar fascia with hypertonic saline suggest its contribution to low back pain. Pain 2014; 155: 222–231.

Schleip R, Jäger H, Klingler W. What is 'fascia'? A review of different nomenclatures. J Bodywork Mov Ther 2012; 16: 496–502.

Sobotta J. Atlas de Anatomía Humana. Tomo 1. 21a ed. Madrid: Editorial Médica Panamericana. 2000.

Solow B, Tallgren A. Head posture and craniofacial morphology. Am J Phys Anthropol 1976; 44: 417–435.

Swanson RL. Biotensegrity: A unifying theory of biological architecture with applications to osteopathic practice, education, and research. J Am Osteop Assoc 2013; 113: 34–52.

Taguchi T, Hoheisel U, Mense S. Dorsal horn neurons having input from low back structures in rats. Pain 2008; 138: 119–129.

Takahashi S, Kuribayash i G, Ono T, Ishiwata Y, Kuroda T. Modulation of masticatory muscle activity by tongue position. Angle Orthod 2005; 75: 35–39.

Tesarz J, Hoheisel U, Wiedenhöfer B, Mense S. Sensory innervation of the thoraco-lumbar fascia in rats and humans. Neuroscience 2011; 194: 302–308.

van der Wal J. The architecture of the connective tissue in the musculoskeletal system -an often overlooked functional parameter as to proprioception in the locomotor apparatus. Int J Ther Massage Bodywork 2009; 2: 9–23.

Vaticón D. Sensibilidad Myofascial: El Sistema Craneosacro como la unidad biodinámica. ed. In: Libro de Ponencias XIX Jornadas de Fisioterapia. Madrid: EUF ONCE Universidad Autónoma de Madrid. 2009.

Visscher CM, Huddleston Slater JJ, Lobbezoo F, Naeije M. Kinematics of the human mandible for different head postures. J Oral Rehabil 2000; 27: 299–305.

Ward R. Foundations for Osteopathic Medicine. Philadelphia: Lippincott Williams & Wilkins. 2003.

Westesson PL, Kurita K, Eriksson L, Katzberg RW. Cryosectional observations of functional anatomy of the temporomandibular joint. Oral Surg Oral Med Oral Pathol 1989; 68: 247–251.

Wilson J, Kiely J. The multi-functional foot in athletic movement: extraordinary feats by our extraordinary feet. Human Mov Sci 2016; 17: 15–20.

Yucesoy C. Epimuscular myofascial force transmission implies novel principles for muscular mechanics. Exerc Sport Scienc Rev 2010; 38: 128–134.

Chapter 14
Clinical classification of cranial neuropathies
Harry von Piekartz, Toby Hall

Cranial neural tissue: a component of the peripheral nervous system

The taxonomy of peripheral neural tissue allows the inclusion of all afferent fibers and processes of the nervous system that arise distal to the dorsal horn or the brain stem nucleus (Merskey & Bogduk, 1994; Bereiter et al., 2000). Hence, all cranial neural tissue including the cranial dura can be included in the peripheral neural system. It is interesting to note that nerve roots, spinal and cranial ganglions, as well as spinal and cranial dura are almost identical in their anatomical constitution. Thus, from an anatomical perspective, it is impossible to separate cranial and spinal neural tissue (Murzin & Goriunov, 1979). Functionally, the cranial neural tissue is a continuum with the rest of the peripheral nervous system, with the same physiology and mechanical qualities (Breig, 1978). Just like the rest of the peripheral neural system, the cranial system reacts to mechanical and chemical irritants in a similar neurobiological fashion, including inflammation, altered conduction, and vascularization, as well as changes to connective tissue (Cruccu et al., 2014).

Cranial nociceptive and peripheral neuropathic pain

Dysfunction of the cranial peripheral nervous system is an important factor to consider in musculoskeletal pain conditions including temporomandibular disorders (TMDs) and is the basis for this chapter. The classic form of neural disorder is a peripheral neuropathy such as radiculopathy or peripheral nerve compression, which may induce peripheral neuropathic pain. Such pain has been defined by the International Association for the Study of Pain (IASP) as pain caused by a lesion or disease of the somatosensory system (Jensen et al., 2011).

The fundamental cause of peripheral neuropathic pain is damage to the nervous system itself, but as Zusman (2008) pointed out, nerve damage does not always cause pain, with less than 10% of peripheral nerve injuries associated with significant pain (Marchettini et al., 2006). An example of this in the orofacial region can be seen with hypoglossal nerve damage associated with gradual invasion of the hypoglossal canal from an expanding tumor. The main features include dysfunction in motor control of the tongue (altered endurance, coordination and strength) rather than pain (Gursoy et al., 2014). Conversely and perplexingly, minor nerve injury is capable of causing severe pain (Bove et al., 2003; Dilley et al., 2005; Greening et al., 2005).

The classic examples of neuropathic pain in the orofacial region include trigeminal, mandibular, maxillary, glossopharyngeal, and superior laryngeal neuralgia (Sommer, 2007). In the clinical setting, recommendations based on IASP guidelines regarding the diagnosis of neuropathic pain have been published (Treede et al., 2008) and recently updated (Finnerup et al., 2016).

Other chapters in this book have discussed presentations involving nociceptive pain arising from musculoskeletal structures such as muscles and joints in the orofacial region. Distinguishing between nociceptive pain and peripheral cranial neuropathic pain is important, although separating the two can be difficult on a clinical level (Markman et al., 2004) and even theoretically (Bennett, 2006). Complications arise where both neuropathic pain and nociceptive pain coexist. However, differentiating between peripheral neuropathic and nociceptive pain is important as we believe each condition requires a different treatment approach and each has a differing prognosis (Hans et al., 2007). For example, treatment

Chapter 14

of a medial capsulitis of the TMJ together with an inflamed disc needs a different treatment/management approach if the inferior alveolar nerve (branch of the mandibular nerve) is damaged inducing neuropathic pain. As Forssell et al. (2015) suggested, the diagnostic criteria of cranial neuropathic pain have been poorly defined by the International Headache Society (IHS) and our understanding of the underlying pathophysiological mechanisms are less well understood. The diagnosis and management of these pain disorders is difficult and often inadequate (Woda, 2009; Forssell et al., 2015). Of particular relevance to manual therapists is that patients with some features of neuropathic pain respond less favorably to manual therapy (Jull et al., 2007), particularly neural mobilization (Nee et al., 2013), highlighting the importance of classification of neuropathic pain.

Neural disorders

A further complication in the management of orofacial and other musculoskeletal pain conditions is that pain may be associated with a neural disorder without neurologic conduction loss (Dilley et al., 2005). This kind of pain, usually termed peripheral nerve sensitization (PNS), is explained by an inflammatory process affecting the connective tissue elements of a peripheral nerve, or axons themselves (Hall & Elvey, 1999). This kind of problem is accompanied by dysfunction of the interface tissue surrounding the nerve, which triggers the inflammatory process, sensitizing neural tissue. Consequently, pain may be influenced by certain postures and movements (Nee & Butler, 2006), which mechanically stress the sensitized nerve tissue. For example, patients may experience pain during activities of daily living involving orofacial movements such as chewing, talking, or singing, or with typical head movement such as when shaving the arm pit, putting on shoes, and other sustained neck flexion positions. Such movements and positions challenge mechanically the mechanosensitive cranial neural system (von Piekartz, 2015).

Management of neural pain disorders includes mobilization of the nervous system to decrease pain associated with PNS. However, there is growing evidence that not all peripheral neural disorders respond to such management (Schäfer et al., 2014; Su & Lim, 2016). Carpal tunnel syndrome (CTS) is the most common peripheral neuropathy, yet an old systematic review failed to find convincing evidence of significant therapeutic effects for neural mobilization (Medina McKeon & Yancosek 2008). Considering this evidence, it might seem that neural mobilization for CTS should not be applied. However, the methodology in these trials was weak due to poor subject selection, whereby some patients were not appropriate for this form of intervention, thus reducing the overall effect of therapy. In fact, a more recent randomized clinical trial found that the inclusion of neural mobilization of the median nerve within a multimodal manual therapy approach was equally effective at long term as surgery for the management of CTS (Fernández-de-las-Peñas et al., 2015). Furthermore, positive benefits have also been more recently shown for neural mobilization when compared to a 'keep active approach' (Nee et al., 2012; Ferreira et al., 2016) for individuals with cervicobrachial pain and features of PNS. The most recent review has concluded that neural mobilization may be effective for some conditions, but not for all (Basson et al., 2017).

Mobilization of cranial neural tissue is a newer phenomenon, with few physical therapists using it in management. This is despite clinical evidence supporting the need for cranial neural mobilization. For example, patients after meningitis may have reduced neck flexion associated with neck and face pain (Curtis et al., 2010). Neurosurgeons position the head during suboccipital decompression of the cerebellopontine angle (CPA) in extension (Jannetta et al., 2005), to reduce the stress on these structures. Neck flexion exercise is also given to reduce dural fibrosis in the intracranial occipital region after suboccipital surgery (Barba & Alksne, 1984; Bohman et al., 2014). In a single case study, Geerse and von Piekartz (2015) determined that a young female patient with chronic unilateral headache was misdiagnosed with TMJ arthrosis rather than a neural disorder of the auriculotemporal branch of the mandibular nerve. Specific neural mobilization of the involved nerve and the scar tissue, through upper cervical flexion, was associated with a reduction in headache (Geerse & von Piekartz, 2015).

An explanation for this disparity in treatment response requires an understanding of the basic mechanisms underlying neuropathic and nociceptive pain. Essentially, neural pain disorders can be broadly classified into 3 subgroups (Schäfer et al., 2009b) based on treatment likely to be effective (Schäfer et al., 2011). Each can be identified with careful clinical examination and requires a different management approach. These categories are: 1, neuropathic pain with sensory hypersensitivity; 2, compressive neuropathy; and 3, PNS.

Cranial neuropathic pain with sensory hypersensitivity

Peripheral nerve damage occurs from a variety of insults including physical nerve trauma, metabolic and vascular diseases, infections, neurotoxins, autoimmune insult, and irradiation and may lead to the development of neuropathic pain (Treede et al., 2008). Despite this nerve damage, it is important to recognize that chronic pain does not always occur after nerve injury (Costigan et al., 2009). The prevalence of moderate to severe neuropathic pain has been estimated by survey to be up to 5% in the general population (Bouhassira et al., 2008). It would appear that patients who present with these features respond poorly to any form of manual therapy (Schäfer et al., 2011) including exercise (O'Connell et al., 2013), or even medical intervention (Finnerup, et al., 2007). Hence early identification is essential for appropriate management.

Facial neuralgias with a sensory hypersensitivity are not common in daily general practice and therefore not adequately diagnosed by physicians or other therapists (Evers, 2017). Potential examples of such disorders include superior laryngeal, auriculotemporal, glossopharyngeal, or idiopathic trigeminal neuralgia. The classic presentation is stabbing, aching, throbbing or shooting pain, which extends for short episodes lasting seconds or minutes. This pain is not directly related to activity. Early identification is essential for appropriate management (Sommer, 2007).

Neuropathic pain arises from multiple pathophysiological changes in the central and peripheral nervous system. In the peripheral nervous system, these include altered gene expression and changes in ion channels that lead to ectopic activity. Indeed, stimulus-independent, spontaneous pain is a common feature of this form of pain. Peripheral input then causes synaptic facilitation and loss of inhibition at multiple levels of the nervous system, ultimately inducing central amplification (Decosterd et al., 2002). Over time this may lead to neuronal cell death and aberrant synaptic connectivity, providing the structural basis for persistently altered processing of both nociceptive and innocuous afferent input. Through a process of altered gene transcription, A fibers then behave more like C fibers, and non-noxious input now drives central sensitization (Decosterd et al., 2002). Once these changes have occurred, the input arising from normally innocuous activity such as light touch, joint movement, or muscle contraction is perceived as painful and may produce and/or maintain central sensitization and sensory hypersensitivity (Campbell & Meyer, 2006). These widespread and deep changes to the central and peripheral nervous systems lie towards the extreme end of the chronic neuropathic pain continuum, and for the purposes of classification are defined as neuropathic pain with sensory hypersensitivity (NPSH).

The diagnosis of neuropathic pain is based on key clinical features. The presence of the following four criteria increases the confidence in diagnosis (Treede et al., 2008):

1. Pain within a distinct neuroanatomically plausible distribution, for example facial dysesthesia during shaving or a shooting line of pain from

proximal to distal in the mandible, consistent with the mandibular nerve;

2. A history consistent with a lesion or a disease affecting the somatosensory system, for example after tooth extraction on the background of a whiplash-associated disorder several years ago;

3. Demonstration of altered bedside neurological function such as facial skin conduction changes with unilateral anesthesia, lack of endurance or strength of the mandibular muscles or a 'dry mouth';

4. Demonstration of the relevant lesion or disease by confirmatory test, for example mandibular nerve conduction loss or evidence of nerve compromise on MRI.

This form of pain is usually disabling and characterized by a specific set of positive features in response to increased excitability of the central and peripheral nervous system (mechanical allodynia and abnormal unpleasant sensations such as burning pain or electric shocks) together with negative signs and symptoms associated with lack of nerve conduction, which may distinguish this form of pain from other types of chronic pain (Attal et al., 2008; Baron, 2009; Baron et al., 2009). Positive features (that is, dysesthesia, allodynia, or hyperalgesia while shaving in the region of the mandible) occur within the damaged nerve innervation territory, whereas negative features are generally associated with reduced axonal conductivity of the damaged nerve. This might include anesthesia in the mandible region or lack of muscle endurance. Testing for nerve conduction loss including sensation and motor function (strength, endurance and coordination) would be important in confirming neuropathic pain. In the presence of more severe disorder, which is typical in these cases, it may not be appropriate to undertake pain provocation nerve tests, including those movements that load the peripheral nerve, as well as nerve palpation and neurodynamic testing.

Recognition of the presence of NPSH can also be achieved through the use of screening tools such as the Leeds Assessment of Neuropathic Symptoms and Signs (LANSS) Questionnaire (Bennett, 2001) shown in Table 14.1. Other questionnaires include

Table 14.1

Leeds Assessment for Neuropathic Symptoms and Signs (LANSS) Questionnaire (item score). A score greater than 12 indicates the presence of neuropathic pain.

Item	
1	Does the pain have qualities like pricking, tingling, pins & needles? (yes = 5)
2	Does the skin in the painful area look different, mottled, red/pink? (yes = 5)
3	Does the pain cause the affected area to be abnormally sensitive to touch? (yes = 3)
4	Does your pain come in bursts: electric shocks, shooting, or bursting (yes = 2)
5	Does the painful area feel like the skin temperature has changed, for example hot or burning (yes = 1)
6	Is there evidence of mechanical allodynia? (yes = 5)
7	Is there evidence of pin prick hyperalgesia or hypoalgesia? (yes = 3)

the neuropathic pain questionnaire (Galer & Jensen, 1997), the Douleur Neuropathique 4 (DN4) (Bouhassira et al., 2005), ID Pain (Portenoy, 2006) and the Standardized Evaluation of Pain (StEP) (Scholz et al., 2009). Each tool characterizes neuropathic pain by the presence of positive and negative symptoms and signs and attempts to identify the presence of neuropathic pain in a different way. For example the ID Pain is purely subjective (Portenoy, 2006), whereas the LANSS and DN4 consist of a questionnaire regarding pain description, together with items relating to the neurological examination. The sensitivity and specificity of each questionnaire have been summarized elsewhere (Hall & Elvey 2009). Each tool looks at slightly different items relating to neuropathic pain hence they cannot be used interchangeably, with each tool giving a different interpretation of the presence of neuropathic pain (Walsh et al., 2012).

Understanding the underlying process of NPSH helps us to understand how best to manage these debilitating conditions. As symptoms are associated with abnormal afferent processing of sensory information in the central nervous system, management should be directed at the abnormal processing of afferent input and not at mobilization of the nervous system.

Compressive neuropathy

Compression inducing damage of the peripheral nervous system does not necessarily cause symptoms, as previously mentioned. Even in the head–face region there may be evidence of neural conduction loss with minimal or no pain, such as in dysarthria, hemifacial spasm, facial paralysis, and diploplia (Haller et al., 2016). The presence of inflammatory mediators combined with compression appears to be the important factor in the development of symptoms. The prevalence of asymptomatic nerve compromise in the craniofacial region has been investigated in the CPA. For example there is evidence of microvascular compression of the trigeminal nerve in the CPA in healthy people, to a rate that was almost the same incidence as reported in symptomatic people with trigeminal neuralgia (Peker et al., 2009). Another example is compression of the mental or inferior alveolar nerves, which causes a 'numb chin syndrome' (NCS) in some people without pain in the lower face (Smith et al., 2015). Hence, as is the case with any other body region, imaging evidence of nerve compression should be interpreted with caution, and only if the findings are consistent with the clinical evaluation.

Clinically however, we find some patients with significant imaging and clinical signs of compression neuropathy (CN), correlated with significant pain but with an absence of positive features, and such patients test negative on neuropathic screening tools such as the LANSS scale (Schäfer et al., 2011; Moloney et al., 2013; Schäfer et al., 2014; Tampin et al., 2013). These patients fit the IASP criteria for neuropathic pain and fall under the category of 'definite neuropathic pain' according to other published guidelines (Treede et al., 2008). However, patients with CN appear to respond differently to physical intervention such as a manual therapy when compared with individuals with NPSH, presumably because of a difference in underlying pain mechanisms.

Classically, patients with features of CN present with signs of a loss of neurological conduction. In other body regions, nerve conduction loss is confirmed by the clinical evaluation of deep tendon reflexes, muscle power, skin sensation tests and vibration perception. However, this depth of analysis is not so easily available in the craniofacial region and a more comprehensive examination is required. In addition to these typical clinical findings, radiologic and electrodiagnostic evidence of CN consistent with the clinical findings would also be informative if available. As imaging by itself is not that useful in diagnosis, a combination of all these factors is likely to improve diagnostic accuracy (Haig et al., 2007).

The classic example of CN in the orofacial region is trigeminal neuralgia, which is characterized by paroxysmal, shock-like pain localized to the divisions of one or more branches of the trigeminal nerve. This is often associated with vascular compression of the sensory portion of the trigeminal nerve by an aberrant loop of artery or vein (Marinkovic et al., 2007; Marinkovic et al., 2009). Evidence for a compression element is shown by the positive effects of decompression surgery (Lovely & Jannetta, 1997). Furthermore, the severity of trigeminal nerve atrophy is related to clinical outcomes after surgical decompression (Leal et al., 2014). The vascular contact progressively compresses the trigeminal nerve root, causing symptoms to develop gradually over time inducing deformation, demyelination or remyelination (Marinkovic et al., 2009). Although pain is not always a feature of trigeminal nerve root compression, clearly changes to the ultrastructure and immunohistochemistry of the trigeminal nerve in patients with pain suggest evidence of compressive neuropathy (Marinkovic et al., 2009). Under these circumstances, there may be minimal evidence of axonal mechanosensitivity on clinical tests that lengthen the nerve (Olmarker et al., 1989; Amundsen et al., 1995) and minimal positive symptoms (Schäfer et al., 2009a).

Patients with pain associated with peripheral nerve or nerve root compression typically present with symptoms associated with activity or postures that increase compression of the involved neural structures. In the classic example of cervical foraminal stenosis, neck extension and ipsilateral lateral flexion or rotation, either in a single plane or when combined are typically provocative. These movements further reduce the space around the nerve root (Takasaki et al., 2009). This is also seen in cranial neural tissue. For example if cranial nerve tissue is compressed in the suboccipital area, then upper cervical extension may be provocative (Barba & Alksne, 1984). Another example is when an ipsilateral crossbite or lateral movement of the mandible towards the symptomatic side induces compression of trigeminal branches (Assaf et al., 2014). For these movements to compress neural structures there must be a reduction in the volume of the nerve space to begin with, which usually occurs through some degenerative process, or space-occupying lesion.

In the case of trigeminal CN, nerve conduction loss is difficult to diagnose and is based on a range of clinical indicators. At present, there is no clear clinical diagnostic test to determine if the trigeminal nerve is compressed and diagnosis is based on other typical clinical findings including pain description, location, and distribution, together with imaging evidence of CN. Unfortunately simple tools such as the neuropathic pain screening tool and painDETECT questionnaire (PD-Q) appear unsuitable in diagnostic workup in orofacial pain (Elias et al., 2014). Specialized electrodiagnostic tests may be useful in differential diagnosis (Jaaskelainen, 2004) and include the blink reflex, corneal reflex, jaw-jerk, recordings of trigeminal somatosensory-evoked potentials and sensory neurography for damage of myelinated sensory fibers. Thermal quantitative sensory testing may be also useful in detection of trigeminal small-fiber dysfunction, but is time consuming in daily practice and the equipment relatively expensive.

Table 14.2 outlines a grading system for the identification of neuropathic pain with features of CN based on an evidence-based guideline (Treede et al., 2008). If all four criteria are met, a definitive diagnosis of neuropathic pain can be made, and the source of nerve compression of musculoskeletal origin identified to rule out other forms of nerve damage such as diabetic neuropathy. Unfortunately, criterion 4 is not normally available to the clinician when examining most patients. MRI for example is the gold standard test to identify cranial nerve compression, particularly for the extracranial critical zones and variety of cranial nerve anastomoses, but it is not always available. An example of a classic CN is 'Eagle Syndrome', which is caused by compression of the glossopharyngeal nerve (IX), and is often misdiagnosed. The clinical presentation is described in the following case. A 38-year old female with a dry mouth, swallowing problems and a dull pain in the mandibular–sternocleidomastoid triangle fulfils criterion 1. The problem increased slowly after an upper respiratory tract infection two months previously. Six months prior to this, she had the right wisdom teeth extracted, fulfilling criterion 2. Examination revealed decreased activity of the soft palate on the right side (over the palatoglossal arch) during swallowing, as well as dysesthesia in the posterior part of the tongue. Weakness or lack of endurance of movement of the tongue fulfils criterion 3. A lateral X-ray revealed an increased right styloid process which could potentially compress the glossopharyngeal nerve (IX), providing evidence for criterion 4. Therefore, after surgical resection of the styloid process the symptoms of dry mouth and tongue dysesthesia, as well as decreased activity of the soft palate improved.

Peripheral nerve sensitization

Under some circumstances peripheral nerve injury or disease does not cause nerve damage sufficient to induce conduction loss, but the nerve becomes inflamed. In this situation, nerve trunk connective tissue becomes sensitized, which might explain pain arising from minor nerve damage (Zusman, 2008). Although the disorder involves the nerve trunk, the pain is nociceptive, as damage of the conducting elements does not occur per se. This is an important distinction, particularly when considering the use of neural mobilization techniques, as will become apparent later in this chapter.

One explanation for the pain in this situation is the nervi nervorum which provides a sporadic plexus of sensory nerves, that innervate the connective tissue layers of nerve trunks (Bove & Light 1995; Bove & Light, 1997). The basic function of the nervi nervorum is protection from excessive mechanical stress, as they respond to excessive stretch and focal pressure of the nerve they innervate (Zochodne, 1993; Bove & Light, 1997). Under normal circumstances, minimal responses are evoked by elongation of nerve tissue (Dilley et al., 2005). However, inflammatory mediators sensitize the nervi nervorum which may then be a source of nociception, even during small

Table 14.2

A grading system for the identification of compression neuropathy (Treede et al., 2008).

	Criteria	Explanation
1	Pain with a distinct neuroanatomically plausible distribution	A region corresponding to a peripheral innervation territory in the CNS
2	A history suggestive of a relevant lesion or disease affecting the peripheral or central somatosensory system	The suspected lesion is associated with pain, in a manner consistent for the condition
3	Demonstration of the distinct neuroanatomically plausible distribution by at least one confirmatory test	Neurologic signs concordant with the distribution of pain. May be supplemented by laboratory and objective tests for subclinical abnormalities
4	Demonstration of the relevant lesion or disease by at least one confirmatory test	Confirms the presence of the suspected lesion, such as imaging studies (MRI etc.)

movements that might occur during activities of daily living. For example, sensitization of the trigeminal or mandibular nerves may induce pain during movements such as eating, teeth cleaning, and yawning among others. Recently, in an excellent overview article, Chichorro et al. (2017) suggested that chronic orofacial pain may arise from long-term changes in afferent input to the brain by cranial PNS as well as changes in brain structure and modulatory pathways. Collectively, these changes result in amplification of nociception that promotes and sustains craniofacial chronic pain states (Chichorro et al., 2017).

Apart from sensitization of the nervi nervorum explaining nerve trunk pain, it has been also suggested that inflammation from the adjacent tissues may infiltrate the nerve connective tissue layers to the axons themselves (Eliav et al., 1999). These inflammatory mediators invoke physiological changes to the nerve as a result of cytokine production (Eliav et al., 2009), inducing pain (Bennett, 2006; Zusman, 2008). This process explains mechanosensitivity of inflamed nerves (Eliav et al., 1999; Bove et al., 2003; Dilley et al., 2005). Despite the physiological changes to axonal mechanosensitivity, the axons appear to conduct normally (Dilley et al., 2005). Hence this condition fails to fulfill the cardinal sign of neuropathy, which is altered axonal conduction and neurological deficit. When more extreme forms of inflammation occur with associated nerve swelling and hypoxia, structural nerve damage may occur with associated changes in nerve conduction (Gazda et al., 2001; Kleinschnitz et al., 2005). Thus, there appears to be a sliding scale of nerve injury associated with different degrees of nerve inflammation. It has also been suggested that chronic focal nerve inflammation inducing ongoing C fiber discharge, may also explain the development of complex regional pain syndrome (Bove, 2009).

In animal experimental models, it has been shown that only a proportion of Aδ and C fibers develop axonal mechanosensitivity. In these models, the responsive mechanosensitive fibers fire at only 3% stretch (Dilley et al., 2005). Potentially, even small movements of the orofacial region may be enough to induce movement of sufficient magnitude to evoke a pain response if the orofacial neural tissue is sensitized. Disruption to axoplasmic flow and axonal transport at the inflamed nerve site (Dilley & Bove, 2008a; Dilley & Bove, 2008b) are believed to be the major mechanisms underlying mechanosensitivity of axons. In addition, changes occur in the type and density of ion channels which results from altered ion channel expression in the cell body (Costigan & Woolf, 2000; Campbell & Meyer, 2006). The result is that some axons generate impulses to mechanical stimuli when they would normally not. Mechanosensitization of axons and nervi nervorum following nerve inflammation, is referred to as peripheral nerve sensitization (PNS). The presence of PNS may be detected through careful clinical examination of neurodynamic tests and nerve trunk palpation.

Pathophysiological changes in non-neural tissues adjacent to the peripheral nerve may induce physiological and physical changes of the nerve and the development of PNS, which can be identified through careful assessment (Hall & Elvey 1999; Nee & Butler, 2006). Cranial neural tissues may be inherently vulnerable to abnormal neural dynamics and consequent inflammation due to the unique relationships to cranial non-neural structures. Some examples are mentioned below:

1. Cranial dural tissue connections with cranial nerves: The cranial dura has a protective role for the brain and it has a rich vascularization and sensory innervation from the trigeminal and upper cervical dorsal root ganglia (Zhao et al., 2016). The internal layers are strongly connected with the occiput and strongly bound together with nerves that run through the skull floor including the oculomotor (III), trigeminal (V), vestibulocochlear (VII), glossopharyngeal (IX),

vagus (X) and hypoglossal (IX) nerves (Wilson-Pauwels et al., 2013).

2. Topography of the brainstem: The brainstem lies clearly dorsal to the head/neck flexion–extension axis and 10 of the 12 cranial nerves arise from the dorsolateral side of the brainstem (Breig, 1978). During upper cervical flexion, the brainstem angulates 6° to 32° and it moves in a dorsocranial direction which means that head motions (particularly upper cervical flexion and lateral flexion) induces elongation and mechanical stress of intracranial neural tissue (Doursounian et al., 1989).

3. Intracranial zones susceptible to dynamic changes:

   A. Nerve entry zones: Cranial nerves arising from the dorsolateral side of the brainstem have a number of anastomoses, which are embedded in cranial arteries, some of which are connected to each other by connective tissue. Some examples include branches of the trigeminal, oculomotor, vestibular, and facial nerves (Demski, 1993; Brown et al., 2000).

   B. Cerebellopontine angle (CPA): This cerebrospinal fluid-filled space includes the nerve entry zones bounded by the pons, cerebellum and the temporal bone. This region is vulnerable to pressure increases, for example with aneurysm, minor benign tumors, or fibrosis of connective tissue (Schessel et al., 1993; Koperer et al., 1999).

   C. Cavernous sinus: This tunnel is formed on the ventrolateral side of the cranium and extends from the sphenoid–temporal bone, around dural tissue. The tunnel includes the carotid artery, oculomotor, trochlear, and ophthalmic nerves as well as the maxillary division of the trigeminal nerve (Wilson-Pauwels et al., 2013).

4. Extracranial zones susceptible to dynamic changes: The extracranial part of cranial neural

tissue has a great variability and anastomoses, which may explain misdiagnosis of patients with head and face pain (Shoja et al., 2014, 2014b). An example is the extensive variability in the distribution of the trigeminal nerve from the brainstem through the CPA, Meckel's cave, cavernous sinus through into the peripheral divisions (Graff-Radford et al., 2015). Variability in the supra- and infraorbital foramina for the ophthalmic and maxillary nerve divisions, as well as variations of the head of the mandible/TMJ disc distance, may induce abnormal movement of associated cranial neural tissue and may predispose individuals to PNS and neuropathic pain (Pedulla et al., 2009).

Clinical reasoning for assessment and treatment

Nerve trunk inflammation and consequent PNS may be associated with a range of musculoskeletal disorders including TMD and orofacial pain and should be evaluated for as a routine aspect of clinical examination (Nee & Butler, 2006). Nerve inflammation can explain nerve pain in the absence of significant fascicular damage. The presence of nerve mechanosensitivity is important for pain provoked by neurodynamic tests. The presence of nerve damage per se does not necessarily evoke a positive response. Indeed, the absence of a positive response to a neurodynamic test has been associated with more severe dysfunction of unmyelinated fibers (Baselgia et al., 2017). Hence, neurodynamic tests are unlikely to be helpful in identifying fascicular damage, but should be helpful in identifying mechanosensitivity of the nerve associated with inflammatory changes.

A diagnosis of cranial PNS is established through comprehensive examination by a process of neurodynamic tests to induce mechanical loading on the cranial neural system. We propose the following three categories of tests to load different parts of the system (including nerve trunks) to determine the presence of a cranial PNS disorder:

Category 1. The most fundamental tests which mechanically challenge the brainstem and nerve entry zones as well as the tissues in the CPA by upper cervical flexion/extension.

Category 2. These tests are relatively simple and can be used to screen a broad spectrum of patients with cranial dysfunction and pain with a cranial neural involvement. These are the 'key' cranial nerves including the trigeminal (V), facial (VII), vestibulocochlear (VIII), accessory (XI) and hypoglossal (XII) nerves (von Piekartz, 2007).

Category 3. These tests evaluate the remaining cranial nerves which are no less important but are encountered in certain specific pathologies and symptoms. These tests are for the olfactory (I), optic (II), oculomotor (III), trochlear (IV), abducens (VI), glossopharyngeal (IX) and vagus (X) nerves (von Piekartz, 2007).

It should be considered that reliability and preliminary validity of the classification system to differentiate different types of nerve problems has been demonstrated to be good in patients with low back related leg pain (Schäfer et al., 2008, 2009a, 2009b, 2011, 2014) and in patients with upper limb pain (Moloney et al., 2015). To date, no studies have investigated the reliability or clinical utility in orofacial pain disorders, hence much further validation is required.

An overview of the decision-making process to test cranial neural tissue mechanosensitivity in patients with craniofacial pain is shown in Figure 14.1. A clinical example of the testing process to identify cranial PNS can be seen in the following example. A 32-year old female patient developed a suprahyoid scar (Figure 14.2) after surgery to remove a tumor in the submandibular region resulting in possible adhesions of the branches of the glossopharyngeal and/or

vagus nerves (X). Her main complaint was difficulty talking for longer than 15 minutes, which provoked a dull ventral throat pain and a growing 'close' feeling in the throat, and she also suffered from dysphagia and dysarthria. There was no evidence of altered conduction (negative for CN) and LANSS scale results were negative. A neurologist reported no evidence of neuropathy. Assessment revealed hypersensitivity to light touch skin sensation over the skin on the right ventral aspect of the throat and right mandibular region. The skin was less movable over the subcutaneous fascia in this area. The pharyngeal branch of the vagus nerve was thicker on palpation than the other side and more sensitive to touch on the right (VAS 8/10) compared to the left side (VAS 2/10) and reproduced the ventral neck pain (VAS 4/10) and altered throat sensation (Figure 14.3). Neurodynamic testing of the vagus nerve was positive with symptom reproduction on the right side together with asymmetry in range and end feel between testing the left and right sides (Figure 14.4). The neurodynamic test comprised upper cervical flexion and contralateral lateral-flexion with cervical extension and anterior posterior movement of the sternum (inspiration and expiration). In this case there were sufficient clinical features to support a diagnosis of PNS affecting the cranial neural tissue, principally affecting the vagus nerve. Treatment included neural mobilization in the form of neural gliding techniques and neural exercise. This treatment was provided in combination with techniques targeting the associated musculoskeletal tissues. The aim of the intervention was to gradually desensitize the neural tissue to a normal level of mechanosensitivity, thereby relieving pain and improving function.

Summary of assessment and management

Although management of cranial neuropathies is not the scope of this chapter, the authors wanted to provide some critical comment on the use of neural mobilization in the management of musculoskeletal

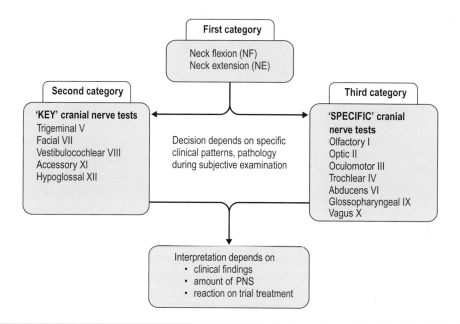

First category

Neck flexion (NF)
Neck extension (NE)

Second category

'KEY' cranial nerve tests
Trigeminal V
Facial VII
Vestibulocochlear VIII
Accessory XI
Hypoglossal XII

Decision depends on specific
clinical patterns, pathology
during subjective examination

Third category

**'SPECIFIC' cranial
nerve tests**
Olfactory I
Optic II
Oculomotor III
Trochlear IV
Abducens VI
Glossopharyngeal IX
Vagus X

Interpretation depends on
• clinical findings
• amount of PNS
• reaction on trial treatment

Figure 14.1

Overview of testing for cranial neural tissue mechanosensitivity in patients with craniofacial pain. PNS, peripheral nerve sensitization.

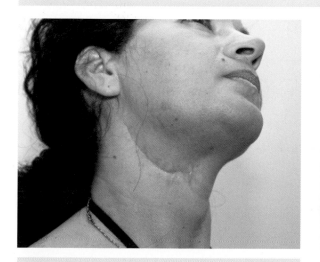

Figure 14.2

A 32-year-old female with PNS of the vagus nerve following a tumor resection in the submandibular region.

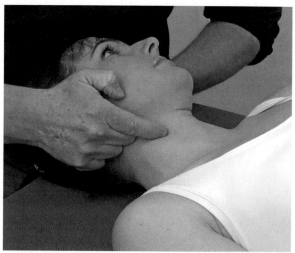

Figure 14.3

Palpation of the pharyngeal branches of the vagus nerve.

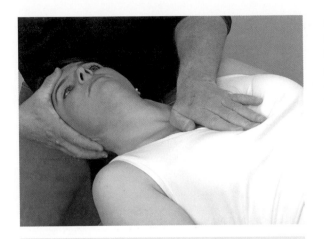

Figure 14.4
Neurodynamic test of the vagus nerve.

disorders such as those seen in orofacial pain. Neural mobilization is a maturing aspect of manual therapy, but its implementation must be carefully considered to be effective. It may appear ineffective in undifferentiated pain conditions (Salt et al., 2016), but useful in carefully selected patients (Nee et al., 2012). A rationale for classification of neural tissue pain disorders into subgroups, with the goal of identifying potential patients suitable for neural mobilization has been given based on neurophysiology and nociceptive mechanisms (Figure 14.5). To determine which category the patient falls into requires a comprehensive examination process. Although patients with orofacial pain may well have features that could be assigned to all categories, the classification system is hierarchical and therefore groups mutually exclusive. The order of diagnosis should be NPSH,

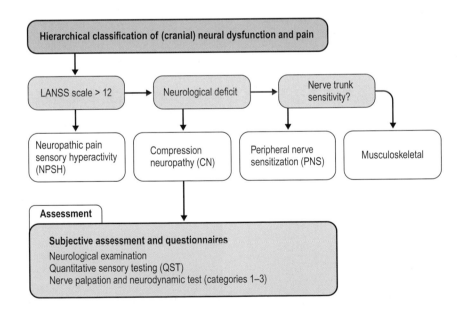

Figure 14.5
Hierarchical classification of cranial neural pain disorders into specific neural subgroups with proposed assessments (modified after Schäfer et al., 2009b). LANSS, Leeds Assessment of Neuropathic Symptoms and Signs.

CN, PNS and musculoskeletal pain. In the absence of a positive LANSS test (Table 14.1; positive score greater than or equal to 12), the next priority is CN. A diagnosis of PNS is based on an absence of NPSH and CN, and on the presence of signs of mechanosensitive neural tissue. This is the group most likely to respond to neural mobilization techniques. Finally, in the absence of any feature suggesting a neural disorder, patients would be classified as having musculoskeletal pain. The authors strongly support this strategy of classification in patients with neurogenic disorders affecting the head and the face region, although further research is required to determine the validity of this system.

References

Amundsen T, Weber H, Lilleas F et al. Lumbar spinal stenosis: Clinical and radiologic features. Spine 1995; 20: 1178–1186.

Assaf AT, Jurgens TP, Benecke AW et al. Numb chin syndrome: a rare and often overlooked symptom. J Oral Facial Pain Headache 2014; 28: 80–90.

Attal N, Fermanian C, Fermanian J et al. Neuropathic pain: are there distinct subtypes depending on the aetiology or anatomical lesion? Pain 2008; 138: 343–353.

Barba D, Alksne JF. Success of microvascular decompression with and without prior surgical therapy for trigeminal neuralgia. J Neurosurg 1984; 60: 104–107.

Baron R. Neuropathic pain: a clinical perspective. Handb Exp Pharmacol 2009; 194: 3–30.

Baron R, Tolle TR, Gockel U, Brosz M, Freynhagen R. A cross-sectional cohort survey in 2100 patients with painful diabetic neuropathy and postherpetic neuralgia: Differences in demographic data and sensory symptoms. Pain 2009; 146: 34–40.

Baselgia LT, Bennett DL, Silbiger RM, Schmid AB. Negative neurodynamic tests do not exclude neural dysfunction in patients with entrapment neuropathies. Arch Phys Med Rehabil 2017; 98: 480–486.

Basson A, Olivier B, Ellis R, Coppieters M, Stewart A, Mudzi W. The effectiveness of neural mobilization for neuro-musculoskeletal conditions: A systematic review and meta-analysis. J Orthop Sports Phys Ther 2017 doi: 10.2519/jospt.2017.7117.

Bennett GJ. Can we distinguish between inflammatory and neuropathic pain. Pain Res Manage 2006; 11: S11A–S15A.

Bennett M. The LANSS Pain Scale: the Leeds assessment of neuropathic symptoms and signs. Pain 2001; 92: 147–157.

Bereiter DA, Hirata H, Hu JW. Trigeminal subnucleus caudalis: beyond homologies with the spinal dorsal horn. Pain 2000; 88: 221–224.

Bohman LE, Pierce J, Stephen JH, Sandhu S, Lee JY. Fully endoscopic microvascular decompression for trigeminal neuralgia: technique review and early outcomes. Neurosurg Focus 2014; 3: E18.

Bouhassira D, Attal N, Alchaar H et al. Comparison of pain syndromes associated with nervous or somatic lesions and development of a new neuropathic pain diagnostic questionnaire (DN4). Pain 2005; 114: 29–36.

Bouhassira D, Lanteri-Minet M, Attal N, Laurent B, Touboul C. Prevalence of chronic pain with neuropathic characteristics in the general population. Pain 2008; 136: 380–387.

Bove G, Light A. Unmyelinated nociceptors of rat paraspinal tissues. Journal of Neurophysiology 1995; 73: 1752–1762.

Bove G, Light A. The nervi nervorum: Missing link for neuropathic pain? Pain forum 1997; 6: 181–190.

Bove GM. Focal nerve inflammation induces neuronal signs consistent with symptoms of early complex regional pain syndromes. Exp Neurol 2009; 219: 223–227.

Bove GM, Ransil BJ, Lin HC, Leem JG. Inflammation induces ectopic mechanical sensitivity in axons of nociceptors innervating deep tissues. J Neurophysiol 2003; 90: 1949–1955.

Breig A. Adverse mechanical tension in the central nervous system: Relief by functional neurosurgery. Stockholm, Almquist and Wiksell; 1978.

Brown H, Hidden G, Ledroux N, Poitevan L. Anatomy and blood supply of the lower four cranial and cervical nerves: relevance to surgical neck dissection. Proc Soc Exp Biol Med 2000; 223: 352–361.

Campbell JN, Meyer RA. Mechanisms of neuropathic pain. Neuron 2006; 52: 77–92.

Chichorro JG, Porreca F, Sessle B. Mechanisms of craniofacial pain. Cephalalgia 2017; 37: 613–626.

Costigan M, Woolf CJ. Pain: molecular mechanisms. J Pain 2000; 1: 35–44.

Costigan M, Scholz J, Woolf CJ. Neuropathic pain: a maladaptive response of the nervous system to damage. Annu Rev Neurosci 2009; 32: 1–32.

Cruccu G, Pennisi EM, Antonini G et al. Trigeminal isolated sensory neuropathy (TISN) and FOSMN syndrome: despite a dissimilar disease course do they share common pathophysiological mechanisms? BMC Neurol 2014; 14: 248.

Curtis S, Stobart K, Vandermeer B, Simel DL, Klassen T. Clinical features suggestive of meningitis in children: a systematic review of prospective data. Pediatrics 2010; 126: 952–960.

Decosterd I, Allchorne A, Woolf CJ. Progressive tactile hypersensitivity after a peripheral nerve crush: non-noxious mechanical stimulus-induced neuropathic pain. Pain 2002; 100: 155–162.

Demski LS. Terminal nerve complex. Acta Anat 1993; 148: 81–95.

Dilley A, Bove GM. Disruption of axoplasmic transport induces mechanical sensitivity in intact rat C-fibre nociceptor axons. J Physiol 2008a; 586: 593–604.

Dilley A, Bove GM. Resolution of inflammation-induced axonal mechanical sensitivity and conduction slowing in C-fiber nociceptors. J Pain 2008b; 9: 185–192.

Dilley A, Lynn B, Pang SJ. Pressure and stretch mechanosensitivity of peripheral nerve fibres following local inflammation of the nerve trunk. Pain 2005; 117: 462–472.

Doursounian L, Alfonso JM, Iba-Zizen MT et al. Dynamics of the junction between the medulla and the cervical spinal cord: an in vivo study in the sagittal plane by magnetic resonance imaging. Surg Radiol Anat 1989; 11: 313–322.

Elias L, Yilmaz Z, Smith J et al. PainDETECT: a suitable screening tool for neuropathic pain in patients with painful post-traumatic trigeminal nerve injuries? Int J Oral Maxillofac Surg 2014; 43: 120–126.

Eliav E, Herzberg U, Ruda MA, Bennett JG. Neuropathic pain from an experimental neuritis of the rat sciatic nerve. Pain 1999; 83: 169–182.

Eliav E, Benoliel R, Herzberg U, Kalladka M, Tal M. The role of IL-6 and IL-1beta in painful perineural inflammatory neuritis. Brain Behav Immun 2009; 23: 474–484.

Evers S. Facial pain: Overlapping syndromes. Cephalalgia 2017; 37: 705–713.

Fernández-de-las-Peñas C, Ortega-Santiago R, de la Llave-Rincón AI et al. Manual physical therapy versus surgery for carpal tunnel syndrome: A randomized parallel-group trial. J Pain 2015; 16: 1087–1094.

Ferreira G, Stieven F, Araujo F, Wiebusch M, Rosa C, Plentz R, Silva M. Neurodynamic treatment did not improve pain and disability at two weeks in patients with chronic nerve-related leg pain: a randomised trial. J Physiother 2016; 62: 197–202.

Finnerup NB, Otto M, Jensen TS, Sindrup SH. An evidence-based algorithm for the treatment of neuropathic pain. MedGenMed 2007; 9: 36.

Finnerup NB, Haroutounian S, Kamerman P et al. Neuropathic pain: an updated grading system for research and clinical practice. Pain 2016; 157: 1599–1606.

Forssell H, Jaaskelainen S, List T, Svensson P, Baad-Hansen L. An update on pathophysiological mechanisms related to idiopathic oro-facial pain conditions with implications for management. J Oral Rehabil 2015; 42: 300–322.

Galer BS, Jensen MP. Development and preliminary validation of a pain measure specific to neuropathic pain: the Neuropathic Pain Scale. Neurology 1997; 48: 332–338.

Gazda LS, Milligan ED, Hansen M et al. Sciatic inflammatory neuritis (SIN): behavioral allodynia is paralleled by peri-sciatic proinflammatory cytokine and superoxide production. J Peripher Nerv Syst 2001; 6: 111–129.

Geerse WK, von Piekartz HJ. Ear pain following temporomandibular surgery originating from the temporomandibular joint or the cranial nervous tissue? A case report. Man Ther 2015; 20: 212–215.

Graff-Radford S, Gordon R, Ganal J, Tetradis S. Trigeminal neuralgia and facial pain imaging. Curr Pain Headache Rep 2015; 19: 19.

Greening J, Dilley A, Lynn B. In vivo study of nerve movement and mechanosensitivity of the median nerve in whiplash and non-specific arm pain patients. Pain 2005; 115: 248–253.

Gursoy M, Orru E, Blitz AM, Carey JP, Olivi A, Yousem D. Hypoglossal canal invasion by glomus jugulare tumors: clinico-radiological correlation. Clin Imaging 2014; 38: 655–658.

Haig AJ, Geisser ME, Tong H et al. Electromyographic and magnetic resonance imaging to predict lumbar stenosis, low-back pain, and no back symptoms. J Bone Joint Surg Am 2007; 89: 358–366.

Hall T, Elvey RL. Nerve trunk pain: physical diagnosis and treatment. Man Ther 1999; 4: 63–73.

Hall T, Elvey RL. Evaluation and treatment of neural tissue pain disorders. In: Donatelli R, Wooden M (ed). Orthopaedic physical therapy. New York, Churchill Livingstone; 2009.

Haller S, Etienne L, Kovari E, Varoquaux AD, Urbach H, Becker M. Imaging of neurovascular compression syndromes: Trigeminal neuralgia, hemifacial spasm, vestibular paroxysmia, and glossopharyngeal neuralgia. AJNR Am J Neuroradiol 2016; 37: 1384–1392.

Hans G, Masquelier E, De Cock P. The diagnosis and management of neuropathic pain in daily practice in Belgium: an observational study. BMC Public Health 2007; 7: 170.

Jaaskelainen SK. Clinical neurophysiology and quantitative sensory testing in the investigation of orofacial pain and sensory function. J Orofac Pain 2004; 18: 85–107.

Jannetta PJ, McLaughlin MR, Casey KF. Technique of microvascular decompression. Technical note. Neurosurg Focus 2005; 18: E5.

Jensen TS, Baron R, Haanpaa M et al. A new definition of neuropathic pain. Pain 2011; 152: 2204–2205.

Jull G, Sterling M, Kenardy J, Beller E. Does the presence of sensory hypersensitivity influence outcomes of physical rehabilitation for chronic whiplash?: A preliminary RCT. Pain 2007; 129: 28–34.

Kleinschnitz C, Brinkhoff J, Sommer C, Stoll G. Contralateral cytokine gene induction after peripheral nerve lesions: dependence on the mode of injury and NMDA receptor signaling. Brain Res Mol Brain Res 2005; 136: 23–28.

Koperer H, Weinsberger D, Jodicke A, Boker D. Postoperative headache after the lateral suboccipital approach: craniotomy versus craniectomy. Minim Invasive Neurosurg 1999; 42: 175–178.

Leal PR, Barbier C, Hermier M, Souza M, Cristino-Filho G, Sindou M. Atrophic changes in the trigeminal nerves of patients with trigeminal neuralgia due to neurovascular compression and their association with the severity of compression and clinical outcomes. J Neurosurg 2014; 120: 1484–1495.

Lovely TJ, Jannetta PJ. Microvascular decompression for trigeminal neuralgia. Surgical technique and long-term results. Neurosurg Clin N Am 1997; 8: 11–29.

Marchettini P, Lacerenza M, Mauri E, Marangoni C. Painful peripheral neuropathies. Curr Neuropharmacol 2006; 4: 175–181.

Marinkovic S, Todorovic V, Gibo H et al. The trigeminal vasculature pathology in patient with neuralgia. Headache 2007; 47: 1334–1339.

Marinkovic S, Gibo H, Todorovic V, Antic B, Kovacevic D, Milisavljevic M, Cetkovic M. Ultrastructure and immunohistochemistry of the trigeminal peripheral myelinated axons in patients with neuralgia. Clin Neurol Neurosurg 2009; 111: 795–800.

Markman J, Dukes E, Siffert J, Griesing T. Patient flow in neuropathic pain management: Understanding existing patterns of care. Eur J Neurol 2004; 11: 135–136.

Medina McKeon JM, Yancosek KE. Neural gliding techniques for the treatment of carpal tunnel syndrome: a systematic review. J Sport Rehabil 2008; 17: 324–341.

Merskey H, Bogduk N. Classification of chronic pain: Descriptions of chronic pain syndromes and definitions of pain terms. Seattle, IASP; 1994.

Moloney N, Hall T, Doody C. Sensory hyperalgesia is characteristic of nonspecific arm pain: a comparison with cervical radiculopathy and pain-free controls. Clin J Pain 2013; 29: 948–956.

Moloney NA, Hall TM, Leaver AM, Doody CM. The clinical utility of pain classification in non-specific arm pain. Man Ther 2015; 20: 157–165.

Murzin VE, Goriunov VN. [Study of the strength of the adherence of the dura mater to the bones of the skull]. Zh Vopr Neirokhir Im N N Burdenko 1979; 4: 43–47.

Nee R, Butler DS. Management of peripheral neuropathic pain: Integrating neurobiology, neurodynamics, and clinical evidence. Phys Ther Sport 2006; 7: 36–49.

Nee RJ, Vicenzino B, Jull GA, Cleland JA, Coppieters MW. Neural tissue management provides immediate clinically relevant benefits without harmful effects for patients with nerve-related neck and arm pain: a randomised trial. J Physiother 2012; 58: 23–31.

Nee RJ, Vicenzino B, Jull GA, Cleland JA, Coppieters MW. Baseline characteristics of patients with nerve-related neck and arm pain predict the likely response to neural tissue management. J Orthop Sports Phys Ther 2013; 43: 379–391.

O'Connell NE, Wand BM, McAuley J, Marston L, Moseley GL. Interventions for treating pain and disability in adults with complex regional pain syndrome. Cochrane Database Syst Rev 2013; 4: CD009416.

Olmarker K, Rydevik B, Holm S, Bagge U. The effects of experimental graded compression on blood flow in spinal nerve roots. A vital microscopic study on porcine cauda equina. J Orthop Res 1989; 7: 817–823.

Pedulla E, Meli GA, Garufi A, Mandala ML, Blandino A, Cascone P. Neuropathic pain in temporomandibular joint disorders: case-control analysis by MR imaging. AJNR Am J Neuroradiol 2009; 30: 1414–1418.

Peker S, Dincer A, Necmettin Pamir M. Vascular compression of the trigeminal nerve is a frequent finding in asymptomatic individuals: 3-T MR imaging of 200 trigeminal nerves using 3D CISS sequences. Acta Neurochir 2009; 151: 1081–1088.

Portenoy R. Development and testing of a neuropathic pain screening questionnaire: ID Pain. Curr Med Res Opin 2006; 22: 1555–1565.

Salt E, Kelly S, Soundy A. Randomised controlled trial for the efficacy of cervical

lateral glide mobilisation in the management of cervicobrachial pain. Open J Ther Rehabil 2016; 4: 132–145.

Schäfer A, Hall T, Briffa K, Ludtke K, Mallwitz J. QST profiles of subgroups of patients with low back related leg pain – do they differ? International Association for the Study of Pain, Glasgow; 2008.

Schäfer A, Hall T, Briffa K, Ludtke K, Mallwitz J. Changes in somatosensory profiles in subgroups of patients with sciatica after 4 weeks of manual therapy: an observational cohort study. International Association for the Study of Pain, Glasgow, IASP press; 2009a.

Schäfer A, Hall T, Briffa K. Classification of low back-related leg pain: a proposed patho-mechanism-based approach. Man Ther 2009b 14: 222–230.

Schäfer A, Hall T, Muller G, Briffa K. Outcomes differ between subgroups of patients with low back and leg pain following neural manual therapy: a prospective cohort study. Eur Spine J 2011; 20: 482–490.

Schäfer A, Hall T, Rolke R, Treede R, Ludtke K, Mallwitz J, Briffa K. Low back related leg pain: an investigation of construct validity of a new classification system. J Back Musculoskelet Rehabil 2014; 27: 409–418.

Schessel DA, Rowed DW, Nedzelski JM, Feghali JG. Postoperative pain following excision of acoustic neuroma by the suboccipital approach: observations on possible cause and potential amelioration. Am J Otol 1993; 14: 491–494.

Scholz J, Mannion RJ, Hord DE et al. A novel tool for the assessment of pain: validation in low back pain. PLoS Med 2009; 6: e1000047.

Shoja MM, Oyesiku NM, Griessenauer CJ et al. Anastomoses between lower cranial and upper cervical nerves: a comprehensive review with potential significance during skull base and neck operations. Part I: trigeminal, facial, and vestibulocochlear nerves. Clin Anat 2014a; 27: 118–130.

Shoja MM, Oyesiku NM, Shokouhi G et al. A comprehensive review with potential significance during skull base and neck operations. Part II: glossopharyngeal, vagus, accessory, and hypoglossal nerves and cervical spinal nerves 1-4. Clin Anat 2014b; 27: 131–144.

Smith, RM, Hassan A, Robertson CE. Numb chin syndrome. Curr Pain Headache Rep 2015; 19: 44.

Sommer C. Neuralgic and idiopathic pain: Pathophysiology and management. In: Türp J, Sommer C, Hugger A (eds). The puzzle of orofacial pain: Integrating research into clinical management. Basel, Karger; 2007. Pp 153–165.

Su Y, Lim EC. Does evidence support the use of neural tissue management to reduce pain and disability in nerve-related chronic musculoskeletal pain?: A systematic review with meta-analysis. Clin J Pain 2016; 32: 991–1004.

Takasaki H, Hall T, Jull G, Kaneko S, Iizawa T, Ikemoto Y. The influence of cervical traction, compression, and spurling test on cervical intervertebral foramen size. Spine 2009; 34: 1658–1662.

Tampin B, Slater H, Briffa NK. Neuropathic pain components are common in patients with painful cervical radiculopathy, but not in patients with nonspecific neck-arm pain. Clin J Pain 2013; 29: 846–856.

Treede RD, Jensen TS, Campbell JN et al. Neuropathic pain: redefinition and a grading system for clinical and research purposes. Neurology 2008; 70: 1630–1635.

von Piekartz HJM. Craniofacial pain: Neuromusculoskeletal assessment, treatment and management. Edinburgh, Butterworth-Heinemann; 2007.

von Piekartz HJM. Kiefer, Gesichts- und Zervikalregion: Neuromuskuloskeletale Untersuchung, Therapie und Mangagement. Berlin, Thieme Georg Verlag; 2007.

von Piekartz HJM. Untersuchung und Behandlung des kranialen Nervengewebes. In von Piekartz HJM (ed). Kiefer, Gesichts-und Zervikalregion: Neuromuskuloskeletale Untersuchung, Therapie und Management. Georg Thieme Verlag; 2015: 392–465.

Walsh J, Raby M, Hall T. Agreement and correlation between the self-report Leeds Assessment of Neuropathic Symptoms and Signs and Douleur Neuropathique 4 questions neuropathic pain screening tools in subjects with low back-related leg pain. J Manipulative Physiol Ther 2012; 35: 196–202.

Wilson-Pauwels L, Stewart P, Akeson E, Spacey S. Cranial nerves: Function and dysfunction. PMPH-USA, PMPH; 2013.

Woda A. A dysfunctional pain group in addition to the neuropathic and nociception/inflammatory groups of orofacial pain entities? J Orofac Pain 2009; 23: 89–90.

Zhao J, Bree D, Harrington MG, Strassman AM, Levy D. Cranial dural permeability of inflammatory nociceptive mediators: Potential implications for animal models of migraine. Cephalalgia 2016; pii: 0333102416663466.

Zochodne D. Epineural peptides: A role in neuropathic pain. Can J Neurolog Sci 1993; 20: 69–72.

Zusman M. Mechanisms of peripheral neuropathic pain: Implications for musculoskeletal physiotherapy. Phys Ther Rev 2008; 13: 313–323.

Chapter 15

Therapeutic exercise, postural training and motor control in temporomandibular disorders

Susan Armijo-Olivo, Cristina Lozano-López, Elisa Bizetti Pelai, Laurent Pitance, Ambra Michelotti, Blanca Codina García-Andrade

Introduction

Therapeutic exercise is one of the most commonly used approaches to treat musculoskeletal pain and associated disorders, including temporomandibular disorders (TMDs). The use of therapeutic exercise has grown enormously in physiotherapy due to its benefits to treat conditions such as low back pain, neck pain, cervicogenic headache, and osteoarthritis among others (Armijo-Olivo et al., 2016; Fransen et al., 2015; Gross et al., 2016). Therapeutic exercise has been considered a cornerstone for the rehabilitation of musculoskeletal disorders (Philadelphia Panel, 2001). Exercise treatment aims to restore normal function by altering sensory input, reducing inflammation, decreasing pain and muscular activity, as well as improving coordination and strengthening of muscles, and promoting the repair and regeneration of tissues (Taylor et al., 2007). Although the effects of therapeutic exercise on pain are not fully understood, its application is widely used (Armijo-Olivo et al., 2016; Fransen et al., 2015; Gross et al, 2016). Emerging evidence has highlighted that treatment for chronic musculoskeletal pain conditions, including exercises that target not only the peripheral musculoskeletal system but also cortical neuroplastic changes caused by chronic pain, provide the greatest potential for rehabilitation success (Pelletier et al., 2015). Besides its effects on function and health, therapeutic exercise is known to have some pain-relieving effects (Sokunbi et al., 2007, 2008) and specific motor control exercises targeted to the neck can enhance the neural control of the cervical spine in individuals with neck involvement such as patients with TMD.

It has been highlighted that any exercise program should restore the patient's key functional deficits. This function-oriented approach is meaningful for patients and facilitates compliance with the exercises. In addition, therapeutic exercise should be implemented early in the rehabilitation process and has to be free of pain to avoid exacerbation of symptoms and fear avoidance behavior (O'Leary et al., 2009).

Exercises are widely prescribed by clinicians treating TMDs because of the 'self-management character' of the treatment and amelioration of coping for the patient. In order to perform correctly any exercise program, it is very important to motivate and carefully instruct the patient, to achieve good compliance.

In this chapter we will describe specific exercises for the orofacial region, specifically the jaw, and also we will describe exercises for the neck, which are generally used in subjects with TMD and orofacial pain due to the close relationship between the stomatognathic system and the cervical spine (Armijo Olivo et al., 2006) and the neck musculoskeletal impairments seen in subjects with TMD (Armijo-Olivo et al., 2010, 2011, 2012; Olivo et al., 2010). It is hoped that this chapter helps clinicians working with patients with TMD to plan a treatment protocol and provide guidance in their treatment using therapeutic exercises.

Jaw exercises

Patients with TMD present abnormal temporomandibular joint (TMJ) movement patterns and jaw functional limitations. These dysfunctional movement patterns are mainly the result of reorganized jaw muscle activity, specifically in chronic TMD patients with severe symptomatology (Mapelli et al., 2016). Dysfunction and craniofacial pain, among others, cause psychological dysfunction in these patients. Exercises are useful to change the experience of pain in TMDs, decreasing fear avoidance, kinesiophobia and catastrophizing behaviors (Nijs et al., 2013). Exercise induces physiological changes: it reduces the overall sensitivity on the central nervous system with a modified pain output; and also, it produces an induced endogenous analgesia effect (it is thought to occur due to a release of endogenous opioids and activation of spinal inhibitory mechanisms) (Littlewood et al., 2013). Although different therapeutic exercises have different mechanisms of action, the general objective of exercises is to allow healing and prevent further injury to the musculoskeletal system (Durham et al., 2016).

Jaw exercises involve the active participation of patients in their own management. For this reason they are included as a component of a self-management program for TMDs. Education, self-massage, thermal therapy, dietary advice and nutrition, parafunctional behavior identification, monitoring and avoidance are embraced also in self-management. When patients perform jaw exercises, they feel motivated and they feel responsible of their treatment (Durham et al., 2016; Lindfors et al., 2017). A qualitative study looking at patients' experiences of therapeutic jaw exercises in the treatment of masticatory myofascial pain concluded that patients consider jaw exercises as a useful treatment due to their simplicity and effectiveness (Lindfors et al., 2017).

There is still a lack of consensus about dosage or duration of the exercises. For now, it has been recommended to do exercises until the 'pain limit' or tolerance, that is, patients must not feel pain when exercising. However, a recent investigation has shown that protocols using exercises into pain for chronic musculoskeletal pain offer a small but significant benefit over pain-free exercises in the short term (Smith et al., 2017). There is evidence to support that therapeutic exercise is effective across a diverse range of physiotherapy practices, specifically when it is individualized or targeted (Taylor et al., 2007). Exercises, mainly postural corrections and jaw exercises, seem to be beneficial for patients with myogenous and arthrogenous TMDs, although, the overall level of evidence is low (Armijo-Olivo et al., 2016; Medlicott & Harris, 2006).

In this section, we will describe a protocol of jaw exercises which has been used to restore mobility, improve proprioception, and to decrease pain in subjects with TMD. Also, we explain aspects of education that should be considered by the clinician when treating patients with TMD.

General jaw exercises

Jaw exercises are usually combined with other physical therapy techniques such as joint mobilizations or manipulations, and physical agents for the management of patients with TMD. The principal aims of these treatments are to increase jaw range of movement and to decrease pain intensity (Medlicott & Harris, 2006). In the case of subjects in an acute phase or intense pain, it is recommended to do first slow and controlled active or passive exercises and, when the symptomatology decreases, strengthening exercises of the masticatory muscles can be performed.

In patients with TMD, the TMJ can be very sensitive. For this reason, patients are taught to progressively load the joint using frequent exercises with small number of repetitions (Armijo-Olivo & Gadotti, 2016). Although there is no consensus about dosage of exercises, some authors, such as Rocabado (1979) designed a 6 x 6 x 6 protocol: six exercises performed six times a day, with six repetitions of each exercise. Other clinicians prefer that the patient perform one or two exercises each hour, doing a few repetitions of each one. Also, it has been suggested to do the exercises in conjunction with an already established routine (for example tooth brushing) to enhance adherence of the patient to the program (Lindfors et al., 2017). It is important for these patients to avoid any movements or parafunctions that might aggravate the condition (Bae & Park, 2013; Durham et al., 2016; Nascimento et al., 2013).

Jaw exercises can be divided into active or passive jaw movements, stretching exercises, and proprioceptive exercises.

Active jaw movements

There is evidence supporting the use of active exercises to reduce muscle spasm and pain, to improve muscle strength and resistance, and to restore muscle function and motor control (Armijo-Olivo & Gadotti, 2016). At the beginning, active jaw movements are performed with the help of a mirror to provide visual feedback on the position of the jaw and to facilitate their execution. Then, patients can perform the exercises without the need of the mirror.

A. Active mouth movements without resistance

The most common jaw exercises are the active mouth opening, laterotrusive movements, and protrusive movements (Bae & Park, 2013; Niemelä et al., 2012). To perform these active exercises, the patients can start with their jaw in the middle range position of mouth opening for a few seconds, doing the movements in a slow and controlled way. During the open mouth exercise, the tip of the tongue should remain coupled to the palate in order to establish a limit of the opening movement, especially if the patients have TMJ hypermobility. These movements are usually used to enhance relaxation of the jaw muscles, to improve lubrication of the TMJ, and to obtain controlled and symmetrical mandibular mobility as well as to help control pain through the stimulation of joint receptors (de Felício et al., 2010; Haketa et al., 2010). These exercises are easy to perform and patients are advised to do them during the day in their daily routine (Figure 15.1). Also subjects are encouraged to perform lateral and protrusive movement of the jaw in this position.

B. Control TMJ rotation

Another variant of the active mouth opening is to perform an active mouth opening movement with control of the TMJ rotation (Mulet et al., 2007).

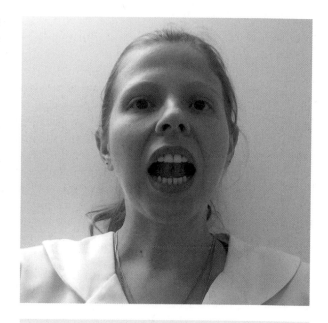

Figure 15.1
Active mouth movement without resistance.

To perform it, the patient locates the index fingers over the TMJ and opens and closes the mouth, stopping if he/she feels that the condyle ('ball') of the joint is moving forward against the fingers. The patient holds his/her tongue placed on the soft palate while doing the exercise. This exercise is indicated primarily for subjects with arthrogenous TMDs because it aids the subject to be aware of the proper manner of executing habitual jaw functions such as chewing, yawning or swallowing. Also, it is useful for patients with myogenous and mixed TMDs to improve their motor control which is decreased in these conditions.

C. Active mouth movements with resistance

Active jaw exercises can also be made with resistance using the patient's own fingers or they can be done by the therapist. To do these exercises, the patient must place his/her index finger over, under or beside the chin, depending on the desired movement, to apply a low resistance. In this case, the aims of these exercises are to recruit the highest possible number of muscular motor units from the masticatory muscles and improve strength. Also, graded contractions with a low load for longer periods of time could be helpful to increase endurance. There is evidence, from other pathologies, that dynamic resistance training correlates with improved joint strength, increased neuromuscular performance and better performance of functional tasks (Yadav & Attrey, 2017).

In general, there is not much information about dosages. These exercises are performed according to the patient's tolerance and loading management principles. The 6×6×6 Rocabado's protocol would be applicable for these exercises as well (Rocabado, 1979).

D. Mandibular body-condylar cross-pressure chewing technique

The 'mandibular body-condylar cross-pressure chewing technique' is a modification of a chiropractic technique. It is an active self-mobilization exercise where the patient places his/her hand (pisiform) on the ipsilateral TMJ and the heel of the other hand is kept beside the contralateral side of the chin. Then, the subject opens and closes the mouth exerting pressure over the contacts with his/her hands. If it is tolerable, the pressure should be increased with each successive opening (Figure 15.2). This exercise can be done five times on both sides. The aim of this exercise is to stimulate and stretch the joint capsule and relax the masticatory muscles. Despite limited studies of this technique, it might be recommended for all TMD patients, mainly for arthrogenous cases due to its effect on the joint capsule (Kalamir et al., 2010, 2012, 2013).

E. Active movements using the tongue as 'starter' of the movement

These exercises can be performed to stimulate jaw mobility especially if there is a limitation in the range of motion or if the patient has a fear of movement. The patient can stick out his/her tongue forward or to the right and left sides to induce protruding/opening or lateral jaw movements. In this case, the practitioner should insist more on tongue movement instead of jaw movement when instructing the patient to perform these exercises. These exercises are performed according to the patient's tolerance.

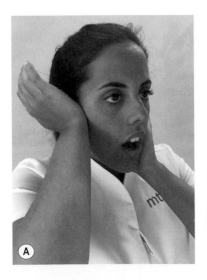

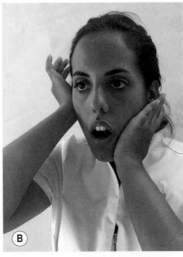

Figure 15.2
Mandibular body-condylar cross-pressure chewing technique.

Passive-assisted jaw movements

Some devices such as the TheraBite jaw motion rehabilitation system® (Atos Medical AB, Hörby, Sweden), Dynasplint (Stubblefield et al., 2010) or tongue depressors can be used to passively assist jaw movements. These devices aim to improve the coordination of jaw movements and to increase range of motion. These devices are reported to be effective to improve range of motion and decrease pain intensity in subjects with arthrogenous and/or myogenous TMD. Subjects with myogenous TMD have shown greater reduction in pain intensity than subjects with arthrogenous TMD (Kraaijenga et al., 2014; Maloney et al, 2002).

A. Passive jaw movements using a TheraBite® device

TheraBite® is a passive jaw mobilization system that can be used by the patient without the help of a medical professional. It consists of two mouthpieces, attached to plastic handles. The mouthpieces are inserted between the upper and lower teeth. The patient's mouth can be opened by pressing together the plastic handles that force the mouthpieces to separate. The device must be held in the patient's preferred hand. The use of a TheraBite® device has been reported to reduce pain intensity and improve range of motion. The TheraBite® is a high-torque appliance that provides a short-duration passive stretch (Maloney et al., 2002). Some studies have determined that this device offers faster and better functional improvement than classic physical therapy when used to treat acute myogenic TMD (Satomi et al., 2013).

The program must be personalized according to the patients' symptomatology. The common dosage is 7-7-7; this means, seven movements, maintained for seven seconds, performed seven times per day. The regimen will vary depending on the aim, for example, if the objective is to induce more stretching, it would be beneficial to maintain 30 seconds for each repetition.

A mechanically assisted jaw mobilization can be done using stacked tongue depressors as well. For its performance, the patient places a tongue depressor between the upper and lower teeth on both sides. Then, the patient must add tongue depressors to gently force the mouth open and to achieve a moderate stretch. Although there are few studies concerning the dosage of this exercise, it could be convenient to do the assisted exercise between 3–5 times a day, with a pause of two seconds at the maximum possible mouth open position (Ren et al., 2013). The principal aim of this technique is to increase the range of motion of the jaw.

B. Self-mobilization with movement (MWM)

Brian Mulligan introduced MWM, a manual therapy technique combining passive accessory mobilization of the joint performed by the therapist combined with active movement performed by the patient. The principles of the technique have been adapted to the TMJ for painful limitation of mandibular depression or jaw closure (González-Iglesias et al., 2013; Vicenzino et al., 2011). If the manual therapy technique is effective, the therapist teaches self-MWM exercises to the patient. The patient uses his hand, or his fingers to passively mobilize the TMJ in the joint articular plane and performs actively the previously painful or limited movement. A slight passive overpressure can be added at the end of the movement. The technique should be performed without pain. This technique is indicated for limitation of the jaw movement by pain or resistance. The recommended dosage is three sets of 6–10 repetitions.

Stretching

The aim of stretching is to allow movements in the periarticular structures to restore the lubrication efficiency between collagen fibers and stimulate the glycol-aminoglycan synthesis (Carmeli et al., 2001). Stretching is beneficial for both arthrogenous and myogenous TMDs. To self-stretch the jaw muscles, the subject opens the mouth slowly until he/she experiences an initial tension sensation. Then, the patient opens the jaw wide with the aid of their thumb and index fingers (Figure 15.3). The subject is required to maintain this stretching at least for 30 seconds if tolerable, to cause changes in the soft tissues (Michelotti et al., 2004; Niemelä et al., 2012).

Stretching of the jaw muscles can be facilitated by the contract agonist-relax antagonist technique. This technique is based on the principle of reciprocal inhibition; when a muscle is actively contracted, its antagonists are consequently relaxed. Therefore, the aim of this technique is to relax the jaw muscles. For example, in order to facilitate mouth opening, the subject is required to resist the jaw opening movement for 5–10 seconds with a low-load resistance. This movement is thought to cause relaxation of the jaw closing muscles (Kalamir et al., 2010, 2012, 2013). Thus, after the contraction of the jaw opening muscles, the subject is instructed to open their mouth and use the self-stretching technique to improve

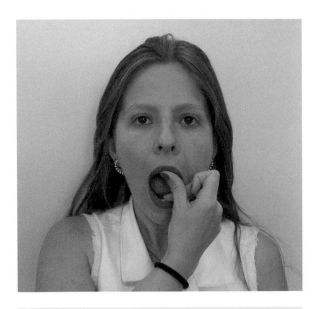

Figure 15.3
Self-stretching in mouth opening.

mouth opening, holding the stretch for 30 seconds if possible. The same principle can be used for lateral movements of the jaw. This technique can be done 3–5 times during a session according to the tolerance of each patient.

Proprioceptive exercises

Jaw proprioception provides information about TMJ position and movement in space. Proprioception gathers information from the muscle afferents, the joint mechanoreceptors and the cutaneous receptors. When there is a TMJ disease, proprioception is impaired affecting the normal biomechanics of the jaw. Proprioceptive exercises are designed to improve motor control increasing mechanoreceptor sensitivity. Also, these exercises can help to recover the viscoelastic properties of the muscular tissue, enhance oxygenation, and increase body temperature. The repeated positioning of the TMJ in specific spatial positions induces changes in the cortex as well (Ju et al., 2011).

The aim of proprioceptive exercises is to improve coordination and to retrain the impaired masticatory muscle contraction patterns which can cause an abnormal distribution of loads to the TMJ and reinforce abnormal equilibrium between muscular groups (Armijo-Olivo & Gadotti, 2016).

A. Guided opening movements

Guided mouth opening and closing exercises can help to improve the coordination of the jaw. Patients must perform the exercise in front of a mirror using a paper covering half of his/her face or drawing a vertical line on the mirror to maintain the lower dental midline parallel and avoid abnormal patterns of contraction. Also, to enhance the coordination of the muscles and the stomatognathic functions, patients can perform mobility exercises for the tongue, lips, and cheeks (Michelotti et al., 2004). These exercises can also be done with the tongue on the roof of the palate (Figure 15.4).

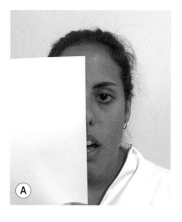
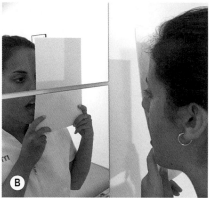

Figure 15.4
Guided opening movements. Lateral view (A); frontal view (B).

B. Rhythmic stabilization

A well-known exercise is rhythmic stabilization that is based on proprioceptive neuromuscular facilitation. One of the functions of this technique is to control the integrity of the muscles. This technique is based on those exercises that reduce the activity of the muscle spindle to a minimum level. The exercise consists of placing the index fingers over the chin and thumbs under the chin to hold the position while the tongue is kept in a resting position. Then, the patient must apply resistance to jaw opening, jaw closing and resistance to jaw lateral movements. The resistance must not allow the jaw to move. Each contraction must be held for 6 seconds, alternating the frequency of 5 contractions between the agonist and antagonist muscles. As this technique is mainly aimed at the muscular system, it should be indicated for patients with myogenous and mixed TMDs (Mulet et al., 2007).

C. Hyperboloid

The Hyperboloid is a mastication device invented by a Brazilian dentist (patent no. 8901216-0) and is registered as a mastication apparatus at the National Institute of Intellectual Property. It has a hyperbolic shape and is made of soft, nontoxic, odorless, tasteless silicone. Its hardness and texture are compatible with the ideal force applied during mastication.

The Hyperboloid is thought to produce proprioceptive excitation in the dentoalveolar nerve, spindles, and Golgi tendon organs. This device has been designed to improve coordination of jaw movements and muscle strength during the movements (Armijo-Olivo & Gadotti, 2016; Giannasi et al., 2014). The patient can perform protrusion and lateral deviation holding the device between central incisors (Figure 15.5). The evidence of Hyperboloid in the research literature is limited. More studies investigating its effects on subjects with TMD are clearly necessary.

Education and counseling

Self-care or self-management approaches are commonly used as initial treatment for patients with TMD. Recently, a Delphi study was conducted with a team of 11 international experts in the field of TMD aiming to identify the components of self-management for TMD. They found that a standard self-management program should be composed of education, self-exercise therapy, thermal modalities, self-massage therapy, diet and nutrition advice, and education about parafunctional behavior (Durham et al., 2016).

There is evidence showing the effectiveness of counseling and self-management programs for improving spontaneous pain, muscle tenderness on palpation, and maximum opening with and without

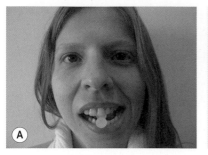
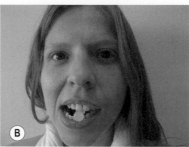
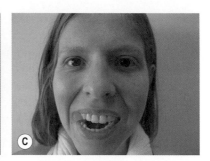

Figure 15.5

Exercises with the Hyperboloid in left (A) and right (B) lateral deviation, and lateral side (C).

pain in patients with TMD (de Freitas et al., 2013). It has been reported that when these programs are associated with posture training and physical therapy they could provide better results than when used alone.

Education should focus on the diagnosis and good prognosis of TMD. Education includes also the bio-psychosocial aspect of TMD etiology, the importance of the conservative treatment approach and the risks of invasive and irreversible treatment. Anatomy and function of the TMJ should also be explained. Advice regarding sleep practice and limited use of analgesics along with nutritional advice are provided to patients. The notion of pain-free mastication is preferred to soft-diet recommendation. In addition, bilateral mastication is encouraged in these patients (Armijo-Olivo & Gadotti, 2016; Orlando et al., 2007). Further, the therapist can explain normal jaw muscle function and inform that overuse of these muscles could be related to the complaint. For this reason, patients must pay attention to their jaw muscle activity and the parafunctional behaviors that exacerbate their pain. They must identify, monitor and avoid parafunctions and stomatognathic system overloading, such as tooth clenching and grinding, gum chewing, resting the jaw on the hand, and excessive mandibular movement. The therapist should teach the patient the relaxed resting position of the jaw and the masticatory muscles without any teeth contacts. Preferably lips should be together with nose breathing. The patient should be encouraged to maintain the resting position of the jaw when she/he is awake. For some patients, biofeedback can be helpful to make them adopt a new position with relaxation of the masticatory muscles (Craane et al., 2012; Gavish et al., 2006; Kalamir et al., 2012, 2013). Readers are referred to Chapter 18 of this textbook for specific information on neuroscience education.

Positive lifestyle habits such as avoiding caffeine and performing physical exercise should be recommended for TMD patients as well. Patients must practice and be mindful of their responsibilities during and after treatment.

Cervical spine exercises

The literature has shown that a strong relationship between neck disability and jaw dysfunction exists (Olivo et al., 2010). This is thought to happen due to the close anatomical, biomechanical, and neurological connections between the neck and the stomatognathic system, especially at the level of the trigeminocervical nucleus (Armijo Olivo et al., 2006; Sessle, 1999). In addition, it has been demonstrated that TMDs are highly associated with neck pain, cervicogenic headache, and whiplash-associated disorders

(Armijo Olivo et al., 2006). These musculoskeletal disorders are characterized by an abnormal function of the cervical flexor and extensor musculature (Jull et al., 2008). Several studies have specifically reported that subjects with TMD present abnormalities of endurance and performance of the cervical flexor and extensor muscles (Armijo-Olivo et al., 2010, 2011, 2012). For example, it has been reported that individuals with TMD presented with reduced cervical flexor/extensor muscle endurance while performing flexor and extensor muscle endurance tests when compared to healthy individuals. Furthermore, patients with mixed TMD presented with steeper negative slopes at several times during the extensor muscle endurance test than healthy subjects indicating a greater fatigability of these muscles (Armijo-Olivo et al., 2012). Also, subjects with TMD exhibited poor performance when carrying out the Craniocervical Flexion Test (CCFT) (Armijo-Olivo et al., 2011) presenting increased electromyographic activity of the superficial neck flexors (Armijo-Olivo et al., 2011). These results highlight the fact that alterations of the endurance capacity of the flexor and extensor cervical muscles could be implicated in the musculoskeletal disturbances observed in individuals with TMD. Therefore, in clinical practice, treatment of the TMD commonly should include therapies and exercises targeted to the cervical spine along with therapies targeted to the jaw.

The evidence testing therapies targeted to the neck are just emerging; however, they have great potential. As mentioned in the Chapter 10, only two studies (Calixtre et al., 2016; La Touche et al., 2009) have tested neck exercises combined with neck manual therapy techniques in subjects with a diagnosis of TMD. These studies showed that treatment directed to the cervical spine may be beneficial in decreasing pain intensity in the masticatory muscles and increasing pain-free mouth opening in patients with myofascial TMD. These results indicated that treating cervical muscular impairments in subjects with TMD could help decrease symptoms and improve quality of life of these individuals and thus cervical treatment strategies should be used in these patients.

In summary, neck motor control exercises seem to improve pain and level of dysfunction in patients with cervical involvement such as TMD, headache, and neck pain (Calixtre et al., 2016; Jull et al., 2002, 2004, 2009; La Touche et al., 2009). Thus, cervical motor control exercises are one of the most promising choices to treat patients with TMD (Armijo-Olivo et al., 2016). However, it is important to emphasize that, to the best of our knowledge, the literature does not have a randomized controlled trial, with an adequate methodology, that has tested the effectiveness of exercises directed to the cervical level in isolation in patients with TMD.

In this section, we will describe a protocol of neck exercises which has been used to target motor control at the cervical level in subjects with neck involvement. The effectiveness of this protocol has been extensively tested in the literature for patient populations such as cervicogenic headache and neck pain (Falla et al., 2007, 2013; Jull et al., 2002, 2004, 2008, 2009; La Touche et al., 2009) and has the potential to decrease symptoms in subjects with TMD, based on the results of recent studies (Calixtre et al., 2015; La Touche et al., 2009). These exercises can be performed in isolation or in conjunction with jaw exercises in people with TMD.

Cervical muscle training

For training cervical muscles, two approaches have been proposed (Jull et al., 2009; O'Leary et al., 2009). One of them involves low-load contractions targeting motor control (Falla et al., 2013) and the other focuses in general strengthening and endurance exercises for the neck muscles (Berg et al., 1994; Jordan & Manniche, 1996). It has been highlighted that both regimens have positive effects on patients and they can be used at different times of the rehabilitation process (O'Leary et al., 2009). Low-load intensity exercises and motor control exercises must be applied at the initial stages of the condition when subjects' pain and disability may impede high-load exercises; while high-intensity, global exercises involving a greater number of muscles must be used after re-education of and coordination between the deep and postural neck muscles have been established.

Jull et al. (2002) and Falla et al. (2013) have proposed an exercise protocol to target cervical muscle impairments in patients with cervical involvement and cervicogenic headache (Jull et al., 2002, 2004, 2009; La Touche et al., 2009). This exercise protocol is generally delivered in eight weeks and consists of progressive exercises for neck flexors and extensors for 30–45 minutes twice a week as described below (Falla et al., 2007, 2013). This protocol can be divided in several phases and it is targeted to the neck flexor and extensor muscles.

Neck flexors training

The first phase of the neck flexors training consists on the re-education of the craniocervical flexion movement using an incremental craniocervical flexion movement in a relaxed, supine position, by using a pressure biofeedback sensor located behind the neck of the subject. This exercise targets the deep flexors of the upper cervical region, the longus capitis and colli (Armijo-Olivo et al., 2011) rather than the superficial flexors, sternocleidomastoid and anterior scalene muscles.

The correct craniocervical flexion movement is extremely important for the exercise program (Jull et al., 2004). The clinician must teach the patient how to perform the movement correctly and to control and/or eliminate any compensation strategy, such as neck retraction, excessive cervical flexion, and/or jaw clenching. The patient nods the head gently and slowly as if saying 'yes' so that the sensor measures the level of pressure exerted by the subject. The starting level of pressure is set at 22mmHg and then can be progressed until 30mmHg. For the treatment to be progressed, the craniocervical flexion movement must be performed correctly, with precision in each

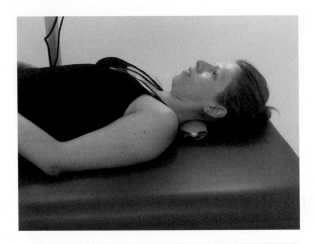

Figure 15.6
Training craniocervical flexion movement.

target level (Falla, 2004; Jull et al., 2004; O'Leary et al., 2007). The objective is to achieve 10mmHg above the baseline without compensation or contraction of the superficial neck flexor muscles. The movement needs to be done 10 times perfectly to proceed to the next level (Figure 15.6). If the patient has difficulties in performing the nodding movement correctly, the clinician can advise him/her to look down before starting the nodding movement. Moreover, the therapist can also suggest to the patient to perform the movement while breathing out (Cagnie et al., 2008).

Training of the holding capacity of the deep neck flexors

After the patient is able to perform the craniocervical flexion movement correctly, the clinician must teach the patient how to perform the craniocervical flexion movement slowly and in a controlled manner, with the head and neck in a neutral position. As mentioned above, during the task, patients should be guided by feedback from a pressure unit placed behind the neck to monitor the slight flattening of the cervical lordosis, which occurs with the contraction of the longus colli. Once the correct craniocervical flexion motion is achieved, the patient can begin holding progressively increasing ranges of craniocervical flexion using feedback from the pressure unit placed behind their neck. The feedback is provided by a screen placed in front of the patient's eye to avoid compensatory movements (Figure 15.7).

Each patient must initially perform craniocervical flexion to sequentially reach five pressure targets in 2 mmHg increments from a baseline of 20 mmHg to the final level of 30 mmHg. The clinician identifies the target level that the patient can hold steadily for 5 seconds without resorting to retraction, without

dominant use of the superficial neck flexor muscles, and without a quick, jerky craniocervical flexion movement to start the program. For each target level, the contraction duration should be increased to 10 seconds, and the patient is trained to perform 10 repetitions with brief rest periods between each contraction (5 seconds). Once one set of 10 repetitions of 10 seconds is achieved at one target level, the exercise should be progressed to train the next target level up to the final target of 10 repetitions of 10 seconds at 30 mmHg.

High-load training of the flexor muscles

At later stages of rehabilitation, patients can be instructed to train their flexor muscles using a higher load exercise with the head weight as the load. The patients must perform repetitions of a head lift for flexors, which are performed initially seated upright leaning backwards against a wall and then progressing to the supine position as able (Figure 15.8). The head lift needs to be preceded with craniocervical flexion followed by cervical flexion to just clear the head from the supporting surface and the craniocervical flexion position must be maintained

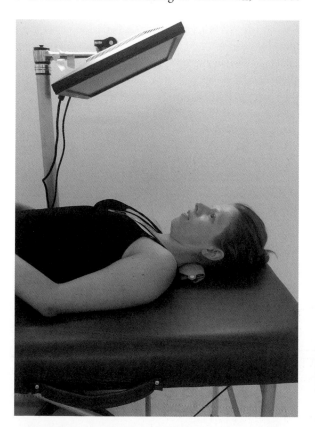

Figure 15.7
Training of the holding capacity of the deep neck flexors.

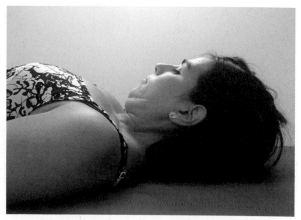

Figure 15.8
High-load training of cervical flexor muscles.

throughout the exercise (one set of 5 repetitions with a 1–2 second holding time only). The number of repetitions and sets must be increased as permitted by the patient's response to the exercise, and an endurance element must be incorporated by increasing the time the position is held, depending on the patient's progress.

Patients also are instructed to train their cervical flexor muscles in different positions. They progress the exercises to the sitting and upright positions. The first part of this next stage consists of moving the head and cervical spine into an extension movement in the sitting or upright position. This phase of the movement involves an eccentric contraction of the cervical flexor muscles. Any compensation, such as chin retraction or cervical retraction, should be discouraged. After this, subjects are required to come back to neutral position of the cervical spine. This phase is done by contracting concentrically the cervical flexor muscles. It is important to check that the movement is initiated at the level of the craniocervical region rather than having a dominant action of the sternocleidomastoid. The clinician can progress this exercise by increasing the range of the head extension movement as the control improves; and second, by adding isometric hold exercises in different parts of the range of cervical returning movement (concentric flexion) to improve the cervical flexion synergy through functional ranges of extension (Figure 15.9).

Training of the deep cervical extensor muscles

Cervical extensor muscles participate in neck control, and thus they should be trained to ensure proper movement at the cervical spine. In order to train the cervical extensors, the patient could start the movements in either sitting or upright position and progress to prone on elbows position and four-point kneeling position.

To target the suboccipital muscles, patients must be instructed to let the head and neck move into flexion, and then to return to the starting position to train the eccentric/concentric function of the cervical extensors. The clinician must teach the patient how to perform the movement. Attention should be given to the position of the head and neck and also the scapula. Chin poking, for example, is one of the most common compensations seen with this movement, and indicates excessive craniocervical extension, which usually is caused by dominance of the superficial muscles (for example semispinalis capitis).

Also, it is important to train the rectus capitis posterior major and minor muscles in recognition of their key proprioceptive function, their role in supporting and controlling the upper cervical joints, and evidence of the changes that can occur in these muscles with neck pain involvement. The patient performs a craniocervical extension and flexion (head nodding) exercise whilst maintaining the

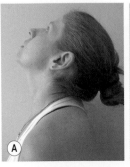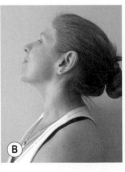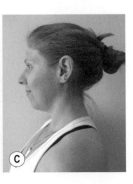

Figure 15.9
Retraining of the cervical flexor muscles in upright position. (A) Beginning of the motion in extension; (B) mid-range; (C) end of exercise.

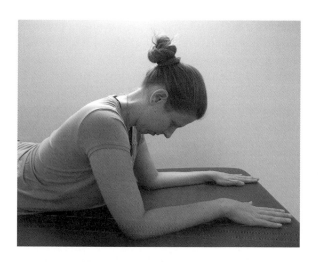

Figure 15.10
Training of the cervical extensor muscles, favoring craniocervical flexion movement and maintaining the lower cervical spine in neutral position.

mid and lower cervical spine in its neutral position (Figure 15.10).

Another exercise facilitates the obliquus capitis superior and inferior and is a rotation movement of less than 40 degrees to focus rotation to the upper cervical region (10 repetitions for each movement should be done).

Retraining of the deep lower cervical extensors of the cervical spine

This exercise is a progression of the exercises described above and should be performed in a similar way, but with the patient in four-point kneeling position. The participants must perform higher load exercises with head weight as the load, focusing on training the deep cervical extensors, and the semispinalis cervicis/multifidus group. Initially the patient should perform up to 15 repetitions of neck extension whilst maintaining their head in a neutral position. The range of cervical extension through which the extensor

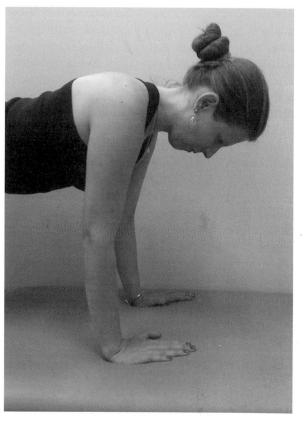

Figure 15.11
Retraining of the deep lower cervical extensors of the cervical spine.

muscles are trained should be progressively increased. The number of repetitions and sets must also be increased as permitted by the patient's response to the exercise, and an endurance element could be incorporated by increasing the time the position is held, depending on progress (Figure 15.11).

Co-contraction of the neck flexors and extensors combined with arm and leg movements

Once the patient is able to achieve an appropriate pattern of contraction of the cervical flexors and extensors, then this type of exercise is started. For example, in the four-point kneeling position, the patient first performs upper cervical flexion while keeping the lower cervical spine in a neutral position. This configuration is maintained by the patient, who is encouraged to keep the spine and the rest of the body stabilized. When the patient can perform the movement correctly and hold the position for at least 10 seconds, 10 times, then the exercise can be progressed. For example, arm and leg movements can accompany the cervical control. In this case, subjects are asked to raise an arm and maintain the stability of the body, as well as the stability of the cervico-thoracic system. The patient then raises a leg. These movements are alternated (right arm, left leg; then left arm, right leg) until the patient can maintain and perform the correct movement pattern. This exercise can be done on an exercise ball to increase instability and therefore increase the challenge to the spinal stabilization system.

Retraining of scapular position

Subjects suffering neck pain and associated disorders such as TMD present postural alterations of the head and neck and the scapular regions. It is important for clinicians to teach patients to feel the correct position and movement of the scapula and re-educate the axioscapular muscles. Thus, it is necessary to activate all of the musculature that controls the scapular position (that is, the low and mid trapezius, serratus anterior, levator scapulae, and rhomboid muscles). However, before retraining can begin, lengthening and relaxation of the hyperactive and tight muscles to maintain the biomechanical environment and to allow re-education of muscular function of the cervical spine is recommended. Thus, stretching of the upper trapezius, sternocleidomastoid, the levator scapulae, pectoralis minor, and pectoralis major must be performed. Pectoralis muscle tightness for example limits scapular motion and should be addressed before the re-education of the axioscapular muscles. The unilateral corner stretch is a classic self-stretch of the pectoralis minor muscle. In a standing position, the patient abducts his/her humerus up to 90° with the elbow flexed to 90° and places the palm on a flat planar surface. Then, the patient creates a horizontal abduction by rotating the trunk away from the elevated arm, maximizing the stretch across the chest (Borstad & Ludewig, 2006). In order to maximize the upper trapezius stretching, the neck of the patient needs to be inclined to the opposite side, with head rotated to the same side (face looking at the same side), and a flexion movement of the neck performed until the patient feels tension but not pain. The position needs to be held for at least 20–30 seconds and repeated three times. This can be done passively by the therapist and can be taught to the patient, so she/he can perform it themselves. Similarly for the stretching of the sternocleidomastoid, the patient should bring the ear towards the opposite shoulder, then turn the head to the opposite side and the face to the same side, so that the nose is pointing towards the ceiling at about a 45° angle; then bring the right hand down and reach towards the floor to get more of a stretch. The position needs to be held for at least 20–30 seconds and repeated for three times.

Training the endurance capacity of the scapular stabilizers

Training of the endurance capacity of the scapular stabilizers consists of maintaining the correct position of the scapula for at least 10 seconds. The clinician must ensure that the patient acquires the adequate skills in achieving the desired scapular motion and posture; in order to do this, the clinician could provide tactile cues to the patient to facilitate the action and endurance. Once the patient has learned to correctly control the scapula position and motion, the exercises should focus on movement repetitions with the goal to facilitate new patterns of automatic scapular position and movement behavior. A way to progress these exercises is to change the patient from the side-lying position to the prone position and then to sitting position. The patient can use gravity resistance to train the endurance of the scapular muscles. Patients are taught to incorporate and practice scapular control training into problematic functional daily activities relevant to their disorders such as for example computer working (Cagnie et al., 2014; Falla, 2004; Jull et al., 2004; O'Leary et al., 2007).

Retraining scapular control with arm movement and load

Retraining scapular control with arm movement and load has the objective of maintaining the position of the scapula while performing movements with the arm. This is accomplished by doing exercises within a small range of motion (≤60°) while holding the correct position of the scapula. Closed chain exercises can be used to progress the difficulty of these exercises. The patient can perform both concentric and eccentric control exercises of the scapula while maintaining the cervical spine in neutral position, in prone, 'on elbows' or four-point kneeling position. This exercise should be done to retrain the holding capacity of the serratus anterior, while keeping the position in intermediate ranges for 10 seconds. The goal is to perform the movement 10 times perfectly (Jull et al., 2004; O'Leary et al., 2007).

Posture re-education exercise

The relationship between head and neck posture and TMD has been a matter of debate for many years. Physical therapists have commonly used cervical-head posture re-education techniques to address postural abnormalities in patients with neck involvement. However, the evidence is still poor and a strong relationship between TMD and posture has not been established. Despite this controversy, a recent systematic review (Armijo-Olivo et al., 2016) found that postural training was one of the interventions recommended to restore or optimize the alignment of the craniomandibular system and to reduce pain in patients who have TMDs with muscular involvement (that is, myogenic TMD). Also, it has been suggested that postural training should be

based on individual needs (Jull et al., 2004). Patients who report posture as an aggravating factor, and who report an improvement of symptoms when performing postural corrections, could use postural correction to improve symptoms. Thus, clinicians who work with patients with TMD having postural abnormalities as an aggravating factor could consider these recommendations for treating these subjects in clinical practice. One study found that a very easy postural exercise could help reduce the superficial activity of cervical muscles and target the deep

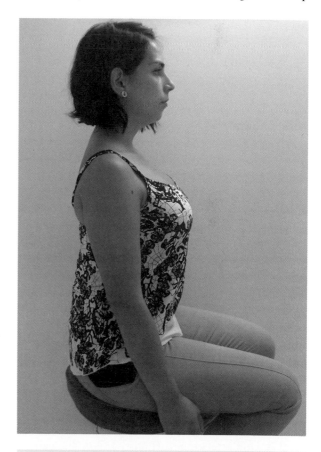

Figure 15.12
Postural exercise to recruit deep cervical flexors and decrease the activity of superficial flexors.

muscles (Beer et al., 2012). The exercise is performed in sitting position, the patient assumes an upright posture in a neutral lumbopelvic position and then gently lengthens the cervical spine by imagining lifting the base of the skull from the top of the neck. Postural control of the scapula is frequently added to this posture exercise. The clinician must teach the patient how to perform the movement correctly. The postural exercise could be done in the clinic (the patient keeps the position for 10 seconds and repeats this posture 5 times) and in the patient's home or work environment (holding the position for 10 seconds ideally every 15–20 minutes throughout their waking day) (Figure 15.12).

C1-C2 self-SNAGs exercises

Evidence shows a decrease in upper cervical (C1-C2) mobility measured by the cervical flexion rotation test in patients with TMD (Greenbaum et al., 2017; von Piekartz et al., 2016; Grondin et al., 2015). Moreover, research shows the utility of upper cervical mobilization for TMD (Calixtre et al., 2016; La Touche et al., 2009). Recently, C1-C2 self-sustained natural apophyseal glide (SNAG) in conjunction with other upper cervical mobilization and exercises have shown effectiveness in reducing pain and headache impact in patients with TMD (Calixtre et al., submitted). In patients with a positive cervical flexion rotation test, C1-C2 self-SNAGs can be prescribed to patients using a cervical self-SNAG strap. The thin rubber-covered strap is positioned on the posterior arch of C1 and drawn horizontally forward across the face. The purpose of the strap is to facilitate C1-C2 rotation. While putting tension in the strap, the patient is asked to rotate the head in the same direction as found to be limited on the cervical flexion rotation test (Figure 15.13). The patient

holds the end range rotation for about 3 seconds and returns to the neutral head position while keeping tension in the strap. The exercise is repeated 3 times several times a day. The exercise should not cause symptoms other than a stretching sensation (Hall et al., 2007). Self-SNAGs C1-C2 increase upper cervical range of motion in rotation. Their efficacy still needs to be further studied in patients with TMD.

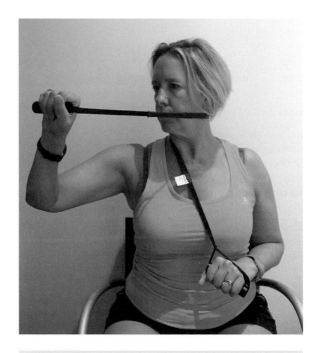

Figure 15.13

Self-application of C1–C2 self-sustained natural apophyseal glide (SNAG) for cervical right rotation. Force is applied to the C1 level via horizontal pressure from the strap. At the same time, the subject actively turns her head to the right.

References

Armijo-Olivo S, Gadotti I. Temporomandibular Disorders. In: Magee DJ, Zachazewski JE, Quillen W, Manske RC. Pathology and Intervention in Musculoskeletal Rehabilitation. 2nd ed. London: Elsevier; 2016. Pp. 119–156.

Armijo Olivo S, Magee DJ, Parfitt M, Major P, Thie NM. The association between the cervical spine, the stomatognathic system, and craniofacial pain: a critical review. J Orofac Pain 2006; 20: 271–287.

Armijo-Olivo S, Fuentes JP, da Costa BR et al. Reduced endurance of the cervical flexor muscles in patients with concurrent temporomandibular disorders and neck disability. Man Ther 2010; 15: 586–592.

Armijo-Olivo S, Silvestre R, Fuentes J et al. Electromyographic activity of the cervical flexor muscles in patients with temporomandibular disorders while performing the craniocervical flexion test: a cross-sectional study. Phys Ther 2011; 91: 1184–1197.

Armijo-Olivo S, Silvestre RA, Fuentes JP et al. Patients with temporomandibular disorders have increased fatigability of the cervical extensor muscles. Clin J Pain 2012; 28: 55–64.

Armijo-Olivo S, Pitance L, Singh V, Neto F, Thie N, Michelotti A. Effectiveness of manual therapy and therapeutic exercise for temporomandibular disorders: Systematic review and meta-analysis. Phys Ther 2016; 96: 9–25.

Bae Y, Park Y. The effect of relaxation exercises for the masticator muscles on Temporomandibular Joint Dysfunction (TMD). J Phys Ther Sci 2013; 25: 583–586.

Beer A, Treleaven J, Jull G. Can a functional postural exercise improve performance in the cranio-cervical flexion test? A preliminary study. Man Ther 2012; 17: 219–224.

Berg HE, Berggren G, Tesch PA. Dynamic neck strength training effect on pain and function. Arch Phys Med Rehabil 1994; 75: 661–665.

Borstad JD, Ludewig PM. Comparison of three stretches for the pectoralis minor muscle. J Shoulder Elbow Surg 2006; 15: 324–330.

Cagnie B, Danneels L, Cools A, Dickx N, Cambier D. The influence of breathing type, expiration and cervical posture on the performance of the cranio-cervical flexion test in healthy subjects. Man Ther 2008; 13:232–238.

Cagnie B, Struyf F, Cools A, Castelein B, Danneels L, O'leary S. The relevance of scapular dysfunction in neck pain: a brief commentary. J Orthop Sports Phys Ther 2014; 44: 435–439.

Calixtre BL, Oliveira AB, Ramalho de Sena Rosa L, Armijo-Olivo S, Visscher C, Alburquerque Sendín F. Effects of upper cervical mobilizations and neck exercises on pain, mandibular function, and headache impact in women with TMD. A single-blinded randomized controlled trial (Submitted).

Calixtre LB, Moreira RFC, Franchini GH, Alburquerque-Sendín F, Oliveira AB. Manual therapy for the management of pain and limited range of motion in subjects with signs and symptoms of temporomandibular disorder: a systematic review of randomised controlled trials. J Oral Rehabil 2015; 42: 847–861.

Calixtre LB, Grüninger BL da S, Haik MN, Alburquerque-Sendín F, Oliveira AB. Effects of cervical mobilization and exercise on pain, movement and function in subjects with temporomandibular disorders: a single group pre-post test. J Appl Oral Sci 2016; 24: 188–197.

Carmeli E, Sheklow SL, Bloomenfeld I. Comparative study of repositioning splint therapy and passive manual range of motion techniques for anterior displaced temporomandibular discs with unstable excursive reduction. Physiotherapy 2001; 87: 26–36.

Craane B, Dijkstra PU, Stappaerts K, De Laat A. One-year evaluation of the effect of physical therapy for masticatory muscle pain: a randomized controlled trial. Eur J Pain 2012; 16: 737–747.

Durham J, Al-Baghdadi M, Baad-Hansen L et al. Self-management programmes in temporo-mandibular disorders: results from an international Delphi process. J Oral Rehabil 2016; 43: 929–936.

de Felício CM, de Oliveira MM, da Silva MAMR. Effects of orofacial myofunctional therapy on temporomandibular disorders. Cranio J Craniomandib Pract 2010; 28: 249–259.

de Freitas RFCP, Ferreira MÂF, Barbosa G a. S, Calderon PS. Counselling and self-management therapies for temporomandibular disorders: a systematic review. J Oral Rehabil 2013; 40: 864–874.

Falla D. Unravelling the complexity of muscle impairment in chronic neck pain. Man Ther 2004; 9: 125–133.

Falla D, Jull G, Russell T, Vicenzino B, Hodges P. Effect of neck exercise on sitting posture in patients with chronic neck pain. Phys Ther 2007; 87: 408–417.

Falla D, Lindstrøm R, Rechter L, Boudreau S, Petzke F. Effectiveness of an 8-week exercise programme on pain and specificity of neck muscle activity in patients with chronic neck pain: a randomized controlled study. Eur J Pain 2013; 17: 1517–1528.

Fransen M, McConnell S, Harmer AR, Van der Esch M, Simic M, Bennell KL. Exercise for osteoarthritis of the knee: a Cochrane systematic review. Br J Sports Med 2015; 49: 1554–1557.

Gavish A, Winocur E, Astandzelov-Nachmias T, Gazit E. Effect of controlled masticatory exercise on pain and muscle performance in myofascial pain patients: A pilot study. Cranio 2006; 24: 184–190.

Giannasi LC, Freitas Batista SR, Matsui MY et al. Effect of a hyperbolide mastication apparatus for the treatment of severe sleep bruxism in a child with cerebral palsy: long-term follow-up. J Bodywork Mov Ther 2014; 18: 62–67.

González-Iglesias J, Cleland JA, Neto F, Hall T, Fernández-de-las-Peñas C. Mobilization with movement, thoracic spine manipulation, and dry needling for the management of temporomandibular disorder: A prospective case series. Physiother Theory Pract 2013; 29: 586–595.

Greenbaum T, Dvir Z, Reiter S, Winocur E. Cervical flexion-rotation test and physiological range of motion – A comparative study of patients with myogenic temporomandibular disorder versus healthy subjects. Musculoskelet Sci Pract 2017; 27: 7–13.

Grondin F, Hall T, Laurentjoye M, Ella B. Upper cervical range of motion is impaired in patients with temporomandibular disorders. Cranio J Craniomandib Pract 2015; 33: 91–99.

Gross AR, Paquin JP, Dupont G et al. Exercises for mechanical neck disorders: A Cochrane review update. Man Ther 2016; 24: 25–45.

Haketa T, Kino K, Sugisaki M, Takaoka M, Ohta T. Randomized clinical trial of treatment for TMJ disc displacement. J Dent Res 2010; 89: 1259–1263.

Hall T, Chan HT, Christensen L, Odenthal B, Wells C, Robinson K. Efficacy of a C1-C2 self-sustained natural apophyseal glide (SNAG) in the management of cervicogenic headache. J Orthop Sports Phys Ther 2007; 37: 100–107.

Jordan A, Manniche C. Rehabilitation and spinal pain. J Neuromusculoskel Syst 1996; 4: 89–93.

Ju Y-Y, Liu Y-C, Cheng H-YK, Chang Y-J. Rapid repetitive passive movement improves knee proprioception. Clin Biomech 2011; 26: 188–193.

Jull G, Trott P, Potter H et al. A randomized controlled trial of exercise and manipulative therapy for cervicogenic headache. Spine 2002; 27: 1835–1843.

Jull GA, Falla DL, Treleaven JM, Sterling MM, O'Leary SP. A therapeutic exercise approach for cervical disorders. London: Churchill Livingstone-Elsevier; 2004.

Jull GA, O'Leary SP, Falla DL. Clinical assessment of the deep cervical flexor muscles: the craniocervical flexion test. J Manipulative Physiol Ther 2008; 31: 525–533.

Jull GA, Falla D, Vicenzino B, Hodges PW. The effect of therapeutic exercise on activation of the deep cervical flexor muscles in people with chronic neck pain. Man Ther 2009; 14: 696–701.

Kalamir A, Pollard H, Vitiello A, Bonello R. Intra-oral myofascial therapy for chronic myogenous temporomandibular disorders: a randomized, controlled pilot study. J Man Manip Ther 2010; 18: 139–146.

Kalamir A, Bonello R, Graham P, Vitiello AL, Pollard H. Intraoral myofascial therapy for chronic myogenous temporomandibular disorder: a randomized controlled trial. J Manipulative Physiol Ther 2012; 35: 26–37.

Kalamir A, Graham PL, Vitiello AL, Bonello R, Pollard H. Intra-oral myofascial therapy versus education and self-care in the treatment of chronic, myogenous temporomandibular disorder: a randomised, clinical trial. Chiropr Man Ther 2013; 21: 17.

Kraaijenga S, van der Molen L, van Tinteren H, Hilgers F, Smeele L. Treatment of myogenic temporomandibular disorder: a prospective randomized clinical trial, comparing a mechanical stretching device (TheraBite®) with standard physical therapy exercise. Cranio J Craniomandib Pract 2014; 32: 208–216.

La Touche R, Fernández-de-las-Peñas C, Fernández-Carnero J et al. The effects of manual therapy and exercise directed at the cervical spine on pain and pressure pain sensitivity in patients with myofascial temporomandibular disorders. J Oral Rehabil 2009; 36: 644–652.

Lindfors E, Hedman E, Magnusson T, Ernberg M, Gabre P. Patient experiences of therapeutic jaw exercises in the treatment of masticatory myofascial pain: a qualitative study. J Oral Facial Pain Headache 2017; 31: 46–54.

Littlewood C, Malliaras P, Bateman M, Stace R, May S, Walters S. The central nervous system – an additional consideration in "rotator cuff tendinopathy" and a potential basis for understanding response to loaded

therapeutic exercise. Man Ther 2013; 18: 468–472.

Maloney GE, Mehta N, Forgione AG, Zawawi KH, Al-Badawi EA, Driscoll SE. Effect of a passive jaw motion device on pain and range of motion in TMD patients not responding to flat plane intraoral appliances. Cranio 2002; 20: 55–66.

Mapelli A, Zanandréa Machado BC, Giglio LD, Sforza C, De Felício CM. Reorganization of muscle activity in patients with chronic temporomandibular disorders. Arch Oral Biol 2016; 72: 164–171.

Medlicott MS, Harris SR. A systematic review of the effectiveness of exercise, manual therapy, electrotherapy, relaxation training, and biofeedback in the management of temporomandibular disorder. Phys Ther 2006; 86: 955–973.

Michelotti A, Steenks MH, Farella M, Parisini F, Cimino R, Martina R. The additional value of a home physical therapy regimen versus patient education only for the treatment of myofascial pain of the jaw muscles: short-term results of a randomized clinical trial. J Orofac Pain 2004; 18: 114–125.

Mulet M, Decker KL, Look JO, Lenton PA, Schiffman EL. A randomized clinical trial assessing the efficacy of adding 6 x 6 exercises to self-care for the treatment of masticatory myofascial pain. J Orofac Pain 2007; 21: 318–328.

Nascimento MM, Vasconcelos BC, Porto GG, Ferdinanda G, Nogueira CM, Raimundo RC. Physical therapy and anesthetic blockage for treating temporomandibular disorders: a clinical trial. Med Oral Patol Oral Cirugia Bucal 2013; 18: e81-e85.

Niemelä K, Korpela M, Raustia A, Ylöstalo P, Sipilä K. Efficacy of stabilisation splint treatment on temporomandibular disorders. J Oral Rehabil 2012; 39: 799–804.

Nijs J, Roussel N, Paul van Wilgen C, Köke A, Smeets R. Thinking beyond muscles and joints: therapists' and patients' attitudes and beliefs regarding chronic musculoskeletal pain are key to applying effective treatment. Man Ther 2013; 18: 96–102.

O'Leary S, Falla D, Hodges PW, Jull G, Vicenzino B. Specific therapeutic exercise of the neck induces immediate local hypoalgesia. J Pain 2007; 8: 832–839.

O'Leary S, Falla D, Elliott JM, Jull G. Muscle dysfunction in cervical spine pain: implications for assessment and management. J Orthop Sports Phys Ther 2009; 39: 324–333.

Olivo SA, Fuentes J, Major PW, Warren S, Thie NMR, Magee DJ. The association between neck disability and jaw disability. J Oral Rehabil 2010; 37: 670–679.

Orlando B, Manfredini D, Salvetti G, Bosco M. Evaluation of the effectiveness of biobehavioral therapy in the treatment of temporomandibular disorders: a literature review. Behav Med Wash DC 2007; 33: 101–118.

Pelletier R, Higgins J, Bourbonnais D. Is neuroplasticity in the central nervous system the missing link to our understanding of chronic musculoskeletal disorders? BMC Musculoskelet Disord 2015; 16: 25.

Philadelphia Panel. Philadelphia Panel evidence-based clinical practice guidelines on selected

rehabilitation interventions: overview and methodology. Phys Ther 2001; 81: 1629–1640.

Ren W, Ao H, Lin Q, Xu Z, Zhang B. Efficacy of mouth opening exercises in treating trismus after maxillectomy. Chin Med J 2013; 126: 2666–2669.

Rocabado M. Head and Neck Biomechanics: Joint Treatment. Buenos Aires: Intermedica; 1979.

Satomi T, Tanaka T, Kobayashi T, Iino M. Developing a new appliance to dissipate mechanical load on teeth and improve limitation of vertical mouth. J Oral Maxillofac Res 2013; 4: e4.

Sessle BJ. Neural mechanisms and pathways in craniofacial pain. Can J Neurol Sci J Can Sci Neurol 1999;26: S7-S11.

Smith BE, Hendrick P, Smith TO et al. Should exercises be painful in the management of chronic musculoskeletal pain? A systematic review and meta-analysis. Br J Sports Med 2017: bjsports-2016-097383.

Sokunbi O, Watt P, Moore A. Changes in plasma concentration of serotonin in response to spinal stabilisation exercises in chronic low back pain patient. Niger Q J Hosp Med 2007; 17: 108–111.

Sokunbi O, Moore A, Watt P. Plasma levels of beta-endorphin and serotonin in response

to specific spinal based exercises. South Afr J Physiother 2008; 64: 31–37.

Stubblefield MD, Manfield L, Riedel ER. A preliminary report on the efficacy of a dynamic jaw opening device (Dynasplint Trismus System) as part of the multimodal treatment of trismus in patients with head and neck cancer. Arch Phys Med Rehabil 2010; 91: 1278–1282.

Taylor NF, Dodd KJ, Shields N, Bruder A. Therapeutic exercise in physiotherapy practice is beneficial: a summary of systematic reviews 2002-2005. Aust J Physiother 2007; 53: 7–16.

Vicenzino B, Hing W, Hall T, Rivett D. Mobilisation with Movement: the Art and the Science. Elsevier Australia; 2011.

von Piekartz H, Pudelko A, Danzeisen M, Hall T, Ballenberger N. Do subjects with acute/subacute temporomandibular disorder have associated cervical impairments: A cross-sectional study. Man Ther 2016; 26: 208–215.

Yadav M, Attrey P. Effect of dynamic versus isometric resistance exercise on pain and functional ability in elderly patients with osteoarthritis of knee. Indian J Physiother Occup Ther - Int J 2017; 11: 30.

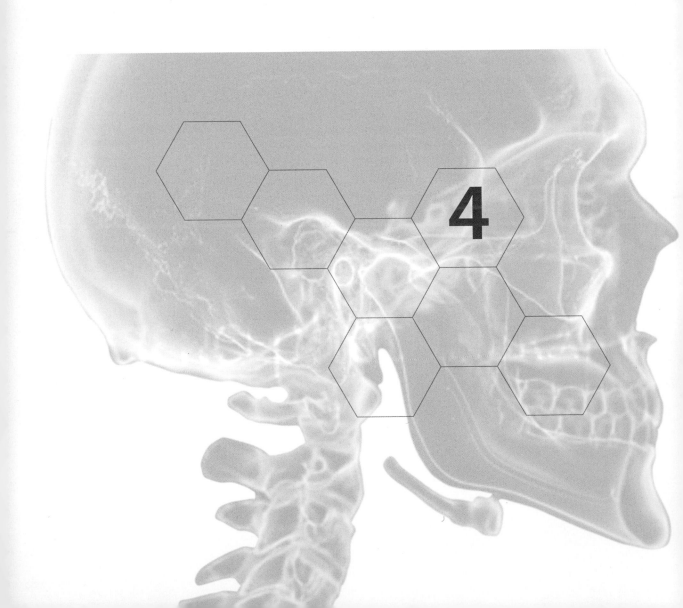

4

PART 4

Other interventions for temporomandibular disorders

Chapter 16

Dry needling for myofascial trigger points in temporomandibular disorders

César Fernández-de-las-Peñas, Juan Mesa-Jiménez

Trigger point dry needling

One of the most popular interventions for the management of trigger points (TrPs) is dry needling (DN). The American Physical Therapy Association (APTA) defines dry needling as a 'skilled intervention using a thin filiform needle (usually an acupuncture needle) to penetrate the skin that stimulates TrPs, muscles, and connective tissue for the management of musculoskeletal disorders' (APTA, 2013). Dry needling falls within the scope of practice of different health professions including medicine, physical therapy, chiropractic, veterinary medicine, acupuncture, or dentistry, dependent on jurisdictions. Each profession uses their discipline-specific philosophy and management approaches to determine when and how dry needling techniques should be applied. In fact, there is a debate as to whether dry needling is acupuncture (Zhou et al., 2015); however, there are several differences between these interventions, for example in the clinical reasoning for their application, the underlying mechanisms, the technique, and philosophy of application, etc. and readers are referred to other texts for this debate. In addition, it is important to note that although acupuncture practitioners may refer to dry needling as 'TrP acupuncture,' this does not imply that dry needling would be the exclusive domain of any discipline. Furthermore, dry needling can be also applied to other structures, such as ligaments, tendons, scar tissue, or fascial adhesions (Dunning et al., 2014); however, this chapter will focus on trigger point dry needling (TrP-DN).

Although TrP-DN can be divided into superficial and deep dry needling (Dommerholt & Fernández-de-las-Peñas, 2013), deep dry needling is the most widely used intervention, particularly the 'fast-in, fast-out' technique (Hong, 1994). This technique consists of inserting the needle into the TrP area until a first local twitch response is obtained. A local twitch response is defined as brief and sudden contraction of the taut band with needle insertion (Dommerholt & Fernández-de-las-Peñas, 2013). Once a first local twitch response is obtained, the needle is moved up and down, with no rotations, to get more local twitch responses. Hong (1994) proposed that local twitch responses should be obtained during the application of the technique for it to be effective. However, we do not know how many local twitch responses are needed for a positive outcome. A recent study has found no clinical differences in pain related to the number of local twitch responses obtained in patients with neck pain (Fernández-Carnero et al., 2017). Nevertheless, in this study, individuals exhibited significant clinical improvement when eliciting the highest number (n=6) of local twitch responses or local twitch responses until exhaustion compared with not eliciting (Fernández-Carnero et al., 2017). Another study suggested that the local twitch response may not be considered necessary for a successful treatment since no differences at one week were observed between patients experiencing local twitch responses and those not experiencing local twitch responses (Koppenhaver et al., 2017). Discrepancies in the published studies have led some authors to question the need for local twitch response during TrP-DN (Perreault et al., 2017).

Due to the invasive nature of the procedure and the use of solid needles, there is a risk of penetrating vital organs and other body structures, such as the lungs, intestines, kidneys, urethra, nerves and arteries, among others. While the incidence of acupuncture-induced pneumothorax is less than 1 per 10,000 cases, the incidence of TrP-DN induced pneumothorax is unknown since only one case report has been published in the literature (Cummings et al., 2014). Therefore, application of

TrP-DN should always be anatomy-driven, since an extensive knowledge of anatomical relations is required (Halle & Halle, 2016). Clinicians must follow guidelines for safe dry needling practice, which includes hand washing, and other measures (ASAP, 2007; McEvoy et al., 2012; Bachmann et al., 2014). A prospective study of the risk of adverse events of TrP-DN showed that the risk of a significant adverse event was lower than 0.04 per cent with approximately 8,000 dry needling treatments (Brady et al., 2014). The most common adverse events were pain during and after needling, bleeding and bruising (Brady et al., 2014). Of particular interest is postneedling induced soreness, which is thought to be a consequence of the neuromuscular damage generated by the repetitive needling insertions into the muscle (Domingo et al., 2013). The presence of postneedling soreness can be associated with a possible reluctance to receive further needling therapy by the patient, generating patient dissatisfaction and reduction in treatment adherence. In fact, it is highly recommended to advise the patient about the presence of soreness after TrP-DN (APTA, 2012). There are some studies investigating potential therapeutic strategies to decrease postneedling soreness. All studies found that application of spray and stretch (Martín-Pintado-Zugasti et al., 2014), ischemic compression (Martín-Pintado-Zugasti et al., 2015) or low-load eccentric exercise (Salom-Moreno et al., 2017) after TrP-DN was effective in the short term (between 6–24 hours) for reducing postneedling soreness in comparison to a wait-and-see group. Interestingly all studies showed that postneedling soreness tended to disappear 48 to 72 hours after TrP-DN without any postneedling intervention suggesting that maybe postneedling soreness is a physiological secondary effect of TrP-DN. Nevertheless, a short-term reduction of postneedling-induced pain may be important for the patient's perception of recovery as those subjects experiencing strong postneedling soreness may refuse to receive further treatments. In fact, this may be related to a prior development of fear of needles, which is often found in patients after previous negative experiences with needles. Nevertheless, it is interesting to note that fear of needles has no impact on the clinical outcomes of dry needling (Joseph et al., 2013).

The scientific evidence for trigger point dry needling

It is almost 40 years since the first paper reporting the use of dry needling for the management of pain was published (Lewit, 1979). Several systematic reviews summarizing the evidence for this intervention were published; however, the last five years of publications have been the most important on this topic as most recent systematic reviews and meta-analyses have confirmed the effectiveness of TrP-DN for the management of pain. For instance, it has been concluded that TrP-DN is effective for the management of pain conditions in the upper (Kietrys et al., 2013) and lower (Morihisa et al., 2016) quadrants. Other meta-analyses concluded that TrP-DN is effective for the management of neck–shoulder pain (Liu et al., 2015) and low back pain (Liu et al., 2017a). One systematic review investigated the effectiveness of TrP-DN just in one muscle, such as the upper trapezius (Cagnie et al., 2015). Another review found positive effects of TrP-DN in multiple body areas, suggesting the broad applicability of this treatment approach for multiple muscle groups (Boyles et al., 2015). Based on current evidence, the Canadian Agency for Drugs and Technologies in Health has accepted the use of dry needling following an appropriate clinical reasoning in the public health system (CADTH, 2016). All reviews concluded that no evidence exists on the long-term effects of TrP-DN (Kietrys et al., 2013; Boyles et al., 2015; Cagnie et al., 2015; Liu et al., 2015; Gattie et al., 2017; Liu et al., 2017a).

Nevertheless, it should be recognized that not all meta-analyses reported positive outcomes for dry needling; one meta-analysis concluded that dry needling was less effective at decreasing pain compared to a placebo (Rodríguez-Mansilla et al., 2016). The review by France et al. (2014) found insufficient evidence to strongly advocate the use of Tr-DN for headaches. This may be related to differences in technique, clinical reasoning, patient populations, TrP diagnostic criteria, and the training received by the clinician applying the technique, among other reasons. An interesting meta-analysis found evidence suggesting that TrP-DN applied by physical therapists was superior to no treatment or sham treatment, but was as equally effective as other physical therapy treatments for short- and mid-term follow-ups for functional outcomes in patients with musculoskeletal pain (Gattie et al., 2017).

It is important to consider that TrP-DN should be applied in combination with other interventions and not just as an isolated therapeutic approach. Téllez-García et al. (2015) found that a combination of TrP-DN and a neuroscience education program was more effective than the neuroscience education program alone for improving pain, related disability, and kinesiophobia in patients with mechanical low back pain. This was also supported by Liu et al. (2017a), who showed moderate evidence supporting the effectiveness of TrP-DN for low back pain, particularly when combined with other therapies. The effectiveness of a multidisciplinary manual therapy program including TrP-DN for temporomandibular disorders (TMDs) has been also proposed (González-Iglesias et al., 2013; Butts et al., 2017).

Several studies have demonstrated that real TrP-DN of the masticatory muscles was more effective than medication or sham needling in patients with TMDs (Fernández-Carnero et al., 2010a; González-Perez et al., 2012; Itoh et al., 2012; González-Perez et al., 2015) or bruxism-related pain (Blasco-Bonora et al., 2017). In fact, point-specific dry needling is more effective than nonpoint-specific needling for the management of TMDs (Dıraçoğlu et al., 2012). The orofacial region is the area where there are more studies comparing the effectiveness of TrP-DN versus other injection therapies. This is an important point as outlined by

Lewit (1979) and Hong (1994) who postulated that there is no effect from the injected substance as it is the mechanical effect of the needle which exerts the main therapeutic mechanisms. Two studies reported no significant differences between botulinum toxin injections, lidocaine injections and TrP-DN in patients with headaches and orofacial pain (Venâncio et al., 2008; 2009). Another study observed no significant differences between injections with saline or anesthetic and TrP-DN in individuals with temporalis muscle pain (Sabatke et al., 2015). In fact, the meta-analysis conducted by Ong and Claydon (2014) found no significant differences between TrP-DN and lidocaine injection at short- and mid-term follow-up periods confirming that the therapeutic effect is related to the needle and not to any particular substance.

Mechanisms of trigger point dry needling

The underlying mechanism by which TrP-DN exerts its therapeutic effects is not completely understood, and both mechanical and neurophysiological mechanisms have been proposed (Dommerholt, 2011; Chou et al., 2012; Cagnie et al., 2013).

From a mechanical point of view, several hypotheses including disruption of the integrity of dysfunctional end plates, increase in sarcomere length, and reduction of the overlap between actin and myosin filaments are proposed. The first hypothesis is based on the fact that TrP-DN reduces end-plate noise at the TrP (Chen et al., 2001; Chou et al., 2009; Hsieh et al., 2011). A recent study has confirmed that TrP-DN decreases the amplitude and frequency of end-plate noise and end-plate spike, which are typical features of spontaneous electrical activity of TrPs, and decreases acetylcholine levels (Liu et al., 2017b). The second mechanical hypothesis may be related to the fact that TrP-DN can improve muscle blood flow and oxygenation (Cagnie et al., 2012). Therefore, it seems that dry needling exerts mechanical effects on the

TrP area, which can start a cascade of mechanisms of action (Cagnie et al., 2013).

From a neurophysiological viewpoint, the application of TrP-DN on subjects with chronic pain may reduce both peripheral and central sensitization by removing the source of peripheral nociception (TrP), by modulating spinal efficacy in the dorsal horn and by activating central inhibitory pain pathways. In fact, TrP-DN may act at different levels in this process. First, the insertion of a needle into the human body is likely to have a physiological effect, such as a release of endorphins, a change in pain thresholds, or an expectancy of a positive outcome. Real needling and so-called sham procedures can activate cortical brain areas involved in sensorimotor processing, and deactivate brain regions that are more active during rest than during other tasks (Napadow et al., 2009). A systematic review found that insertion of a needle in the body produced activation of the sensorimotor cortical network, in the insula, thalamus, anterior cingulate cortex, primary and secondary somatosensory cortex, but also a deactivation of the limbic-paralimbic-neocortical network, in the medial prefrontal cortex, caudate, amygdala, posterior cingulate cortex, and parahippocampal cortex (Chae et al., 2013).

Secondly, it has also been demonstrated that TrP-DN may evoke antinociceptive effects by modulating segmental mechanisms at the spinal cord (Srbely et al., 2010). This spinal cord mechanism is supported by studies reporting remote effects of TrP-DN in muscles anatomically located in the referred pain area of the needled muscle (Hsieh et al., 2007; Fernández-Carnero et al., 2010b). In fact, Hsieh et al. (2011) found that the remote effect of dry needling depends on an intact afferent pathway from the needled site to the spinal cord and a normal spinal cord function at the levels corresponding to the innervation of the proximally affected muscle. More importantly, the remote effect of TrP-DN also involves the reduction of substance P in spinal superficial laminas of the dorsal horn, supporting a spinal cord mechanism in this process (Hsieh et al., 2014).

Finally, the first neurophysiological step is the periphery (Butts et al., 2016). Shah et al. (2005) found an immediate drop in the concentrations of neurotransmitters, such as calcitonin gene-related peptide and substance P, and also several cytokines and interleukins in the extracellular fluid of the local TrP milieu after the insertion of a needle. Hsieh et al. (2012) confirmed these findings observing that TrP-DN modulated the chemical mediators associated with pain and inflammation, such as substance P, β-endorphin, and tumor necrosis factor α (TNFα); however this study also reported that these effects on chemical concentrations with TrP-DN were dose dependent. Immediately after dry needling the levels of β-endorphin and TNFα increased, while the levels of substance P decreased. The longer-term application of needling also caused changes in the levels of cyclooxygenase-2 (COX-2), vascular endothelial growth factor (VEGF), inducible nitric oxide synthase (iNOS), and hypoxia-inducible factor 1-alpha (HIF-1α). The increase in substance P, COX-2, and TNFα levels may be associated with more tissue damage (Hsieh et al., 2012). Therefore, it seems that the mechanisms and effects of TrP-DN actions depend on the location of the needle, the depth of the insertion, the number of insertions, the needle forces and motions used, and whether or not a local twitch response is elicited.

Trigger point dry needling for patients with temporomandibular disorders

This section provides basic guidance on TrP-DN for the craniocervical muscles most commonly affected in patients with TMDs (Fernández-de-las-Peñas et al., 2010). It should be considered that this chapter does not constitute a qualification to use TrP-DN in clinical practice. These are general guidelines, which should be adhered to. Once the TrP is identified, the clinician must visualize its location in a three-dimensional perspective and appreciate the depth and presence of neighboring structures before considering the application of the procedure. If needed, anatomical landmarks should be identified and marked, including the margins of the muscle and any relevant bony structure (Halle & Halle, 2016). There is an ongoing debate as to whether disinfection of the skin or the use of gloves is necessary or not and guidelines vary in different countries and regions (ASAP, 2007; McEvoy et al., 2012; Bachmann et al., 2014).

The length of the needle will depend on the targeted muscle and the fat in the area and/or patient. TrP-DN is usually applied with needles in tubes. The tube is placed on the skin overlying the TrP and the needle is quickly tapped into the skin. The tube is removed, and the needle is moved in and out of the TrP by drawing the needle back to the subcutaneous tissue and redirecting it (fast-in and fast-out technique). The tip of the needle can be considered as an extension of the clinician's hand. In fact, the clinician must know where in the area the needle is and which structures will be encountered. Well-developed kinesthetic perception and clinical skills will permit the clinician to appreciate changes in structures and accurately identify when the needle penetrates the skin, the subcutaneous connective tissue and fascial layers, the muscle, and ultimately the TrP area (Dommerholt & Fernández-de-las-Peñas, 2013). Following the procedure, hemostasis is recommended to prevent or minimize local bleeding.

Dry needling of the masseter muscle

The superficial layer originates at the inferior aspect of the zygomatic process whereas the deep layer originates in the upper mandibular ramus and the coronoid process. Both layers insert into the angle and lateral surface of the mandible. The superficial layer refers pain to the eyebrow, the maxilla, the mandible, and the teeth, whereas the deep layer spreads pain deep into the ear and to the temporomandibular joint

(TMJ) area (Simons et al., 1999). For the needling procedure, the patient lies in supine. The muscle is usually needled with a flat palpation, although pincer palpation maybe also possible. The needle is inserted perpendicular to the TrP for both superficial (Figure 16.1) and deep (Figure 16.2) layers.

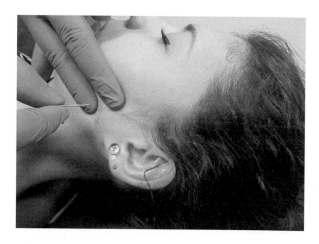

Figure 16.1
Dry needling of the superficial masseter.

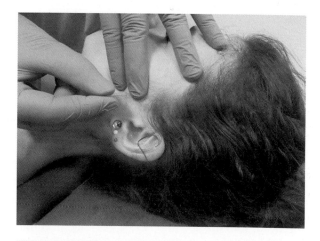

Figure 16.2
Dry needling of the deep masseter.

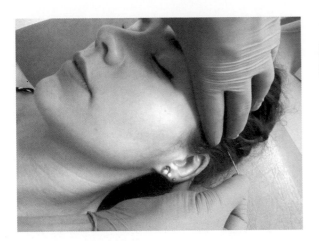

Figure 16.3
Dry needling of the temporalis.

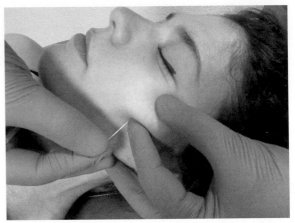

Figure 16.4
Dry needling of the zygomatic muscle (pincer palpation).

Dry needling of the temporalis muscle

The temporalis originates at the temporal fossa and inserts into the anterior border of the mandibular coronoid process and into the anterior border of the ramus of the mandible. TrP in this muscle refers deep pain to the head causing temporal headache and maxillary toothache (Simons et al., 1999). For the needling procedure, the patient lies in supine. The muscle is needled with a flat palpation. The needle is perpendicularly inserted into the skin toward the temporalis fossa (Figure 16.3). Clinicians should be aware of the anatomical trajectory of the superficial temporal artery.

Dry needling of the zygomatic muscle

The zygomatic muscle originates at the zygomatic bone and inserts into the muscles of the mouth, namely the orbicularis oris, levator, and depressor anguli oris. This muscle refers pain around the zygomatic bone, close to the nose and up to the forehead (Simons et al., 1999). For the needling procedure, the patient lies in supine. The muscle can be needled with a pincer or flat palpation. With a flat palpation, the needle is inserted perpendicular to the skin toward the zygomatic bone (Figure 16.4).

Dry needling of the medial pterygoid muscle

The medial pterygoid originates at the medial surface of the lateral pterygoid plate of the sphenoid bone, the maxillary tuberosity, and the pyramidal process of the palatine bone, and inserts into the lower back part of the medial surface of the ramus and angle of the mandible. TrPs in the medial pterygoid refer pain to the maxilla, mandible, teeth, ear, and TMJ (Simons et al., 1999). For the needling procedure, the patient lies in supine. The lower part of the muscle can be needled over the medial surface of the angle of the mandible. With a flat palpation, the needle is fixed between the index and middle fingers of the non-needling hand and inserted into the skin at a shallow angle toward the medial surface of the ramus and angle of the mandible (Figure 16.5).

Dry needling of the lateral pterygoid muscle

The superior head of the lateral pteygoid originates at the infratemporal surface of the greater wing of the sphenoid bone, whereas the inferior head originates at the lateral surface of the lateral pterygoid plate. Both heads insert at the internal surface of the neck of the mandible and the intraarticular disc of the TMJ. The referred pain from this muscle spreads to the maxilla and then deeper to the TMJ (Simons et al., 1999). Due to the clinical relevance of this muscle for the TMJ,

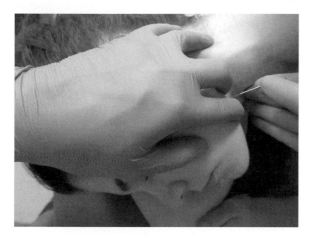

Figure 16.5
Dry needling of the medial pterygoid.

a specific dry needling procedure was developed (Mesa-Jiménez et al., 2015). For the needling procedure, the patient is positioned in side-lying. The dry needling approach uses two needles of 50 to 60 mm in length, one inserted over the zygomatic process posterior to the zygomatic arch (superior head) and the other inserted below the zygomatic process between the mandibular condyle and the coronoid process (inferior head) (Figure 16.6) (Mesa-Jiménez et al., 2015).

Dry needling of the digastric muscle

The anterior belly originates at the inferior border of the mandible, close to its symphysis, whereas the posterior belly originates at the mastoid notch of the temporal bone at the digastric groove. Both bellies are joined together by a common tendon that is indirectly anchored to the hyoid bone through a fibrous loop. TrPs in the anterior belly refer pain to the lower teeth and the tongue, whereas the posterior belly refers pain to the upper part of the mastoid process of the temporal bone (Simons et al., 1999). For the needling procedure, the patient lies in supine. For

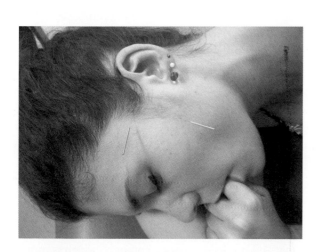

Figure 16.6
Dry needling of the lateral pterygoid.

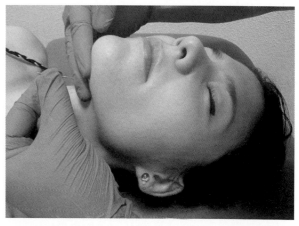

Figure 16.7
Dry needling of the anterior belly of the digastric muscle.

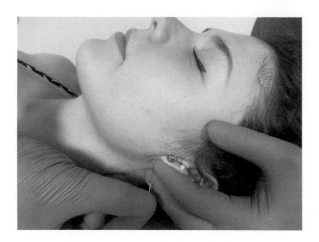

Figure 16.8
Dry needling of the posterior belly of the digastric muscle.

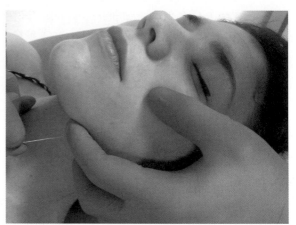

Figure 16.9
Dry needling of the mylohyoid muscle.

the anterior belly, the head and neck of the patient are slightly extended for better access to the muscle. The needle is fixed between the index and middle fingers of the non-needling hand, and inserted perpendicularly toward the lower part of the mandible (Figure 16.7). For the posterior belly the needle is inserted perpendicular to the mastoid notch (mastoid process) toward the transverse process of the atlas (Figure 16.8). Caution must be exercised to avoid needling through the muscle.

Dry needling of the mylohyoid muscle

The mylohyoid muscle originates along the entire length of the mylohyoid line of the mandible and inserts into the anterior lower border of hyoid bone and medial raphe. TrPs in this muscle refer pain to the tongue (Simons et al., 1999). For the needling procedure, the patient lies in supine. The needle is fixed between the index and middle fingers of the non-needling hand, and perpendicularly inserted approximately at the midline between the symphysis of the mandible (needling of anterior belly of the digastric muscle) and the angle of the mandible (needling

of the medial pterygoid) (Figure 16.9). Caution must be exercised to avoid needling through the muscle.

Dry needling of the upper part of the trapezius muscle

The upper part (descending fibers) of the trapezius originates at the external occipital protuberance, the medial third of the superior nuchal line of the occipital bone, the ligamentum nuchae, and the spinous process of C7, and inserts into the posterior border of the lateral third of the clavicle. TrPs in the upper part of the trapezius refer pain ipsilaterally to the posterior-lateral region of the neck, behind the ear, and to the temporal region. For the needling procedure, the patient lies in supine. The upper trapezius is needled with a pincer palpation. The needle is inserted perpendicular to the skin and directed toward the finger of the non-needling hand. The needle can be inserted from anterior to posterior or posterior to anterior (Figure 16.10). The most common serious adverse event is penetrating the lung, and producing a pneumothorax, which is minimized by needling strictly between the fingers holding the muscle in a pincer grasp, with needling directed toward the finger of the non-needling hand.

Dry needling of the sternocleidomastoid muscle

The sternal head originates at the anterior surface of the manubrium sterni and the clavicular head at the superior border and anterior surface of the medial third of the clavicle. Both heads insert into the

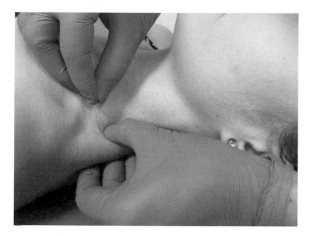

Figure 16.10
Dry needling of the upper part of the trapezius.

mastoid process of the temporal bone. TrPs in this muscle refer pain to the vertex, the occiput, the eye, the forehead and deep into the ear, inducing frontal headache (Simons et al., 1999). For the needling procedure, the patient lies in supine. The sternocleidomastoid muscle is needled with a pincer palpation. The needle is inserted perpendicular to the skin and directed toward the finger of the non-needling hand (Figure 16.11). The carotid artery and the jugular vein lie medial to the muscle. Lift the sternocleidomastoid muscle away from the carotid artery, and needle between the fingers holding the muscle in a pincer grasp, directing the needle as described above, to avoid needling the artery and vein.

Dry needling of the obliquus capitis inferior muscle

The obliquus capitis inferior originates at the spinous process of the axis (C2) and attaches to the transverse process of the atlas (C1). The referred pain elicited by TrPs in this muscle is perceived as deep pain spreading from the occiput toward the region of the orbit (Simons et al., 1999). For the

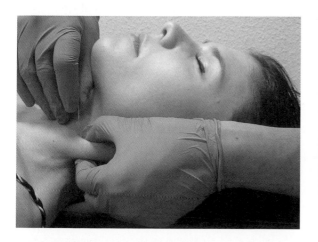

Figure 16.11
Dry needling of the sternocleidomastoid muscle.

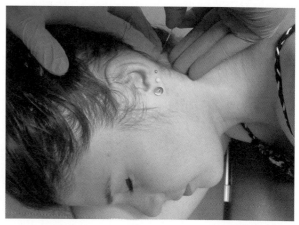

Figure 16.12
Dry needling of the obliquus capitis inferior muscle.

needling procedure, the patient is positioned in side-lying. The muscle is needled at a point midway between the transverse process of C1 and the spinous process of C2. The needle is inserted perpendicular to the skin directly in the medial half of the muscle toward the patient's opposite eye in a slightly cranial–medial direction (Figure 16.12). Clinicians should avoid directing the needle strictly cranially or too laterally to prevent inadvertent penetration of the vertebral artery.

References

APTA – American Physical Therapy Association. Physical therapists & the performance of dry needling: An educational resource paper. Alexandria, VA: APTA Department of Practice and APTA State Government Affairs; 2012. Available: http://www.apta.org/StateIssues/DryNeedling/ResourcePaper/ [Nov 20, 2017].

APTA – American Physical Therapy Association. Description of dry needling in clinical practice: an educational resource paper. Alexandria, VA: APTA Public Policy, Practice, and Professional Affairs Unit; 2013. Available: http://www.apta.org/StateIssues/DryNeedling/ClinicalPracticeResourcePaper/ [Nov 20, 2017].

ASAP – Australian Society of Acupuncture Physiotherapists. Guidelines for safe acupuncture and dry needling practice. ASAP; 2007. Available: http://combinedhealth.com.au/webfiles/ASAP_Guidelines_2013.pdf [Nov 20, 2017].

Bachmann S, Colla F, Gröbli C, Mungo G, Gröbli L, Reilich P, Weissmann R. Swiss guidelines for safe dry needling. Dry Needling Verband Schweitz; 2014. Available: http://www.dgs-academy.com/fileadmin/documents/Swiss_Guidelines_for_safe_1.7_Dry_Needling.pdf [Nov 20, 2017].

Blasco-Bonora PM, Martín-Pintado-Zugasti A. Effects of myofascial trigger point dry needling in patients with sleep bruxism and temporomandibular disorders: a prospective case series. Acupunct Med 2017; 35: 69–74.

Boyles R, Fowler R, Ramsey D, Burrows E. Effectiveness of trigger point dry needling for multiple body regions: a systematic review. J Man Manip Ther 2015; 23: 276–293.

Brady S, McEvoy J, Dommerholt J, Doody C. Adverse events following trigger point dry needling: a prospective survey of chartered physiotherapists. J Man Manip Ther 2014: 22: 134–140.

Butts R, Dunning J, Perreault T, Mourad F, Grubb M. Peripheral and spinal mechanisms of pain and dry needling mediated analgesia: a clinical resource guide for health care professionals. Int J Phys Med Rehabil 2016; 4: 2.

Butts R, Dunning J, Pavkovich R, Mettille J, Mourad F. Conservative management of temporomandibular dysfunction: a literature review with implications for clinical practice guidelines. J Bodyw Mov Ther 2017; 21: 541–548.

CADTH – Canadian Agency for Drugs and Technologies in Health. Dry Needling and Injection for Musculoskeletal and Joint Disorders: A Review of the Clinical Effectiveness, Cost-Effectiveness, and Guidelines. Ottawa, ON: Canadian Agency for Drugs and Technologies in Health; 2016. Available: https://www.ncbi.nlm.nih.gov/books/NBK395711/ [Nov 20, 2017]

Cagnie B, Barbe T, De Ridder E et al. The influence of dry needling of the trapezius muscle on muscle blood flow and oxygenation. J Manipulative Physiol Ther 2012; 35: 685–691.

Cagnie B, Dewitte V, Barbe T, Timmermans F, Delrue N, Meeus M. Physiologic effects of dry needling. Curr Pain Headache Rep 2013; 17: 348.

Cagnie B, Castelein B, Pollie F, Steelant L, Verhoeyen H, Cools A. Evidence for the use of ischemic compression and dry needling in the management of trigger points of the upper trapezius in patients with neck pain: a systematic review. Am J Phys Med Rehabil 2015; 94: 573–583.

Chae Y, Chang DS, Lee SH et al. Inserting needles into the body: a meta-analysis of brain activity associated with acupuncture needle stimulation. J Pain 2013; 14: 215–222.

Chen JT, Chung KC, Hou CR et al. Inhibitory effect of dry needling on the spontaneous electrical activity recorded from myofascial trigger spots of rabbit skeletal muscle. Am J Phys Med Rehabil 2001; 80: 729–735.

Chou, LW, Hsieh YL, Kao MJ, et al. Remote influences of acupuncture on the pain intensity and the amplitude changes of endplate noise in the myofascial trigger point of the upper trapezius muscle. Arch Phys Med Rehabil 2009; 90: 905–912.

Chou LW, Kao MJ, Lin JG. Probable mechanisms of needling therapies for myofascial pain control. Evid Based Complement Alternat Med 2012; 2012: 705327.

Cummings M, Ross-Marrs R, Gerwin R. Pneumothorax complication of deep dry needling demonstration. Acupunct Med 2014; 32: 517–519.

Dıraçoğlu D, Vural M, Karan A, Aksoy C. Effectiveness of dry needling for the treatment of temporomandibular myofascial pain: a double-blind, randomized, placebo controlled study. J Back Musculoskelet Rehabil 2012; 25: 285–290.

Domingo A, Mayoral O, Monterde S, Santafé MM. Neuromuscular damage and repair after dry needling in mice. Evid Based Complement Alternat Med 2013; 2013: 260806.

Dommerholt J. Dry needling: peripheral and central considerations. J Manual Manipul Ther 2011; 19: 223–237.

Dommerholt J, Fernández-de-las-Peñas C. Trigger Point Dry Needling: An Evidenced and Clinical-Based Approach. 1st ed. London: Churchill Livingstone: Elsevier; 2013.

Dunning J, Butts R, Mourad F, Young I, Flannagan S, Perreault T. Dry needling: a literature review with implications for clinical practice guidelines. Phys Ther Rev 2014; 19: 252–265.

Fernández-Carnero J, La Touche R, Ortega-Santiago R et al. Short-term effects of dry needling of active myofascial trigger points in the masseter muscle in patients with temporomandibular disorders. J Orofac Pain 2010a; 24: 106–112.

Fernández-Carnero J, Ge HY, Kimura Y, et al. Increased spontaneous electrical activity at a latent myofascial trigger point after nociceptive stimulation of another latent trigger point. Clin J Pain 2010b; 26: 138–143.

Fernández-Carnero J, Gilarranz-de-Frutos L, León-Hernández JV et al. Effectiveness of different deep dry needling dosages in the treatment of patients with cervical myofascial pain: A Pilot RCT. Am J Phys Med Rehabil 2017; 96:726–733.

Fernández-de-las-Peñas C, Galán-del-Río F, Alonso-Blanco C, Jiménez-Garcia R, Arendt-Nielsen L, Svensson P. Referred pain from muscle trigger points in the masticatory and neck-shoulder musculature in women with temporomandibular disorders. J Pain 2010; 11: 1295–1304.

France S, Bown J, Nowosilskyj M, Mott M, Rand S, Walters J. Evidence for the use of dry needling and physiotherapy in the management of cervicogenic or tension-type headache: a systematic review. Cephalalgia 2014; 34: 994–1003.

Gattie E, Cleland JA, Snodgrass S. The effectiveness of trigger point dry needling for musculoskeletal conditions by physical therapists: aa systematic review and meta-analysis. J Orthop Sports Phys Ther 2017; 47: 133–149.

González-Iglesias J, Cleland JA, Neto F et al. Mobilization with movement, thoracic spine manipulation, and dry needling for the management of temporomandibular disorder: A prospective case series. Physiother Theory Pract 2013; 29: 586–595.

González-Perez LM, Infante-Cossio P, Granados-Nuñez M, Urresti-Lopez FJ. Treatment of temporomandibular myofascial pain with deep dry needling. Med Oral Patol Oral Cir Bucal 2012; 17: 781–785.

González-Perez LM, Infante-Cossio P, Granados-Nunez M et al. Deep dry needling of trigger points located in the lateral pterygoid muscle: Efficacy and safety of treatment for management of myofascial pain and temporomandibular dysfunction. Med Oral Patol Oral Cir Bucal 2015; 20: 326–333.

Halle JS, Halle RJ. Pertinent dry needling considerations for minimizing adverse effects - part one. Int J Sports Phys Ther 2016; 11: 651–662.

Hong C. Lidocaine injection versus dry needling to myofascial trigger point. The importance of the local twitch response. Am J Phys Med Rehabil 1994; 73: 256–263.

Hsieh YL, Kao MJ, Kuan TS et al. Dry needling to a key myofascial trigger point may reduce the irritability of satellite MTrPs. Am J Phys Med Rehabil 2007; 86: 397–403.

Hsieh YL, Chou LW, Joe YS et al. Spinal cord mechanism involving the remote effects of dry needling on the irritability of myofascial trigger spots in rabbit skeletal muscle. Arch Phys Med Rehabil 2011; 92: 1098–1105.

Hsieh YL, Yang SA, Yang CC, Chou LW. Dry needling at myofascial trigger spots of rabbit skeletal muscles modulates the biochemicals associated with pain, inflammation, and hypoxia. Evid Based Complement Alternat Med 2012; 2012: 342165.

Hsieh YL, Yang SA, Liu SY, Chou LW, Honc CZ. Remote dose-dependent effects of dry needling at distant myofascial trigger spots of rabbit skeletal muscles on reduction of substance P levels of proximal muscle and spinal cords. Biomed Res Int 2014; 2014: 982121.

Itoh K, Asai S, Ohyabu H, Imai K, Kitakoji H. Effects of trigger point acupuncture treatment on temporomandibular disorders: a preliminary randomized clinical trial. J Acupunct Meridian Stud 2012; 5: 57–62.

Joseph L, Mohd Ali K, Ramli A et al. Fear of needles does not influence pain tolerance and sympathetic responses among patients during a therapeutic needling. Pol Ann Med 2013; 20: 1–7.

Kietrys DM, Palombaro KM, Azzaretto E et al. Effectiveness of dry needling for upper quarter myofascial pain: A systematic review and meta-analysis. J Orthop Sports Phys Ther 2003; 43: 620–634.

Koppenhaver SL, Walker MJ, Rettig C et al. The association between dry needling-induced twitch response and change in pain and muscle function in patients with low back pain; a quasi-experimental study. Physiotherapy 2017; 103: 131–137.

Lewit, K 1979. The needle effect in the relief of myofascial pain. Pain 6: 83–90.

Liu L, Huang QM, Liu QG, Ye G, Bo CZ, Chen MJ, Li P. Effectiveness of dry needling for myofascial trigger points associated with neck and shoulder pain: a systematic review and meta-analysis. Arch Phys Med Rehabil 2015; 96: 944–955.

Liu L, Huang QM, Liu QG, Thitham N, Li LH, Ma YT, Zhao JM. Evidence for dry needling in the management of myofascial trigger points associated with low back pain: a systematic review and meta-analysis. Arch Phys Med Rehabil 2017a; Jul 6. pii: S0003-9993(17)30452–5.

Liu QG, Liu L, Huang QM, Nguyen TT, Ma YT, Zhao JM. Decreased spontaneous electrical activity and acetylcholine at myofascial trigger spots after dry needling treatment: a pilot study. Evid Based Complement Alternat Med 2017b; 2017: 3938191.

Martín-Pintado Zugasti A, Rodríguez-Fernández ÁL, García-Muro F, et al. Effects of spray and stretch on post-needling soreness and sensitivity after dry needling of a latent myofascial trigger point. Arch Phys Med Rehabil 2014; 95: 1925–1932.

Martín-Pintado-Zugasti A, Pecos-Martin D, Rodríguez-Fernández ÁL, et al. Ischemic compression after dry needling of a latent myofascial trigger point reduces post-needling soreness intensity and duration. PM R 2015; 7: 1026–1034.

McEvoy J, Dommerholt J, Rice D, Holmes L, Grobli C, Fernández-de-las-Penas C. Guidelines for Dry Needling Practice. Dublin: Irish Society of Chartered Physiotherapists; 2012. Available: http://www.colfisiocv.org/sites/default/files/Guidelines%20for%20Dry%20Needling%20Practice%20ISCP%202012.pdf [Nov 19, 2017].

Mesa-Jiménez JA, Sánchez-Gutiérrez J, de-la-Hoz-Aizpurua JL, Fernández-de-las-Peñas C. Cadaveric validation of dry needle placement in the lateral pterygoid muscle. J Manipulative Physiol Ther 2015; 38: 145–150.

Morihisa R, Eskew J, McNamara A, Young J. Dry needling in subjects with muscular trigger points in the lower quarter: A systematic review. Int J Sports Phys Ther 2016; 11: 1–14.

Napadow V, Dhond RP, Kim J et al. Brain encoding of acupuncture sensation - coupling on-line rating with fMRI. Neuroimage 2009; 47: 1055–1065.

Ong J, Claydon LS. The effect of dry needling for myofascial trigger points in the neck and shoulders: a systematic review and meta-analysis. J Bodyw Mov Ther 2014; 18: 390–398.

Perreault T, Dunning J, Butts R. The local twitch response during trigger point dry needling: is it necessary for successful outcomes? J Bodyw Mov Ther 2017; 21: 940–947.

Rodríguez-Mansilla J, González-Sánchez B, De Toro García A et al. Effectiveness of dry needling on reducing pain intensity in patients with myofascial pain syndrome: a meta-analysis. J Tradit Chin Med 2016; 36: 1–13.

Sabatke S, Scola RH, Paiva ES, Kowacs PA. Injecction [sic] of trigger points in the temporal muscles of patients with miofascial [sic] syndrome. Arq Neuropsiquiatr 2015; 73: 861–866.

Salom-Moreno J, Jiménez-Gómez L, Gómez-Ahufinger V et al. Effects of low-load exercise on postneedling-induced pain after dry needling of active trigger point in individuals with subacromial pain syndrome. PM R 2017 May 5; pii: S1934–1482(16)31008–5.

Shah JP, Phillips T, Danoff J, Gerber L. An in-vivo microanalytical technique for measuring the local biochemical milieu of human skeletal muscle. J Appl Physiol 2005; 99: 1977–1984.

Simons DG, Travell JG, Simons LS. Travell and Simons' Myofascial Pain and Dysfunction: The Trigger Point Manual. Vol. 1: Upper Half of Body. Baltimore, Williams & Wilkins; 1999.

Srbely JZ, Dickey JP, Lee D, Lowerison M. Dry needle stimulation of myofascial trigger points evokes segmental anti-nociceptive effects. J Rehabil Med 2010; 42: 463–468.

Téllez-García M, de-la-Llave-Rincón AI, Salom-Moreno J, Palacios-Ceña M, Ortega-Santiago R, Fernández-de-las-Peñas C. Neuroscience education in addition to trigger point dry needling for the management of patients with mechanical chronic low back pain: a preliminary clinical trial. J Bodyw Mov Ther 2015; 19: 464–472.

Venâncio Rde A, Alencar FG, Zamperini C. Different substances and dry-needling injections in patients with myofascial pain and headaches. Cranio 2008; 26: 96–103.

Venâncio Rde A, Alencar FG Jr, Zamperini C. Botulinum toxin, lidocaine, and dry-needling injections in patients with myofascial pain and headaches. Cranio 2009; 27: 46–53.

Zhou K, Ma Y, Brogan MS. Dry needling versus acupuncture: the ongoing debate. Acupunct Med 2015; 33: 485–490.

Chapter 17

Acupuncture in temporomandibular disorders

Tom Mark Thayer, Mike Cummings

Introduction

Acupuncture is a traditional therapeutic technique with a long history and strong cultural ties with China and the Far East. The concepts were first formalized by the Yellow Emperor *Hung Ti* around 2,500 BC, and probably reflect observational medicine in the context of the time, and its further development over generations. This has produced a complex system of diagnosis based upon careful history taking and observations, centered around the conceptual framework of chi (also spelled qi or ch'i), the life energy of the body. Disturbances in the chi are considered to lead to ill health, and acupuncture is used as one technique that is considered to improve the flow of the chi, and restore normal health. A number of approaches may be used to improve the flow of the chi, with traditional simple needling probably being the most common, but acupressure techniques, cupping, and moxibustion (burning herbs) are all based on the same traditional principles.

Acupuncture relies on the use of solid filiform needles, inserted into the body at a range of sites to induce changes at those sites that may then lead to symptom resolution. While the traditional concepts may seem flawed to the Western (medically) trained professional, the theoretical modeling of the action of acupuncture is reasonably robust, and some observed outcomes may be supported. Evidence for some acupuncture-based interventions is reasonable, but the contextual response (sometimes referred to as placebo) may be strong, and interpretation can be difficult.

Traditional acupuncture describes a number of meridians, or channels, in which the chi flows around the body to nourish the various organs. History taking and examination is aimed at determining where

flow is disturbed, leading to imbalances of the *yin* and *yang,* or the balancing forces of nature in the organs. Acupuncture needling is then prescribed to enhance the flow of the chi and encourage improved health by improving the balance of the *yin* and *yang.* There is a range of variations of traditional techniques, and many practitioners will expound the benefits of one over the other, yet there seems little to recommend any one approach, and many practitioners will use multiple approaches and therapies to achieve results. In broad terms, there are the general body techniques, muscular trigger point (TrP) focused techniques, and microsystem (or homunculus) techniques, such as ear techniques where all needling is undertaken on the ear alone.

Acupuncture points are generally found lying on the meridians, although some lie outside the classically described meridians. There are said to be 12 paired (left and right) meridians, two midline meridians (one ventral, one dorsal), and six isolated meridians. Each is named, although these names have little or nothing to do with our modern understanding of the organs to which they refer. For example, the Stomach meridian (Figure 17.1) has no direct connection to the stomach, but commences in the lower eyelid, extends around the face, including the muscles of mastication, and runs down the front of the body to the leg and foot. While the meridians are not anatomical structures, and probably represent a construct to explain observed phenomena and responses to stimuli, they do appear to be consistently accessible from an anatomical basis, which probably reflects the consistency of the normal structures, and thus referred symptoms from these.

The Stomach meridian is given a shorthand notation of ST. There are 45 acupuncture points lying on this meridian, and each acupuncture point has a

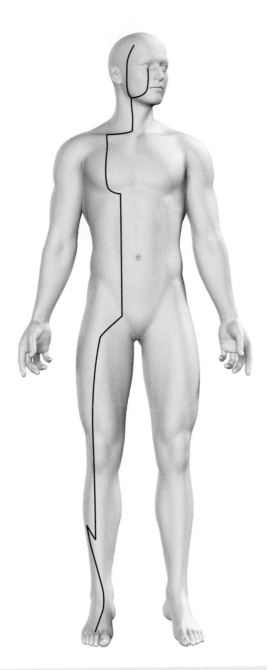

Figure 17.1
Stomach meridian (45 points).

specific site and notation, and these are recorded by notation and meridian, so sites in the masseter muscle are ST5, ST6, and ST7 (Figure 17.2). These points are typically involved in treatment of muscular symptoms of temporomandibular disorders (TMDs). There are also traditional names for each site, so ST6 is also known as *jiache*, and a site in the temporalis muscle, with notation EX2 (Extra 2) is known as *taiyang*. This is a muscular TrP site that is commonly linked with aspects of TMD, and is frequently implicated in headache associated with TMD. Study of the correlation between traditional acupuncture sites, and muscular TrPs, show a significant association, and it seems that this association provides a basis for interpreting TrP sites as acupuncture points, although it should be considered that there is no specific location for muscular TrPs.

Traditional prescribing of acupuncture relates to the clinical findings, and reflects these by using local

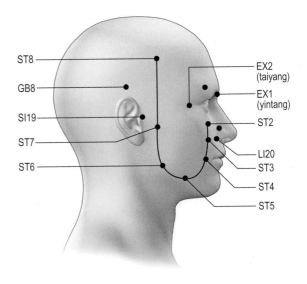

Figure 17.2
Acupuncture points of the head.

sites close to the origin of symptoms, or distant sites for enhancing symptom control. In reality, the sites that are closest to the symptoms are generally best, and in TMDs these tend to be sites in the muscles of mastication. However, in some cases distant sites such as points in the hand or foot may be used, and certainly those lying in the neck and shoulder muscles are often relevant.

Mechanisms

Primary modeling of the action of acupuncture has developed alongside the gate theory of Melzack and Wall (Melzack & Wall, 1965), where stimulus to one area may suppress neurone function in the areas supplied by the same nerves, effectively 'closing the gate' on the transmission of electrical impulses and thus reducing pain. This operates primarily on a segmental basis, with symptom control most easily managed in areas segmentally linked to the acupuncture sites, although there is a degree of vertical overlap as each region is supplied by several spinal nerves. Such neuroanatomic concepts are widely used, from transcutaneous nerve stimulation (TENS) to deep brain stimulation. With acupuncture treatments, the stimulus provided by needling activates afferent neurons, primarily Aδ fibers, thin myelinated neurons that carry the rapid response to initial painful episodes, but the needle action will induce a response from all types of afferent fibers. The afferent fibers then in turn express an inhibitory action via interneurons in the dorsal horn to suppress pain, which is primarily mediated via C-fiber neurons. This mechanism is particularly effective on a segmental basis, but since a single needle insertion through skin and muscle tissues will stimulate more than one segment (often around five segments), and may operate though the cervical or sacral plexus, this can lead to wider action across multiple segments, such that, for example, a point in the hand can suppress symptoms in the shoulder. Studies using functional magnetic resonance imaging (fMRI) demonstrate that brain responses to acupuncture stimulation with deep

tissue sensation (often referred to as *deqi*) include down regulation of many components of the limbic system (Napadow et al., 2016). This might suggest that the responses to acupuncture are mediated centrally as much as peripherally, which may contribute to the use of acupuncture points at quite widely placed sites.

Acupuncture also appears to have both a segmental and a heterosegmental action (meaning action on other segments), with descending control from the brain leading to inhibition of pain from the periphery and modulation of neuronal activity (particularly the inhibitory interneurons) within the spinal cord. The ascending (spinothalamic) and descending (dorsolateral funniculus) pathways thus impact upon pain perception centrally by modulating activity both in the brain and the spinal cord.

Acupuncture points and muscular trigger points

Acupuncture points sometimes appear to have distinctly different functional properties to the surrounding tissues, yet differences cannot be demonstrated histologically. It has been suggested that there may be greater than average innervation or clustering of increased numbers of nerve fibers and receptors at these sites that are commonly in relationship with skeletal muscle and connective tissue (Li et al., 2004; Baldry, 2005). Mechanoreceptors in muscle and skin are also present, as are nociceptors, and all of these may be stimulated by acupuncture needling. Certainly, when palpated, acupuncture sites often seem to be more tender than the surrounding tissues, and this is a primary means of identifying the sites for needling.

Studies suggest that this difference in acupuncture point behavior may be due to different representation in brain activity when the sites are stimulated compared to other tissues, suggesting that the difference between acupuncture points and other tissues, and the way they respond to stimulus, may be a centrally mediated phenomenon (Gu et al., 2015; Li et al., 2016a; Yeo et al., 2016). Alternatively, it may simply be that the increased density of sensory receptors provides increased response to stimulus with consequent downstream impact. Functional magnetic resonance imaging shows modulation of activity within a range of central structures, including the prefrontal cortex, the anterior and posterior insula, the hippocampus, the amygdala, and the periaqueductal gray (PAG). The PAG is involved in the descending regulation of nociception along dorsal horn neurons, through the rostral ventromedial medulla (RVM), involving spinal 5-HT receptors along with α2 adrenoceptors (Yaksh, 1979). The raphe magnus nucleus is part of the RVM, and stimulus here produces a strong inhibition of nociception, forming an important aspect of central mediation of pain (Napadow et al., 2009; Li et al., 2016b; Wang et al., 2016).

Muscular (myofascial) TrPs feature strongly within musculoskeletal problems, and commonly refer pain to distant structures. TrPs and zones within the muscles of mastication are a primary source of pain, referring with characteristic patterns, which have been carefully documented by Travell and Simons (Simons et al., 1999). Careful documentation of the patient's pain patterns may allow mapping of symptoms to muscle groups, and thus diagnosis of pain at distant sites. Pain need not be limited to a TMD, but present as one mimicking conventional dental pain, that is, within the dental structures, and may refer from more distant sites, such as the shoulder, to the facial area.

Muscular TrPs typically form in groups, with opposing points forming in balancing muscles. As a consequence, TrPs in the lateral pterygoid muscle can also commonly accompany TrPs in the masseter muscle. A common clinical presentation for the lateral pterygoid is a complaint of pain in the anterior maxilla described as 'sinus pain', with or without ear pain, with a consequent history of repeated attendances at medical clinics for assessment of these sites. The reality is the patient is presenting with TrPs in the lateral pterygoid muscle that refer to these sites (Figure 17.3), and pain mapping will demonstrate this, thus guiding prescribing. The nature and issues driven by TrPs have been discussed in Chapter 8 of this textbook.

A secondary, and possibly more important, action of acupuncture operates on TrPs and zones to reduce their activity, and thus improve symptoms. When needling a site, the needle changes the local environment by antidromic (reverse) stimulation of small nerves that release trophic neurochemicals promoting actions such as vasodilation and repair. Abnormal and persistent contraction within muscle cells involved in muscle TrPs can be reset by needling,

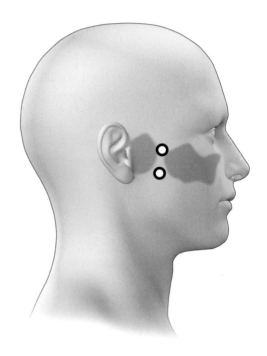

Figure 17.3

Referral pattern from trigger points (TrPs) in the lateral pterygoid muscle.

controlling the metabolic (oxygen) demands of the muscle fibers, and reducing the anaerobic nature of the cellular environment. Needling also potentially releases a number of neurotransmitters, most notably calcitonin gene-related peptide (CGRP), which is a potent vasodilator, at the capillary level. This vasodilation then oxygenates the muscular tissue to relieve pain as consequence of ischemia brought on by parafunctional activity. Vasodilation is evident to the naked eye as the skin surrounding the needle is frequently seen to be red and improved blood flow through the tissues has been demonstrated (Blom, 1993; Cagnie et al., 2012). Parallel work using thermal imaging has shown that a reduction in symptoms brought about by occlusal appliance therapy correlates with an increase in muscle temperature, consistent with increased blood flow (Barão et al., 2011). It is common for patients to report a sensation of warmth during needling. Therefore, as a consequence it may be that the increase in blood flow and oxygenation of the tissues, combined with a reduction in the overall cellular oxygen demand is a very significant factor in managing muscular and myofascial pain.

Technique

Acupuncture relies upon the insertion of fine needles into the tissues, primarily the muscles. The needles vary in length and are gauged as hypodermic needles, but are solid, not hollow. The tip is ground to a fine point, but is not a cutting tip as with hypodermics. In current Western practice, the needles are single use, prepackaged, sterile, and stainless steel. While some practitioners like to use very fine (0.12 mm diameter) needles, practically these can be difficult to use as they have a tendency to bend on insertion, and may be a challenge to insert through fascial layers, particularly with longer lengths. Needles of 0.25 mm have much more structural rigidity, and are more appropriate for deeper needling for muscles such as the lateral pterygoid.

Depth of insertion varies, depending on the site, muscle, and build of the patient. In general most acupuncture in the head and neck can be achieved with 30 mm long needles, but for deeper sites, or patients with a significant amount of body fat, then a greater length of needle may be required, such as 40 or 50 mm. When inserted, patients report a sensation of discomfort (sometimes frank pain with particularly tender muscles), warmth, heaviness, and commonly paresthesia, which may be referred, for example from the upper portion of the masseter muscle (point ST7) (Figure 17.4) to the lateral aspect of the tongue. The sensations felt at the site

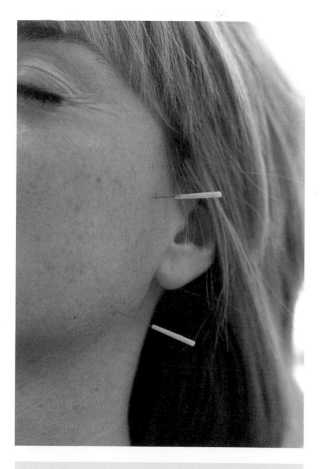

Figure 17.4
Sites ST6 (lower) and ST7 (upper).

Chapter 17

are referred to as the *deqi*, and are considered to be an indicator of effective treatments. Practically, it is observed that failure to achieve a *deqi* response at the site may indicate a poorer response to treatment, or at some sites, incorrect placement. This is based on the clinical experience of the first author.

Twisting of the needle is normally used to increase effectiveness, as this increases the stimulus. Needles may be used both in twisting actions, as well as pushing movements, and depth may vary. Deep stimulation to the periosteum may be used, and provides a very strong stimulus. The variation in types of stimulus allows activation of differing types of receptors at the acupuncture sites. Simple manual stimulation at around 2 Hz is normal. The mechanical action of rotation friction within the skin activates mechanoreceptors and recruits Aδ and Aβ fibers to increase the response and thus improve inhibition of C fibers at the dorsal horn. The increased movement probably also increases the response in the deeper tissues, leading to improved vasodilation, although the opposite response may occur in very sensitive subjects (Sandberg et al., 2005), such as those with fibromyalgia syndrome, for whom a more gentle and superficial approach may be more appropriate.

When needling muscular TrP and zones, the process is the same, but responses are sometimes different. In some cases, when the needle stimulates the TrP, there is a sudden, but usually not painful, contraction of the band of muscle. This TrP 'local twitch response' is usually an indicator of a successful release of the TrP, and relaxation follows quickly; indeed, if required, the needle can be removed as the trigger point has deactivated. TrP dry needling is explained in Chapter 16 of this textbook.

Treatment sessions vary in length. In theory, longer sessions should give improved symptom control, as increased recruitment of neurons can occur at the interneuron site, to increase inhibition of C fibers. Rosted (2001) suggests up to 30 minutes – in reality, there seems to be relatively little increased benefit of 30 minutes' treatment over 10–15 minutes, and certainly hand stimulus of needles for a long period is tiring and time consuming. In fact, the basic science data now seem to show that 10 minutes is enough for adenosine and TNFα effects, but acute modulation of thresholds is maximal at 20 to 30 minutes.

In general, stimulation of needles with an elecrical pulse generator (electroacupuncture or EA) may be employed to provide increased stimulus without hand twisting, and electrical current may be applied across the needles at variable frequencies. This approach is generally not recommended for facial muscles and muscles of mastication, as the facial nerve is recruited at a very low intensity of stimulus. This is most apparent when applying EA near the point ST7. The consequent regular muscle twitching may be disturbing for the patient, although it is not painful.

When to use acupuncture. What is the evidence?

Use of acupuncture for treatment of TMD is based upon a range of decision components, rather like any other treatment planning process. A key factor is the patient's willingness and his or her attitude to acupuncture. Some are keen, some less so. Needle phobias would obviously make acceptance more difficult, but such phobias can be site specific, and many sites that are not visible may be treated quite acceptably as long as the patient cannot see the needles.

In addition, there are alternative methods of stimulating points, such as firm digital pressure (acupressure techniques), which can be particularly effective with TrPs in the neck and temporalis muscles, and other stimuli such as laser stimulators, and electrical stimulators. Low level lasers have become more popular in recent years, and a laser acupuncture technique has been described. Evidence for the effectiveness of this is, however, lacking at present.

Often acupuncture has been deployed in the treatment of chronic and acute pain related to TMDs as a last effort. However, the accumulated scientific material looking at the effectiveness of acupuncture in pain management seems to show a common pattern of effective reduction in pain with improved function. For example, in tension-type headache, a Cochrane review has suggested that acupuncture was as effective as conventional therapies (Linde et al., 2016). A meta-analysis by List & Axelsson (2010) demonstrated positive outcomes with acupuncture for treatment of TMDs, with long-term improvements and success rates as high as conventional therapies, but not more effective. One particular benefit is that there are typically little in the way of side effects, although bruising occasionally occurs, and very rarely a hematoma (typically in the temporalis over which there are relatively large superficial arteries). Effects can be immediate, and it is common to see that pain scores are reduced during the treatment sessions, but responses may be delayed, only appearing after hours or days, and requiring accumulated effects of several visits to become apparent, and while 10–20 per cent of patients appear to fail to respond at all, a majority seem to gain some benefit, although for some this may be short lived.

As a consequence, acupuncture may be prescribed at any stage of therapy, and could be considered as an initial therapy, particularly in patients where myogenous pain is the primary issue. In theory, the muscles may be needled in either acute or chronic phases of TMD, but needling during an acute myospasm will be extremely painful, and in some cases may be best avoided, allowing the initial severe symptoms to settle a little before needling. Alternatively segmentally related sites may be used initially to reduce pain by 'gating' before needling the primary sites at a later appointment.

Of course, TMD problems also involve joint issues, either joint pathologies, such as degenerative disorders, or functional mechanical problems (see Chapter 2), primarily related to meniscal displacement. Acupuncture may offer a degree of pain control in cases of joint damage, as it does with other joints, and may help to improve function as a consequence, if only by a limited amount. It is important to eliminate other significant pathologies of the joint to ensure appropriate therapies are employed.

Meniscal displacement leading to clicking may also be helped with acupuncture, and both the severity and timing of a click may be changed with such an approach. In these cases, needling is aimed toward reducing the displacing forces on the meniscus primarily from the lateral pterygoid muscles (see Chapter 16). Here needles are inserted into the body of the lateral pterygoid muscle and at sites close to the insertions on the neck of the condyle and meniscus to release TrPs and reduce muscle tone. This is combined with needling behind the joint to create an inflammatory response that may 'tighten' the retrodiscal ligaments. Clinically this can be helpful with troublesome clicking, but will not generally eliminate the problem. Typically clicking becomes less prominent, and often appears earlier in the mandibular movement cycle, so that a mid-phase click may become an early-phase click, which would be consistent with the planned approach to the problem.

Therefore, the decision to employ acupuncture relies on a combination of factors; the rationale for prescribing acupuncture is driven by the treatment needs: pain control, to overcome confounding factors for other treatment options, support or enhancement of other approaches to treatment, and psychological symptoms.

Pain control

Acute or chronic pain from TMDs is a primary reason for many patients to seek treatment, and is likewise the primary reason for prescribing acupuncture. This may be as an initial treatment to control symptoms, and can be initiated on the first presenting visit, although in general a planned therapeutic approach is more common. With pain of primarily muscular origin, acupuncture may form the sole treatment, or may be supplemented with other approaches, such as physiotherapy, or an occlusal appliance.

Acute onset pain often responds rapidly to acupuncture, and may improve within a few visits (given the caveat earlier of avoiding a significant myospasm). Chronic pain relief frequently takes longer (four to six visits), and may require retreatments, typically related to poorly controlled personal environmental stress promoting persistent muscle parafunctional activity. Complete elimination of all symptoms may be achieved for some, but for many the outcome is a reduction in symptoms such that these become subclinical and within tolerances.

Confounding factors

For some patients, acupuncture is preferable to other therapies, and some actively seek treatment. For others it proves to be an effective option when there are confounding factors leading to a reduction in tolerance of conventional therapies, such as with patients who struggle with an occlusal appliance, especially those who gag, or those who have been wearing an appliance and have become noncompliant.

In some cases mandibular function may be restricted as a result of muscle derived trismus, or muscular pain. Opening may be limited or painful, and impression-taking for occlusal appliances may be more difficult. Acupuncture prior to impression-taking can improve opening, allowing more accurate impressions. For many cases, this will involve needling immediately prior to taking the impressions, primarily at the most painful sites in the masseter muscle, to reduce pain and thus facilitate opening of the mouth. However, for cases where trismus is more of an issue, as opposed to pain, needling may be required over a few visits to improve function prior to impression taking.

For those who gag, acupuncture can effectively suppress the gag reflex for a large proportion (around

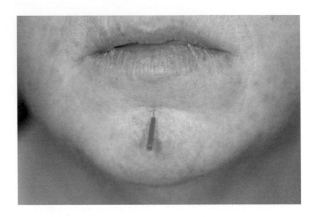

Figure 17.5
Point CV24 for control of gagging.

80 per cent) (Fiske & Dickenson, 2001; Rosted et al., 2006). The response to needling is usually quite rapid (within a few minutes) and facilitates impression-taking, improving the accuracy of impressions and reducing patient stress. Two primary sites are used for this, one on the chin (Figure 17.5), and one at the edge of the ear, and may be used together or independently – although the ear sites are always used bilaterally.

Planned combination therapies

In a proportion of cases, the planned combination of acupuncture with another therapy may enhance the effectiveness of both therapies; typically this is combining occlusal appliance therapy with acupuncture. There are a number of scenarios where this combination is helpful. In some, acupuncture is used as an initiating therapy, for controlling symptoms, while an occlusal appliance is being manufactured; the treatment can then be completed with appliance therapy. Alternatively acupuncture may be used in parallel with appliance therapy, and once symptoms are controlled, it may then be discontinued, relying on the appliance alone (or vice versa). Such an approach may be useful with joint clicking.

For those who show persistent nocturnal bruxism, acupuncture alone is unlikely to maintain control of symptoms with persistent relapses and in such cases appliance therapy at night to reduce bruxism will support the daytime acupuncture therapy. Other therapies such as physiotherapy may combine acupuncture with conventional approaches for symptom control and functional improvement.

In some cases, persistent bruxing that is unresponsive to conventional interventions is a core issue; this may lead to a situation where muscular pain is severe and intractable. While acupuncture may improve sleep patterns, and reduce psychological stress, acupuncture alone is unlikely to solve these symptoms as it cannot control the bruxing at night. In these circumstances, acupuncture may be an initial therapy to reduce symptomatology, which is then followed by botulinum toxin (Botox) treatment to the muscles of mastication – primarily the masseter, and lateral pterygoid. This will reduce the force of contraction by the muscles of mastication. Acupuncture may give a good indicator as to the likely effectiveness of botulinum toxin, and may help to isolate the most symptomatic areas of the muscles by identifying those sites that produce most effective pain control, allowing smaller doses to be used. While botulinum toxin treatment can be very effective in reducing symptoms, the effect will wear off, and the production of antibodies against the toxin progressively reduces effectiveness. Acupuncture may be employed at this point to extend the symptom control.

Psychological symptoms

For many patients, a substantial component of TMD lies in the psychological aspects of the condition. Increased stress and anxiety, as a result of environmental stressors, impact on the patient's tolerance and contribute to the parafunctional drive. Control of this aspect forms a significant component of the overall management plan, and use of suitable psychological interventions is appropriate for many.

Disturbed sleep patterns are a common component of increased psychological stress, and other mental health issues.

A frequently observed function of acupuncture is a sedative or relaxation effect. It is common to see patients becoming clearly relaxed and tired, and occasionally falling asleep in the dental chair! This is probably related to enhanced release of endorphins and serotonin in the central nervous system, leading to the observed relaxation, in addition to increased pain thresholds. The effect may be harnessed to enhance the effect of the primary treatments by

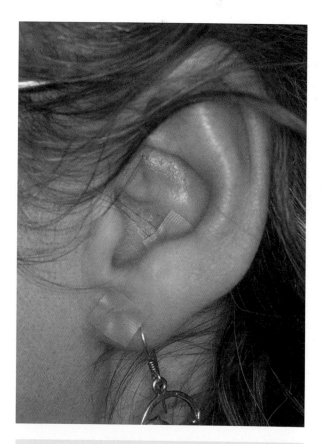

Figure 17.6
Indwelling ear needles for relaxation.

encouraging general relaxation, and thus potentially reducing the stress-related parafunctional drive as well as producing an overall reduction in muscular tone. Enhanced serotonin levels in the central nervous system (CNS) may also help to improve mood, and there is some evidence that acupuncture may be helpful with mild to moderate depression (Wang et al., 2016; MacPherson et al., 2017). Some patients comment that their overall feeling of well-being is improved following acupuncture, and sleep patterns are improved for a few days, probably as a response to increased serotonin levels in the CNS. With some, indwelling ear needles (Figure 17.6) may be placed for several days at a time to reduce the psychological drive to parafunction.

How is acupuncture used?

Acupuncture is relatively simple to use, and prescribing from a Western viewpoint is based upon the pain referral patterns and muscular tenderness. Rosted (2004), in a guide for dentists, has described a number of sites on the head and neck appropriate for use, but needle prescribing is related very much to clinical findings. Prescribing might be considered in stages (Table 17.1):

1. Identify the target muscle or organ, for example the masseter.

2. Identify the acupuncture sites to be treated in the muscle related to pain mapping.

3. Add additional points for specific additional effects, for example relaxation, improved sleep patterns, and increased pain thresholds.

The acupuncture sites are identified, and needles inserted by gentle pushing and twisting, generally at 90 degrees to the skin surface. The needles are inserted to the required depth, or when the patient reports a *deqi* sensation, then rotated clockwise and counterclockwise to stimulate the site. In cases where the primary issue is muscle pain, local needling to the muscles of the head and neck can provide analgesia via gating of pain, and reduced muscle ischemia by reducing muscle tension, switching off TrP sites and improving local blood flow. Needling is aimed toward the primary areas of symptom initiation, identified by examination, and typically these are the muscle attachment zones and any TrP within the muscle.

The sites most implicated are typically the origin and insertion areas of masseter (acupuncture points ST5, ST6, ST7), the body of the lateral pterygoid (ST7), and the anterior fibers of the temporalis (EX2) (Figure 17.7). An additional muscular TrP may also present in the central area of the body of the masseter, which is normally very responsive to needle therapy. Any TrP zone may be treated with acupuncture.

Needling at these sites usually requires insertion of a 30 mm needle, but for the deeper lateral pterygoid

Table 17.1
Stages of prescribing.

TMD	Component of condition	Prescription
Area of body affected	Masseter	Acupuncture sites in masseter muscle ST5, ST6, ST7
Cause	Bruxing	GB2
Stress?	Yes	Relaxation GV20, EX6

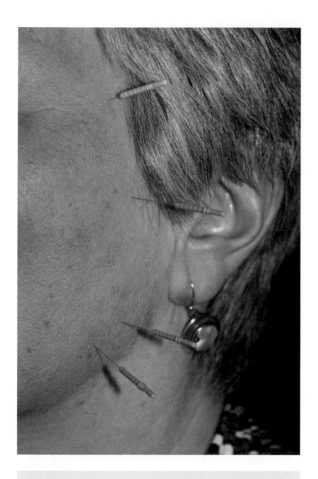

Figure 17.7
Needles in ST5, ST6, ST7, and EX2 (lower to upper) for temporomandibular pain.

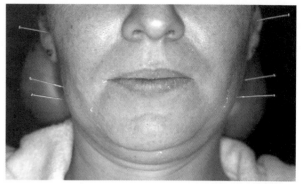

Figure 17.8
Bilateral needling for temporomandibular pain.

trigger points 40 or 50 mm may be needed as the technique requires deeper insertion to effectively pass through the masseter and mandibular notch to reach the muscle. In particularly troublesome sites, double needling (literally placing two needles into the same site) may be advantageous, and this is most noticeable at ST6 (insertion of masseter) and ST7 (origin of masseter).

At sites where the muscles are particularly irritated and painful, needling can be painful and sometimes the site EX2 in the temporalis muscle may be too sore to actually insert a needle. This is managed by use of other local points to desensitize the site that is then treated at a later appointment.

Needling may be unilateral or bilateral, with a slight preponderance for bilateral. However, the sites chosen depend upon the site activity or response to examination, and thus needling may be asymmetrical. Ironically, as the painful areas within the muscles of mastication are fairly consistently troublesome, the prescription is commonly very similar for most patients. From a lateral perspective, the needles often seem to line up in a vertical orientation, and sometimes are placed symmetrically, but this is chance, not design (Figure 17.8). A deeper dry needling approach for the lateral pterygoid muscle is described in Chapter 16.

Examination of the muscles may reveal other sites that are implicated, such as:

- The posterior body of the temporalis muscle (GB8), which is commonly associated with headache.

- The upper attachment of the temporalis muscle (ST8), which is less commonly implicated, but can be useful as an alternative to other temporalis sites.

- Sites within the trapezius muscle that refer to the head and neck.

- Sites within the sternocleidomastoid muscle that refer to the head and face.

In most cases, these represent the formation and activation of muscular TrPs, and in such cases acupuncture should be directed to these sites. This is very prominent in the posterior body of the temporalis (GB8), where the increased bulk of the TrP is easily palpable against the lateral aspect of the skull. The upper portion of the trapezii refers to the occipital and temporal regions, as well as to the angle of the mandible, and is often related to postural issues within the overall diagnostic picture (see Chapter 8). Use of computers is often implicated, but other causes such as whiplash following a traffic collision, or as a response to the psychological trauma, may well initiate or exacerbate TrPs, the event acting as an initiator of bruxism and TMD. Needling to these points will require access to the shoulder and neck, and patients will need to wear appropriate clothing to allow this. Care must be taken to avoid needling toward the lung between the upper ribs. Again treatment in this region may be combined with other physical therapies.

Global pain

Pain centered in the muscles of the head, neck, and shoulder may occur as part of a global pain picture of which TMD is a component. In such cases acupuncture may be a primary therapy to control symptoms of facial pain, but for a significant number of patients physiotherapy is an essential part of the management plan in order to establish effective overall control of the origin of pain in the cervical muscles. In such cases it is necessary to identify the differing aspects of the condition, and direct therapies accordingly; this is sometimes likened to 'peeling the layers of an onion.' Such pain pictures are complex, and may be presenting as part of a wider condition. Amongst these is fibromyalgia, which may present in a localized variant mimicking TMD, but in such cases examination typically shows the entire body of the muscles of mastication are tender, as opposed to the more normal TrP zones, along with muscles that should not normally be affected as part of TMD, such as the buccinator, and the orbicularis oris. Acupuncture may be helpful in some cases for temporary symptom control, but relapse is almost inevitable, and in general such cases are better and properly managed with a multidisciplinary biopsychosocial approach.

Remote acupuncture points

Acupuncture prescribing broadly breaks down to the use of sites local to the problem area, or specific sites more distant termed 'distal points.' Traditional texts describe a number of these, on the limbs, but two stand out as being most important and effective: Large Intestine 4 (LI4) (*hegu*) and Liver 3 (LR3) (*taichong*). Both sites are widely used in acupuncture prescriptions, and form an underpinning component to enhance the use of local points. LI4 lies on the hand, in the first dorsal interosseous muscle, and is easily found by palpation of the web space between the thumb and index finger (Figure 17.9). Needling at this site can be quite uncomfortable, but very effective at increasing overall pain thresholds, along with

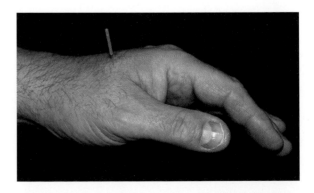

Figure 17.9
Point Large Intestine 4 (LI4).

enhancing other aspects of acupuncture treatments, and amongst other uses may improve pain control following third molar extraction (Lao et al., 1999). The site is easy to access, easy to use, and quite acceptable to patients.

Liver 3 (LR3) lies on the foot in the first dorsal interosseous muscle and may be considered as effectively the corresponding lower limb point LI4. It is also acceptable to patients, but can be quite uncomfortable and sometimes frankly painful. Needling of this site may be challenging to dentists, as it is not on the head, but this is simply a matter of familiarity, and the understanding of the role of the site. Both sites have prominent arteries proximally, at the apex of the space where the metacarpal or metatarsal bones meet, so it is important to avoid angling your needle towards this junction.

The combination of the four sites, (bilateral use of LI4 and LR3) is sometimes called the 'four gates of pain' and can be a very powerful prescription for relief of pain, primarily for those areas supplied by spinal nerves. In the treatment of TMD, the bilateral use of LI4 is most commonly applied, but there is no reason that LR3 should not be used.

These sites seem to be clinically effective, although there may be no direct segmental connection to the origin of pain, such as in the masseter muscle. However, they produce a strong stimulus to the spinal cord, and probably thus impact upon the central nervous system, modifying pain response both peripherally via gating effect in the dorsal root horn, but also by initiating a heterotopic noxious conditioning response that modifies central perception. Gu et al. (2015) using MRI have, however, shown that the brain response to stimulus at LI4 overlaps that from point ST6, which lies in the masseter muscle. Thus stimulus to LI4 could well be expected to impact upon the masseter, and consequently TMD. This recent finding opens up a whole new view on the action and prescribing of acupuncture, and may give some credence and understanding to the therapy when considered in a more traditional format.

Ear acupuncture

An alternative and stand-alone approach is the use of ear acupuncture. This technique relies on the use of acupuncture points placed on the pinna of the ear only and may be used without any body points, but may also be combined with body points during treatment sessions.

The concepts of ear acupuncture are based upon a homunculus where all the points are identified within an abstract representation of the body on the structure of the pinna of the ear. This means that the sites relating to the head are largely centered on the lobe of the ear whereas sites relating to the spine follow along the antihelix and the central organs are clustered around the auditory meatus in the concha. Theoretical understanding of the mechanism of ear acupuncture is much more difficult; however, interestingly most of the central organ sites are supplied by the auditory branch of the vagus nerve and there may therefore be a logical explanation why these sites can be influenced to some extent with ear acupuncture. The remaining parts of the ear are supplied by the auriculotemporal branches of the trigeminal and the cervical nerves and it seems likely that these provide the gating stimulus to the remaining parts of the body and, in the case of TMD, particularly to the muscles of mastication.

Treatment with ear acupuncture is not dissimilar to conventional body acupuncture using small needles applied to the acupuncture points although identification of the points is in some cases more challenging as many lie in a small area and there are variations in site description depending upon the format of ear acupuncture used. The prescription is built up logically using the target organ, then outcome, and then additional effects, and may be quite successful. In Figure 17.10 the patient attended in pain from the right masseter muscle only, and left pain-free following 15 minutes of ear acupuncture.

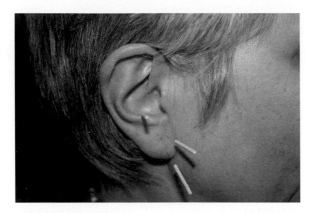

Figure 17.10
Ear needling for temporomandibular pain.

Needling of the ear is typically undertaken using both hands with one supporting the pinna of the ear and the other inserting the needle. Palpation of the ear with a ball burnisher, or the back of the needle handle can be very helpful in identifying tender point sites for needling. Ear acupuncture may be quite uncomfortable especially in the lobe. Physiological response in the lobe with a vigorous vasodilation is typical, and very common. Needles may be rotated intermittently to create adequate stimulus over the treatment session. In rare cases altered sensation may also be perceived in the oral cavity.

In addition, indwelling needles may be left in situ for several days to continue the acupuncture stimulus (Figure 17.6) and this can be applied both for pain relief, with functional improvement, and also for application to reduce anxiety and stress, and may be used prior to a dental appointment for anxious patients (Karst et al., 2007; Rosted et al., 2010; Machalek-Sauberer et al., 2012). This technique can then be translated into the longer term reduction in anxiety and psychological stress and, as a consequence, the same approach may be used to help reduce the drive to abnormal muscular activity in TMDs, using indwelling needles for several days following a

treatment session to enhance the outcome. Bizarrely, acupuncture can be more socially acceptable for some patients in contrast to appropriate psychological therapy such as counseling, cognitive behavioral therapy, or medication. It is important to avoid indwelling needles in patients with valvular heart disease, as there have been several cases of bacterial endocarditis resulting from their use in such patients.

Outcomes and complications

Acupuncture treatment sessions are generally at weekly intervals and last for somewhere around 10 to 20 minutes depending upon the practitioner. In theory, longer treatments should recruit more neurons to suppress pain, but in cases of TMD the deactivation of muscle TrPs may be more important and this deactivation can be achieved quite rapidly with acupuncture. Some practitioners favor multiple visits at two- to three-day intervals but there often seems to be little evidence to show the benefit of this. In some cases responses can be slow and repeating treatment too quickly may not be optimal.

Outcomes for acupuncture therapy can be quite dramatic and many patients may gain significant pain relief and functional improvement over a number of visits (Smith et al., 2007; Shen et al., 2009). Indeed it is common to find that pain is reduced by the time the patient leaves the clinic, and palpation clearly shows reduced tenderness in the masticatory muscles. Generally reported pain from patients using a visual analog scale will show a rapid reduction over the course of the first three or four visits. Although elimination of all symptoms is often impossible, adequate functional improvement and symptom control is satisfactory and patients are substantially more comfortable. This response is typical of acupuncture with musculoskeletal issues but relies upon the control of other aspects of the patient's condition, in particular the psychological axis of TMD (see Chapter 2). The environmental factors leading to the inception of parafunctional activity, and thus symptoms of TMD, are not controlled by acupuncture and therefore if these are not managed relapse will occur with a number of patients. This can be managed by retreatment following reconfirmation of the diagnosis, or alternatively with the provision of other therapies, such as an occlusal splint, as noted above, but long-term management of the psychological aspects should be investigated.

As noted previously, reviews have confirmed the effectiveness of acupuncture in the management of the symptoms of TMDs, both in the short term and long term, but in general report that outcomes are similar but not superior to other therapies (Fernández-Carnero et al., 2010; List & Axelsson, 2010).

Complications from acupuncture vary in significance, but are generally minor and consist of a little bruising. Acupuncture may be used for patients taking anticoagulants, but the risk of bleeding should be explained, and only a limited number of needles placed. Fainting is very occasionally seen and sedation is a common if temporary side effect. Rarely, temporary euphoria or disinhibited behavior may occur. This normally settles rapidly once the needles are removed.

More significant complications, such as incorrect needle placement with penetration of organs (from liver to lung), are uncommon but extensively reported and tend to be related to poorly trained practitioners.

Occasionally the patient may feel unwell following an acupuncture session – normally the first one. Some patients are considered 'strong reactors' and appear to be very sensitive to the effects of acupuncture. For some, the effect dissuades them from further treatments but with others treatment may be continued with significant reduction in the amount of stimulus. This introduces the concept of a 'dose' of acupuncture. The sensitivity of the strong reactor is managed by reducing the dose, and responses can then appear normal. This means reduction in the number of needles, and duration of the session. This might concur with the concept that a longer treatment session may be more effective. In order to reduce the chances of this idiosyncratic response, a small trial of acupuncture may be appropriate in the first treatment session.

Conclusion

The use of acupuncture, as with all treatments, relies upon the appropriate patient choice and information to provide a valid consent for this. However, the general minimal complications that occur from head and neck acupuncture mean that patients can be reassured as to both the efficacy and safety of the technique in managing TMDs, and it can be confidently recommended. The technique should be considered as a primary treatment option, rather than as a rescue option, and is well received by patients.

References

Baldry P. Acupuncture, Trigger Points and Musculoskeletal Pain. 3rd ed. London: Elsevier Churchill Livingstone; 2005.

Barão VA, Gallo AK, Zuim PR, Garcia AR, Assunção W. Effect of occlusal splint treatment on the temperature of different muscles in patients with TMD. J Prosthodont Res 2011; 55: 19–23.

Blom M, Lundeberg T, Dawidson I, Angmar-Månsson B. Effects on local blood flux of acupuncture stimulation used to treat xerostomia in patients suffering from Sjögren's syndrome. J Oral Rehabil 1993; 20: 541–548.

Cagnie B, Barbe T, De Ridder E et al. The influence of dry needling of the trapezius muscle on muscle blood flow and oxygenation. J Manipulative Physiol Ther 2012; 35: 685–691.

Fernández-Carnero J, La Touche R, Ortega-Santiago R et al. Short-term effects of dry needling of active myofascial trigger points in the masseter muscle in patients with temporomandibular disorders. J Orofac Pain 2010; 24: 106–112.

Fiske J, Dickenson C. The role of acupuncture in controlling the gagging reflex using a review of ten cases. Br Dent J 2001; 190: 611–613.

Gu W, Jiang W, He J, Liu S, Wang Z. Blockade of the brachial plexus abolishes activation of specific brain regions by electroacupuncture at LI4: a functional MRI study. Acupunct Med 2015; 33: 457–464.

Karst M, Winterhalter M, Münte S et al. Auricular acupuncture for dental anxiety: A randomized controlled trial. Anaesth Analg 2007; 104: 295–300.

Lao L, Bergman S, Hamilton GR, Langenberg P, Berman B. Evaluation of acupuncture for pain control after oral surgery: a placebo-controlled trial. Acta Otolaryngol Head Neck Surg 1999; 125: 567–572.

Li A, Li XL, Zhang F, Yue JH, Yuan CS, Li K, Zhang QH. A functional magnetic resonance imaging study of the neuronal specificity of an acupoint: acupuncture at Rangu (KI 2) and its sham point. Intern Med J 2016a; 46: 973–977.

Li AH, Zang JM, Xie YK. Human acupuncture points mapped in rats are associated excitable muscle/skin-nerve complexes with enriched nerve endings. Brain Res 2004; 1012: 154–159.

Li Z, Liu M, Lan L, Zeng F et al. Altered periaqueductal gray resting state functional connectivity in migraine and the modulation effect of treatment. Sci Rep 2016b; 6: 20298.

Linde K, Allais G, Brinkhaus B et al. Acupuncture for the prevention of tension-type headache. Cochrane Database Syst Rev 2016; 4: CD007587.

List T, Axelsson S. Management of TMD: evidence from systematic reviews and meta-analyses. J Oral Rehabil 2010; 37: 430–451.

Machalek-Sauberer A, Gusenleitner E, Gleiss A, Tepper G, Deusch E. Auricular acupuncture effectively reduces state anxiety before dental treatment: a randomised controlled trial. Clin Oral Investig 2012; 16: 1517–1522.

MacPherson H, Vickers A, Bland M et al. Acupuncture for Chronic Pain and Depression in Primary Care: A Programme of Research. Southampton, UK: NIHR Journals Library; 2017 Jan. Available: https://www.ncbi.nlm.nih.gov/books/NBK409491/ [Nov 21, 2017].

Melzack R, Wall PD. Pain mechanisms: a new theory. Science 1965; 150: 971–979.

Napadow V, Dhond R, Park K et al. Time-variant fMRI activity in the brainstem and higher structures in response to acupuncture. Neuroimage 2009; 47: 289–301.

Napadow V, Kettner NW, Harris RE. Neuroimaging: a window into human brain mechanisms supporting acupuncture effects. In Filshie J, White A, Cummings M (eds). Medical Acupuncture: A Western Scientific Approach. London: Elsevier; 2016, pp. 59–72.

Rosted P. Practical recommendations for the use of acupuncture in the treatment of temporomandibular disorders based on the outcome of published controlled studies. Oral Dis 2001; 7: 109–115.

Rosted P. Acupuncture for Dentists: 10 Central Treatments. Klim; 2004.

Rosted P, Bundgaard M, Fiske J, Pendersen AM. The use of acupuncture in controlling the gag reflex in patients requiring an upper alginate impression: an audit. Br Dent J 2006; 201: 721–725.

Rosted P, Bundgaard M, Gordon S, Pendersen AM. Acupuncture in the management of anxiety related to dental treatment: a case series. Acupunct Med 2010; 28: 3–5.

Sandberg M, Larsson B, Lindberg L-G et al. Different patterns of blood flow response in the trapezius muscle following needle stimulation (acupuncture) between healthy subjects and patients with fibromyalgia and work-related trapezius myalgia. Eur J Pain 2005; 9: 497–510.

Shen YF, Younger J, Goddard G, Mackey S. Randomized clinical trial of acupuncture for myofascial pain of the jaw muscles. J Orofac Pain 2009; 23: 353–359.

Simons DG, Travell JG, Simons LS. Travell and Simons' Myofascial Pain and Dysfunction: The Trigger Point Manual. Vol. 1: Upper Half of Body. 2nd ed. Baltimore: Lippincott Williams and Wilkins; 1999.

Smith P, Mosscrop D, Davies S, Sloan P, Al-Ani Z. The efficacy of acupuncture in the treatment of temporomandibular joint myofascial pain: a randomised controlled trial. J Dent 2007; 35: 259–267.

Yaksh TL. Direct evidence that spinal serotonin and noradrenaline terminals mediate the spinal antinociceptive effects of morphine in the periaqueductal grey. Brain Res 1979; 160: 180–185.

Yeo S, Rosen B, Bosch P, Noort MV, Lim S. Gender differences in the neural response to acupuncture: clinical implications. Acupunct Med 2016; 34: 364–372.

Wang X, Wang Z, Liu J et al. Repeated acupuncture treatments modulate amygdala resting state functional connectivity of depressive patients. Neuroimage Clin 2016; 12: 746–752.

Chapter 18

Treating the brain in temporomandibular disorders

Harry von Piekartz, Emilio (Louie) Puentedura, Adriaan Louw

Comorbidities associated with orofacial pain

There is evidence demonstrating that the presentation of chronic pain conditions such as low back pain, headache, and orofacial pain share common characteristics (De Leeuw & Klasser, 2013). Pain localization in these conditions often exhibits spreading pain into other areas. Orofacial pain has clear covariate factors (estimated at > 60 per cent) of physical symptoms of other pain disorders and comorbidities in the musculoskeletal system such as arm, low back, hip, and knee pain (Bonato et al., 2017; Turp et al., 1998). This suggests that pain in the face, which has been present for a while, tends to centrally sensitize rapidly.

Furthermore, multistructural somatosensory alterations and changes in the affective and cognitive status may occur. Like any other kind of chronic pain, chronic facial pain may have biological and nonbiological triggers (see Chapter 1). There is evidence supporting the contribution from particular hormonal, psychological and emotional factors, which may be drivers for chronification of facial pain (Svensson & Graven-Nielsen, 2001; Wright, 2000). The duration of face pain (Tjakkes et al., 2010) and nonbiological (psycho-social-emotional) factors seem to be strongly associated with impairments in quality of life in almost 10 per cent of affected patients over the age of 18 (LeResche, 1997). Long-term minor temporomandibular disorders (TMDs) and pain during eating of hard food, chewing, and yawning appear to be associated with mild to moderate depression (Yap et al., 2002). In addition, threat and catastrophizing anxiety disorders, changes in self-efficacy, and sleep disturbance seem to be associated with long-term orofacial pain (Lei et al., 2015; Turner et al., 2005; Turner & Dworkin, 2004).

Somatosensory distortions in patients with temporomandibular disorders

Non-verbal communication changes

One great difference with other body regions is the fact that our face is important for social interaction and interpersonal communication (Ekman, 2007). In some qualitative research studies, it has been shown that patients with orofacial pain have interpersonal communication disturbances. They experienced their pain to be all-embracing, elusive, and difficult to communicate. They lacked words to illustrate their pain and suffering. Even in questionnaires that contained a variety of pain descriptions, the participants found it hard to communicate their pain (Wolf et al., 2008). They felt isolated and showed reduced participation in social life. Dissatisfaction with health care personnel, who provided inadequate information about effective treatments, and difficulties in communicating with care providers are described by the patients themselves (Mohr et al., 2011). Could these communication difficulties be associated with disruption in facial emotion and expression recognition?

Reduced facial expression recognition is a general feature of somatoform disorders (Pedrosa Gil et al., 2009). As an example, Haas et al. (2013) reported that patients with long-term TMD displayed alexithymia (a lack of emotional expression and recognition) and that alexithymic and somatization scores were correlated with deficits in facial expression recognition. This mechanism may even lead to facial dysmorphic disorders (dysfunctional body image, in this case of the person's face) (Buhlmann et al., 2013) or prosopagnosia (a severe deficit in recognizing familiar people from their face) (Chatterjee & Nakayama, 2012). People with orofacial pain take longer than healthy controls to recognize emotions in others. Furthermore, they

Chapter 18

mistake emotions like disgust with fear, and anger with surprise (Haas et al., 2013; von Piekartz & Mohr 2014). Also in left/right facial posture judgment tasks, a person with chronic orofacial pain is less accurate and needs more time compared to healthy controls. There is a strong correlation between the quality (accuracy and speed) of left/right recognition and emotion recognition (von Piekartz & Mohr, 2014). This supports the hypothesis that difficulty in recognizing someone else's emotion from a facial expression reflects deficits in cortical motor processing, rather than cortical emotion processing.

From anecdotal evidence, it is known that patients may perceive pain in the face as 'big or small,' 'asymmetric,' or 'swollen.' Of a mixed group of patients with chronic orofacial pain, such as post-traumatic trigeminal neuropathy, TMD, and persistent idiopathic facial pain, more than 55 per cent reported perceptual distortions of the face (Dagsdottir et al., 2016).

Body image disruption

Based on current evidence, it can be assumed that the neural networks in the premotor cortex, which are necessary for a physiological body schema and for normal function of a body part, are altered in individuals with TMD (Moseley et al., 2012). It is conceivable that neurons of the sensory (S1) and motor (M1) cortex representing the part of the face will be sensitized and disinhibited by pain. This means that neurons will have a higher excitability and be disinhibited even in the surrounding neurotags (Kessler et al., 2007). The clinical consequences are new pain and a changed recognition of the shape and size of the area representing the face – so-called 'smudging' (Moseley et al., 2012). This was investigated with respect to different body regions including the face (Vallence et al., 2013). For example, patients can recognize the affected side as larger or blurred. In the facial region, this could result in a distortion or rigidity of one's own mimicry (Ross et al., 2017). As a consequence, it can affect tactile acuity, the motor control of orofacial–neck activities, and also facial expression. Later, the ability to recognize emotions may change, which may result in pathologies such as alexithymia and prosopagnosia.

Tactile acuity

Accordingly, tactile perception (changes of tactile acuity) seems to be strongly correlated with body image disruptions (MacIver et al., 2008). This is clinically expressed by a change in the two-point discrimination (2PTD) threshold in the affected region (Haggard et al., 2003). In addition, correlations between tactile discrimination and cortical representation in the somatosensory cortex have been identified, showing changes in representation in the sensory homunculus in persistent pain (Wand et al., 2010). A study showed the reference values on a sample of 100 healthy subjects. Vriens and van der Glas (2009) found 2PTD values of 13.1 ± 1.9 mm for the cheek, 6.3 ± 1.4 mm for the upper lip, 5.8 ± 1.5 mm for the lower lip and 8.4 ± 1.9 mm for the mental region. In an unpublished study, there is a significant difference in 2PTD associated with chronic orofacial pain in all described regions from Vriens & van der Glas (2009). A significant difference between left/right discrimination in chronic unilateral head and face pain was also found (Weisbrich et al., 2017).

Motor control

Some research has focused on understanding how pain affects orofacial and neck motor control in the presence of chronic pain (Falla et al., 2004a; Falla et al., 2004b). Specifically, patients with chronic TMD and pain show less accurate recruitment of the masticatory musculature during chewing causing occlusal balancing side interference (Eberhard et al., 2014) and more uncontrolled head movement during mouth opening and chewing (Wiesinger et al., 2013). von Piekartz et al. (2017) found that a battery of eight orofacial and neck motor control tests could differentiate between healthy subjects and subjects with long-term orofacial pain, which may be explained by neuromatrix changes of the (pre)motor cortex neurons.

It may be summarized that persistent orofacial pain is not standing alone, but has a variety of comorbidities (see previous chapters in this textbook). For example, clear cognitive and affective changes may accompany the pain state, which may be expressed as pain threat, catastrophizing, and changes in self-efficacy, sleep disturbances, depression, and cortical tactile, sensory and motor processing disruption. All these factors may be associated with (verbal) communication changes expressed as, for example alexithymia, dysmorphic disorders, and prosopagnosia. These are likely to disturb the individual quality of life (Visscher et al., 2016).

Pain neuroscience education for orofacial pain

It is well established that the various peripheral processes associated with tissue injury and disease states (chemical, thermal and mechanical factors) stimulate nociceptors, and nociceptive information is sent to the brain for processing (Moseley, 2007; Nijs et al., 2013). When faced with threatening information, the brain processes and interprets the threat level via a distributed neuronal network referred to as the pain neuromatrix (Melzack, 2001; Moseley, 2003a). Pain is produced by the brain (Moseley, 2007). Pain is an output, a decision, of the brain, based on the end result of the pain neuromatrix and its interaction with the various neighboring maps, influenced by various biological and psychosocial factors (Puentedura & Louw, 2012). A key element, however, is the concept of threat, especially for patients struggling with orofacial pain. Traditionally threats come in the form of injury, disease or surgery, with the end result of pain, but threats also come from a variety of non-nociceptive-based issues, including altered neuroplasticity, psychosocial factors, etc. (Flor, 2000; Vlaeyen & Linton, 2000). Given the various unique issues patients with orofacial pain struggle with (body image, facial recognition, verbal and nonverbal communication, and left/right discrimination), it could be argued that these patients live with various threats which set them up for a pain experience, even in the absence of a nociceptive event.

This definition of pain, as being an output of the brain based on perception of threat, is of key importance when considering treatments. If pain is produced by the brain based on the perception of threat, then lowering or eliminating threats can have potential therapeutic effects (Gifford, 2014; Moseley, 2007; Gifford, 1998). Lowering threat can be accomplished via a variety of pharmacological and therapeutic treatments. One potential avenue is patient education. In recent years, a new pain-centered educational approach has been designed by physical therapists to alter a person's pain experience, especially for people struggling with chronic pain. This type of education is referred to as pain neuroscience education (PNE) (Louw et al., 2016c; Nijs et al., 2011). In traditional physical therapy educational models, patients are often educated via a biomedical model of their underlying pain experience, which is based on anatomy, pathoanatomy and biomechanical reasons for their pain (Greene et al., 2005; Nijs et al., 2013). Research has shown that patient education using these biomedical models does not only fall short in helping to relieve pain and disability but may in fact induce fear, which increases a pain experience (Louw et al., 2017; Vlaeyen & Linton, 2000). This is especially true for chronic pain. By contrast, PNE focuses on teaching patients more about the underlying neurobiological and neurophysiological processes associated with their pain experience (Moseley et al., 2004; Nijs et al., 2011). It is well established that chronic pain includes complex neurobiological processes such as increased vigilance of the central and peripheral nervous systems (central sensitization, hyperalgesia and allodynia), structural and functional changes in the brain (pain neuromatrix and smudging), and altered immune and endocrine function (cytokine and glial cell activation; cortisol and adrenaline changes) (Melzack, 2001; Moseley, 2007; Woolf, 2007). Patients in pain, especially chronic pain, have a deep desire to know what is going on with them biologically (Louw et al., 2009), and what is truly remarkable is that patients can be properly taught these complex biological processes (Louw et al., 2016b; Moseley, 2003b).

To date, research surrounding PNE has focused on musculoskeletal pain including chronic low back pain, whiplash-associated disorders, fibromyalgia, and chronic fatigue syndrome (Louw et al., 2011; 2016c). Current best evidence provides strong support that PNE positively influences pain ratings, dysfunctions, fear–avoidance, pain catastrophizing, limitations in movement, pain knowledge, and health care utilization in patients struggling with chronic musculoskeletal pain (Louw et al., 2011; 2016c). To date, no specific studies have been conducted on the use of PNE for orofacial pain, but given the common underlying biological processes in the various conditions favorable to PNE, PNE must be considered in the treatment of orofacial pain. If orofacial pain is viewed as a true chronic musculoskeletal issue, the evidence suggests therapists should explore the use of PNE in a multimodal treatment plan for orofacial pain (Louw et al., 2011; 2016c). If, however, orofacial pain is viewed as a neuropathic or idiopathic condition, it can also be argued that PNE should be a clinical consideration. Specific to neuropathic pain, PNE has recently been applied to lumbar radiculopathy (Louw et al., 2014) and also complex regional pain syndrome (Fercho et al., 2017 [submitted for publication]), showcasing similar results as seen in chronic musculoskeletal pain. Aside from the biological plausibility for the use of PNE, the patient also needs to understand why PNE should be considered for orofacial pain. Various qualitative studies have shown that a fundamental question that clinicians must answer for patients is: 'what is wrong with me?' (Gifford, 2014). This basic human inquiry may seem benign but from the perspective of the sufferer seeking help from a health care provider it is a critical initial step in the treatment process. In clinical practice guidelines it is stated that patients should be educated about the nature of their problem and this education should be closely linked to evidence of the biological nature of their problem (Kendall et al., 1997). This may be especially true for chronic pain, which involves complex underlying biological and neuroplastic processes. Additionally, it is important to realize that current pain science treatment for orofacial pain centers around graded motor imagery (GMI) (Moseley, 2006) and a fundamental starting point is patient education. It is inconceivable that advanced treatments such as laterality training, motor imagery, and mirror therapy, should be initiated without first providing the patient with a biologically plausible understanding of his or her problem as well as the intent of the GMI program.

The clinical question is now: How do we teach patients about the complexity of laterality, smudging, facial recognition issues, body image disruption, and so on? PNE is best delivered via one-on-one verbal education using pictures, drawings, metaphors and examples (Louw et al., 2011; 2016a; 2016c). If the current focus of pain science centers on structural and functional shifts in the brain, the PNE metaphor should aim to explain these phenomena and also the proposed plan of care to address the issues. In Appendix 18.1 a metaphor, supported by an image, is used to explain the structural changes in the brain specific to orofacial pain patients (Louw, 2014). This specific metaphor aims to explain neuroplasticity, the homunculus, neglect, smudging, issues with body recognition and GMI. In patients with chronic low back pain receiving manual therapy this metaphor has been shown to be superior to a more traditional biomechanical explanation. Furthermore, the same metaphor has recently been used in a study of complex regional pain syndrome, the results of which showed positive functional shifts in the pain neuromatrix (Fercho et al., 2017 [submitted for publication]).

The PNE metaphors and images used in Appendix 18.1 should allow a patient with orofacial pain to develop a biological understanding of their pain experience. More importantly, they set up the other interventions of the treatment plan. It is imperative to realize education alone is not necessarily sufficient for behavior change in chronic pain (Fordyce, 1987). The various structural and functional brain changes associated with orofacial pain demand tactile manual interventions in addition to PNE. The most recent systematic review of PNE has shown that PNE on its own is not as effective as when it is combined with some form of movement (exercise) or touch (manual therapy) (Louw et al., 2016c). For PNE to succeed, it is therefore imperative to set up the plan of care and explain the various stages of the GMI program. Clinically, as the patient is exposed to various opinions, setbacks, and flare-ups, the PNE message will likely need to be repeated, reinforced, clarified and added to (Louw et al., 2016a).

Treating the face using brain exercises: motor imagery and motor expression

Using the adaptable and changeable qualities of the brain, PNE together with systematic brain exercises may provide an opportunity to restore body image disruption, reduce pain, and improve motor function. There is some strong evidence, for example in chronic regional pain syndrome, that PNE together with systematic brain exercises such as GMI can strongly affect pain and increase activities (Daly & Bialocerkowski, 2009). There is little research available relating to patients with face pain. In a recent explorative mixed method study by Mohr et al. (2017) involving patients with chronic face pain, PNE, GMI, facial motor expression, and sensory retraining of the face were carried out for a training period of six weeks. Their findings demonstrated a clear reduction of pain and its related impairment, alexithymia, and the presence of depression. Together with the results of their interviews, it may be concluded that the therapy combination as mentioned above had a positive effect on pain sensation, increased self-managed pain control and function in subjects with a chronic facial pain state (Mohr et al., 2017).

There are numerous possibilities to apply brain training in the face and head region such as graded motor imagery (implicit, explicit), left/right judgments (laterality retraining), mirror therapy and sensory retraining (motor control and tactile acuity exercises) (Moseley et al., 2012; von Piekartz & Mohr, 2014). Because the quality of left/right discrimination and emotion recognition are strongly related, our focus here will be on motor rehabilitation, motor imagery (MI), and motor expression (ME).

Motor imagery, that is, mental representation of movement without any body movement, has its roots in behavioral and sport rehabilitation research from the end of the twentieth century (Annett, 1995a, 1995b; Dickstein & Deutsch, 2007). The growth of its evidence in sports has expanded to its application in neurological therapy, as for example in Parkinson's disease and post-stroke rehabilitation (Bowering et al., 2013; Schuster et al., 2009; Sharma et al., 2006). It has also been successfully applied in musculoskeletal dysfunctions and pain management of chronic low back pain, neck–arm pain, and foot–leg pain after amputation (MacIver et al., 2008; Schwoebel et al., 2002; Wallwork et al., 2013). Moseley has demonstrated that in chronic regional pain syndrome, the sequence of use, first, of implicit MI (left/right discrimination), then explicit MI (imagined movements) and, at the end, mirroring has better outcomes than other sequences (Moseley, 2004).

This strategy of rehabilitation may also be implemented in patients with face pain by the application of implicit, then explicit facial mimicry training, facial motor expression (real movement or ME) such as isolated muscle chain exercises classified as upper/middle/lower exercises and left/right side exercises. Further, use of the different basic emotions: happiness, sadness, surprise, anger, disgust, and fear, are also appropriate. Mirroring from the unaffected side to the affected side and vice versa, the upper face to the lower face and vice versa.

Normative values for face laterality are: accuracy $>90\%\pm7$, speed of 2.5 seconds ±0.7 and for emotion recognition accuracy $>68\%\pm9$, speed 3.59 seconds ± 0.79 (Grashoff & Klos, 2014). The authors strongly advise starting with mirror therapy in chronic face-pain patients only, when the left/right recognition accuracy and time are almost equal. Clinical experience suggests that implementing mirroring too early on the unaffected side of the face and switching to the affected side may predispose the patient to affective and cognitive dysfunctions and may result in adverse effects. Also, dysynchiria (looking to the virtual part of the face in the mirror and experiencing pain or dysesthesia in the hidden, affected face part) might be an observed phenomenon (Kramer et al., 2008). The advantages of face mirror therapy are: integration of visual motor control exercises (ME) (Figure 18.1) and sensory retraining such as tactile acuity via 2PTD, precise localization, size of touch, sharp versus blunt, and graphesthesia (von Piekartz & Mohr, 2014; Won and Collins, 2012).

Brain exercises as described above have to be performed on a regular basis. They have to be easy to integrate into clinical practice and daily life. Therefore, there are a lot of variations of different applications. Below is an overview of the currently available tools which are reasonably priced.

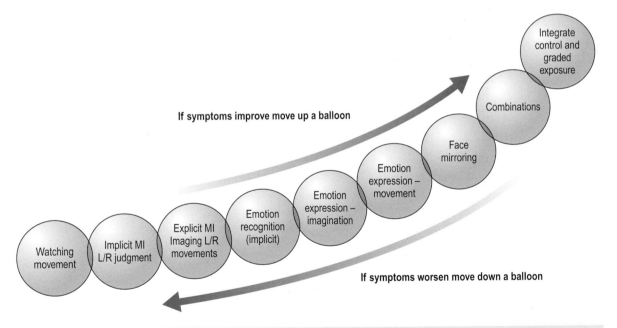

Figure 18.1

An overview of a possible rehabilitation program where face training is integrated. The balloons have an overlap which means that different therapy strategies can be combined by moving one balloon up or down. When symptoms improve and there is reduction in pain, increased motor function, and improved body image, the strategy may be progressed (made longer, with more variations and with the addition of new steps). If symptoms and function should worsen, reduce time, variations and start a step lower. If face mirroring is accepted by the patient, a combination of all strategies is recommended or integration with exercise within the patient's context or in combination with graded exposure. L, left; MI, motor imagery; R, right. (Modified with permission from Moseley et al., 2012.)

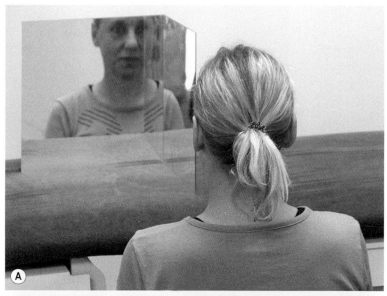

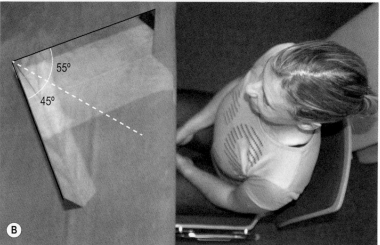

Figure 18.2
Mirror therapy showing the position of two mirrors (each measuring 30 cm by 30 cm) with an angle of 100 degrees towards each other. Patient is facing both mirrors whereby the mirror is rotated followed by a reflection in 55 degrees right and 45 degrees left.

1. Recognise™ Flash Cards, produced by NOI, comprise 24 left and 24 matching right images on dry-erase cards with a whiteboard marker for the hand, foot, knee, back, shoulder, and neck. These are an important tool in the management and rehabilitation of left/right discrimination (laterality) problems. They are useful for varying the challenge to the patient through speed, control over rotation of the images, making up games, and exploring the midline.

2. EmoRec-Cards (Emotion-Recognise-Cards, CRAFTA®) can be used for training the patient to recognize facial expressions and to identify the right and left side of the face. The square cards are printed on both sides. On one side, there is a drawing of a facial expression depicting one of the six basic emotions. The people depicted on these cards differ by age and ethnicity. On the other side, a person is depicted according to the principles

of the GMI program, moving either the right or the left side of the face.

3. Magazines or books are also suitable for assessment and training of laterality recognition. Images of the problematic area, for example hand or face, are selected for laterality recognition and/or emotion recognition. Turning the magazine toward the right, left, or upside down can increase the degree of difficulty. The patient is instructed to mark the appropriate side with a pen.

Digital cameras or smartphones are perfect tools to use to take left/right pictures of the body regions, including the face. Furthermore, these devices allow the recording of the emotions on the day or the different depths of emotions. They can also be used for imitating expressions of left/right and facial expressions.

4. e-health software supports controlling of (physical) health, and may also provide the ideal support for brain exercises.

5. Mirror therapy – this is relatively easy to use for the hand–arm and foot–leg and most clinicians are likely to have a mirror box in the clinic. Special mirror boxes are produced by NOI; they are portable and specially designed for the hand and foot. If you want to mirror the face you need two mirrors on a table. The setup for mirror therapy is shown in Figure 18.2.

6. CRAFTA® Face Mirroring software is advanced software that can be used on IOS or Android devices via the CRAFTA® facial recognition app. Specific isolated face muscle training is also available through this app (ME). The highlight of this program is its face mirroring function with a variety of options (Figure 18.3).

Conclusion

There is evidence to support that head and face pain changes brain functions, which may be expressed in psychoemotional and non-verbal communication

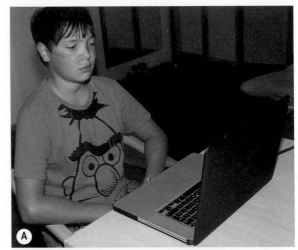

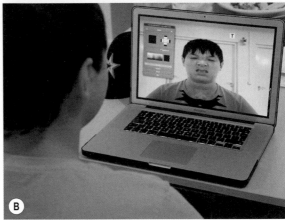

Figure 18.3
User-friendly software with mirroring function used by a male patient after a unilateral face trauma.

changes such as facial expression recognition, body disruption, for example changes in left/right recognition, loss of tactile acuity (two-point discrimination) and changes in fine tuning of orofacial motor control. Individual pain education plans derived from neuroscience (PNE) rather than from biomedical models have been proven to have a satisfactory outcome for patients with chronic musculoskeletal pain but are not well explored for orofacial pain conditions. Based on the evidence of the literature and clinical experience, PNE together with systematic face training by (graded) motor imagery and (graded) motor expression may be an adequate management strategy for the future in patients with TMDs.

References

Annett J. Imagery and motor processes. Br J Psychol 1995a; 86: 161–167.

Annett J. Motor imagery: perception or action? Neuropsychologia 1995b; 33: 1395–1417.

Bonato LL, Quinelato V, De Felipe Cordeiro PC, De Sousa EB, Tesch R, Casado PL. Association between temporomandibular disorders and pain in other regions of the body. J Oral Rehabil 2017; 44: 9–15.

Bowering KJ, O'Connell NE, Tabor A et al. The effects of graded motor imagery and its components on chronic pain: a systematic review and meta-analysis. J Pain 2013; 14: 3–13.

Buhlmann U, Winter A, Kathmann N. Emotion recognition in body dysmorphic disorder: application of the Reading the Mind in the Eyes Task. Body Image 2013; 10: 247–250.

Chatterjee G, Nakayama K. Normal facial age and gender perception in developmental prosopagnosia. Cogn Neuropsychol 2012; 29: 482–502.

Dagsdottir LK, Skyt I, Vase L, Baad-Hansen L, Castrillon E, Svensson P. Reports of perceptual distortion of the face are common in patients with different types of chronic oro-facial pain. J Oral Rehabil 2016; 43: 409–416.

Daly AE, Bialocerkowski AE. Does evidence support physiotherapy management of adult Complex Regional Pain Syndrome Type One? A systematic review. Eur J Pain 2009; 13: 339–353.

de Leeuw R, Klasser GD. Diagnosis and management of TMDs. In: de Leeuw R, Klasser GD (eds). Orofacial Pain: Guidelines for Assessment, Diagnosis, and Management. 5th ed. Chicago, IL: Quintessence Pub Co.; 2013; pp. 127–186.

Dickstein R, Deutsch JE. Motor imagery in physical therapist practice. Phys Ther 2007; 87: 942–953.

Eberhard L, Braun S, Wirth A, Schindler HJ, Hellmann D, Giannakopoulos NN. The effect of experimental balancing interferences on masticatory performance. J Oral Rehabil 2014; 41: 346–352.

Ekman P. Emotions Revealed: Recognizing faces and feelings to improve communication and emotional life (2nd ed.). London: Holt Paperbacks; 2007.

Falla D, Bilenkij G, Jull G. Patients with chronic neck pain demonstrate altered patterns of muscle activation during performance of a functional upper limb task. Spine 2004a; 29: 1436–1440.

Falla DL, Jull GA, Hodges PW. Patients with neck pain demonstrate reduced electromyographic activity of the deep cervical flexor muscles during performance of the craniocervical flexion test. Spine 2004b; 29: 2108–2114.

Fercho KA, Baugh LA, Louw A, Zimney K. Pain neuroscience education effect on pain matrix processing in an individual with complex regional pain syndrome: A single subject research design. 2017 [submitted for publication].

Flor H. The functional organization of the brain in chronic pain. Progress Brain Res 2000; 129: 313–322.

Fordyce WE. Learning processes in pain. In Sternbach RA (ed.) Psychology of Pain 2nd ed. New York: Raven Press; 1987.

Gifford L. Aches and Pain. Cornwall: Wordpress; 2014.

Gifford LS. Pain, the tissues and the nervous system. Physiotherapy 1998; 84: 27–33.

Grashoff M, Klos V. Reference values of facial lateralization and basic emotions and its clinical implementation in chronic facial pain from the CRAFTA Face Recognition Program. University of Applied Science, Osnabruck; 2014.

Greene DL, Appel AJ, Reinert SE, Palumbo MA. Lumbar disc herniation: evaluation of information on the internet. Spine 2005; 30: 826–829.

Haas J, Eichhammer P, Traue HC, Busch V. Alexithymic and somatisation scores in patients with temporomandibular pain disorder correlate with deficits in facial emotion recognition. J Oral Rehabil 2013; 40: 81–90.

Haggard P, Taylor-Clarke M, Kennett S. Tactile perception, cortical representation and the bodily self. Current Biol 2003; 13: R170–173.

Kendall NAS, Linton SJ, Main CJ. Guide to assessing psychosocial yellow flags in acute low back pain: risk factors for long term disability and work loss. Wellington: Accident Rehabilitation & Compensation Insurance Corporation of New Zealand and the National Health Committee; 1997.

Kessler H, Roth J, von Wietersheim J, Deighton RM, Traue HC. Emotion recognition patterns in patients with panic disorder. Depress Anxiety 2007; 24: 223–226.

Kramer HH, Seddigh S, Moseley GL, Birklein F. Dysynchiria is not a common feature of neuropathic pain. Eur J Pain 2008; 12: 128–131.

Lei J, Liu MQ, Yap AU, Fu KY. Sleep disturbance and psychologic distress: prevalence and risk indicators for temporomandibular disorders in a Chinese population. J Oral Facial Pain Headache 2015; 29: 24–30.

LeResche L. Epidemiology of temporomandibular disorders: implications for the investigation of etiologic factors. Crit Rev Oral Biol Med 1997; 8: 291–305.

Louw A. Why You Hurt: Therapeutic Neuroscience Education System. Minneapolis, MN: OPTP; 2014.

Louw A, Louw Q, Crous LCC. Preoperative education for lumbar surgery for radiculopathy. South African J Physiother 2009; 65: 3–8.

Louw A, Diener I, Butler DS, Puentedura EJ. The effect of neuroscience education on pain, disability, anxiety, and stress in chronic musculoskeletal pain. Arch Phys Med Rehabil 2011; 92: 2041–2056.

Louw A, Diener I, Landers MR, Puentedura E. Preoperative pain neuroscience education for lumbar radiculopathy: a multicenter randomized controlled trial with 1-year follow-up. Spine 2014; 39: 1449–1457.

Louw A, Zimney K, O'Hotto C, Hilton S. The clinical application of teaching people about pain. Physiother Theory Pract 2016a; 32: 385–395.

Louw A, Zimney K, Puentedura E. Retention of pain neuroscience knowledge: a multi-centre trial. New Zealand J Physiother 2016b; 44: 91–96.

Louw A, Zimney K, Puentedura EJ, Diener I. The efficacy of pain neuroscience education on musculoskeletal pain: a systematic review of the literature. Physiother Theory Pract 2016c; 32: 332–355.

Louw A, Zimney K, Johnson EA, Kraemer C, Fesler J, Burcham T. De-educate to re-educate: aging and low back pain. Aging Clin Exp Res 2017; 29: 1261–1269.

MacIver K, Lloyd DM, Kelly S, Roberts N, Nurmikko T. Phantom limb pain, cortical reorganization and the therapeutic effect of mental imagery. Brain 2008; 131: 2181–2191.

Melzack R. Pain and the neuromatrix in the brain. J Dental Education 2001; 65: 1378–1382.

Mohr DC, Young GJ, Meterko M, Stolzmann KL, White B. Job satisfaction of primary care team members and quality of care. Am J Med Qual 2011; 26: 18–25.

Mohr G, Moller D, Bochner R, Von Piekartz H. Does orofacial manual therapy and systematic brain training by graded motor imagery and facial expression affect pain perception in patients with chronic unilateral face pain? An explorative mixed-method study. Der Schmerz 2017 [accepted for publication].

Moseley GL. A pain neuromatrix approach to patients with chronic pain. Man Ther 2003a; 8: 130–140.

Moseley GL. Unravelling the barriers to reconceptualisation of the problem in chronic pain: the actual and perceived ability of patients and health professionals to understand the neurophysiology. J Pain 2003b; 4: 184–189.

Moseley GL. Graded motor imagery is effective for long-standing complex regional pain syndrome: a randomised controlled trial. Pain 2004; 108: 192–198.

Moseley GL. Graded motor imagery for pathologic pain. Neurology 2006; 67: 1–6.

Moseley GL. Reconceptualising pain acording to modern pain sciences. Phys Ther Rev 2007; 12: 169–178.

Moseley GL, Hodges PW, Nicholas MK. A randomized controlled trial of intensive neurophysiology education in chronic low back pain. Clin J Pain 2004; 20: 324–330.

Moseley GL, Butler DS, Beames TB, Giles TJ. The Graded Motor Imagery Handbook. Adelaide: Noigroup Publications; 2012.

Nijs J, Paul van Wilgen C, Van Oosterwijck J, van Ittersum M, Meeus M. How to explain central sensitization to patients with 'unexplained' chronic musculoskeletal pain: practice guidelines. Man Ther 2011; 16: 413–418.

Nijs J, Roussel N, Paul van Wilgen C, Koke A, Smeets R. Thinking beyond muscles and joints: therapists' and patients' attitudes and beliefs regarding chronic musculoskeletal pain are key to applying effective treatment. Man Ther 2013; 18: 96–102.

Pedrosa Gil F, Ridout N, Kessler H et al. Facial emotion recognition and alexithymia in adults with somatoform disorders. Depress Anxiety 2009; 26: E26–33.

Puentedura EJ, Louw AA. Neuroscience approach to managing athletes with low back pain. Phys Ther Sport 2012; 13: 123–133.

Ross GB, Sheahan PJ, Mahoney B, Gurd BJ, Hodges P, Graham R. Pain catastrophizing moderates changes in spinal control in response to noxiously induced low back pain. J Biomech 2017; 58: 64–70.

Schuster C, Butler J, Andrews B, Kischka U, Ettlin T. Comparison of embedded and added motor imagery training in patients after stroke: study protocol of a randomised controlled pilot trial using a mixed methods approach. Trials 2009; 10: 97.

Schwoebel J, Coslett HB, Bradt J, Friedman R, Dileo C. Pain and the body schema: effects of pain severity on mental representations of movement. Neurology 2002; 59: 775–777.

Sharma N, Pomeroy VM, Baron JC. Motor imagery: a backdoor to the motor system after stroke? Stroke 2006; 37: 1941–1952.

Svensson P, Graven-Nielsen T. Craniofacial muscle pain: review of mechanisms and clinical manifestations. J Orofac Pain 2001; 15: 117–145.

Tjakkes GH, Reinders JJ, Tenvergert EM, Stegenga B. TMD pain: the effect on health related quality of life and the influence of pain duration. Health Qual Life Outcomes 2010; 8: 46.

Turner JA, Dworkin SF. Screening for psychosocial risk factors in patients with chronic orofacial pain: recent advances. J Am Dental Assoc 2004; 135: 1119–1125.

Turner JA, Brister H, Huggins K, Mancl L, Aaron LA, Truelove EL. Catastrophizing is associated with clinical examination findings, activity interference, and health care use among patients with temporomandibular disorders. J Orofac Pain 2005; 19: 291–300.

Turp JC, Kowalski CJ, O'Leary N, Stohler CS. Pain maps from facial pain patients indicate a broad pain geography. J Dental Res 1998; 77: 1465–1472.

Vallence AM, Smith A, Tabor A, Rolan PE, Ridding M. Chronic tension-type headache is associated with impaired motor learning. Cephalalgia 2013; 33: 1048–1054.

Visscher CM, van Wesemael-Suijkerbuijk EA, Lobbezoo F. Is the experience of pain in patients with temporomandibular disorder associated with the presence of comorbidity? Eur J Oral Sci 2016; 124: 459–464.

Vlaeyen JW, Linton SJ. Fear-avoidance and its consequences in chronic musculoskeletal pain: a state of the art. Pain 2000; 85: 317–322.

von Piekartz H, Mohr G. Reduction of head and face pain by challenging lateralization and basic emotions: a proposal for future assessment and rehabilitation strategies. J Manual Manipulative Ther 2014; 22: 24–35.

von Piekartz H, Stotz E, Both A, Bahn G, Armijo-Olivo S, Ballenberger N. Psychometric

evaluation of a motor control test battery of the craniofacial region. J Oral Rehabil 2017; 44: 964–973.

Vriens J P, van der Glas HW. Extension of normal values on sensory function for facial areas using clinical tests on touch and two-point discrimination. Int J Oral Maxillofac Surg 2009; 38: 1154–1158.

Wallwork SB, Butler DS, Fulton I, Stewart H, Darmawan I, Moseley GL. Left/right neck rotation judgments are affected by age, gender, handedness and image rotation. Man Ther 2013; 18: 225–230.

Wand BM, Di Pietro F, George P, O'Connell NE. Tactile thresholds are preserved yet complex sensory function is impaired over the lumbar spine of chronic non-specific low back pain patients: a preliminary investigation. Physiotherapy 2010; 96: 317–323.

Weisbrich A, Hoffmann M, Von Piekartz H. Tactile discrimination of the skin in patients with unilateral chronic facial pain: a cross-sectional study. J Oral Maxillofac Surg 2017 [submitted for publication].

Wiesinger B, Haggman-Henrikson B, Hellstrom F, Wanman A. Experimental masseter muscle pain alters jaw-neck motor strategy. Eur J Pain 2013; 17: 995–1004.

Wolf JM, Tanaka JW, Klaiman C et al. Specific impairment of face-processing abilities in children with autism spectrum disorder using the Let's Face It! skills battery. Autism Res 2008; 1: 329–340.

Won AS, Collins T. Non-immersive, virtual reality mirror visual feedback for treatment of persistent idiopathic facial pain. Pain Med 2012; 13: 1257–1258.

Woolf CJ. Central sensitization: uncovering the relation between pain and plasticity. Anesthesiology 2007; 106: 864–867.

Wright EF. Referred craniofacial pain patterns in patients with temporomandibular disorder. J Am Dental Assoc 2000; 131: 1307–1315.

Yap AU, Tan KB, Chua EK, Tan HH. Depression and somatization in patients with temporomandibular disorders. J Prosthetic Dentistry 2002; 88: 479–484.

An example of pain neuroscience education applied to orofacial pain		
Story/metaphor	**Image**	**Rationale**
The therapist shows the patient a picture of a hand and asks: 'Is this a left hand or a right hand?' Another hand is shown and the therapist asks: 'How about this one? Is it left or right?' 'Close your eyes and touch your nose with your left index finger.'	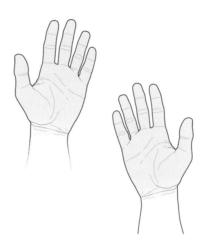	The identification of an unaffected body part is a simple, benign exercise. It engages the patient and draws them into an explanation of neuroplasticity. It is suggested a nonpainful body part is used as a means to stop the patient focusing on the painful body part. Taking vision away allows the patient to consider the question of how one recognizes body parts without seeing them.
Scientists have now shown us that there are areas in your brain that contain maps of the human body. If you look closely, the map has all the parts of the body. Some areas are larger than others. This map is present in all human beings. When life is good and we use body parts, the maps are sharp and crisp and when we show you a hand, you know it is a hand and also whether it is the left or right hand.	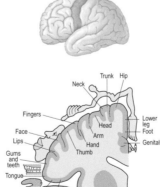	The homunculus is visually stimulating and draws in the patient. It is easy to recognize that there are alterations in the size of various body parts and this will open up further discussion. Showcasing the fact that body maps are plastic allows an early introduction to the ability of the patient's pain to improve. In line with motivational interviewing principles, normalizing this experience allows the patient to realize that he or she is not experiencing anything abnormal, which may ease fear.

Story/metaphor	Image	Rationale

To stay sharp and crisp, the maps need movement, touch, and exercise.

We now know that when body parts are not used, moved or touched, say due to pain, the maps are not exercised enough.

This can be due to pain, fear of pain, having to wear a cast, etc., and is a normal response.

When the body part is not used the map becomes 'smudged' or 'blurred.'

This 'smudging' occurs within a short space of time.

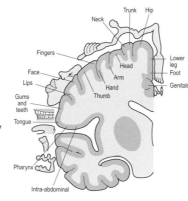

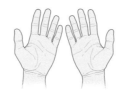

The importance of movement, use, and touch in keeping maps sharp is established.

Linking smudging to pain or fear of pain may help the patient to begin to understand why this happened to him. In a lot of cases people experience pain well after tissues should have healed and do not understand this. This provides a neuroplasticity explanation for the development of pain in the absence of injury, after tissues should have healed.

The fact that changes occur within a short space of time implies smudging can be changed/halted and that time is of the essence.

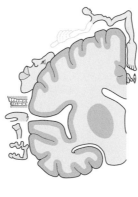

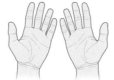

Appendix 18.1

Story/metaphor	Image	Rationale
If the map of a body part becomes smudged or blurred, it confuses the brain because the brain struggles to 'find' the body part. This is why people in pain struggle with distinguishing left from right, recognizing facial expressions and differentiating light touch from stronger pressure, etc. When the brain struggles to find body parts, it will produce pain in the area of the affected body part to protect you. The body's alarm system, the nervous system, typically 'buzzes' at a low level of activity, way below the threshold of the alarm. When threat is perceived the alarm is ramped up and set to 'extra sensitive' to protect you until more information is gathered.	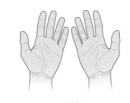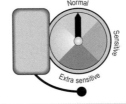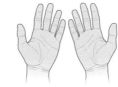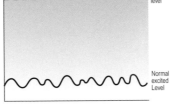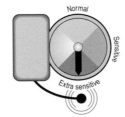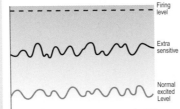	The link between altered plasticity and pain needs to be established. Depicting the nervous system as an alarm system provides a metaphor for central sensitization, hyperalgesia, and allodynia.

Story/metaphor	Image	Rationale
When the alarm system increases its sensitivity, it will have a big impact on your life. Before you experienced pain, you had 'a lot of room' to do many activities or to experience emotions. With the alarm set at extra sensitive, there is little room to do activities or be exposed to emotional events before the alarm goes off. This may make you think there is something seriously wrong, but this is not the case. Your nervous system has become extra sensitive in order to protect you, but this does not necessarily mean something is seriously wrong.		Being able to show patients how this biological process has affected their lives is critical. Patients often equate persistent pain to problems with their tissues. This part of the metaphor shows them how an extra-sensitive alarm system affects their life, with no direct implication of tissue problems. In a number of PNE studies this picture and the accompanying story is ranked as the most important conceptual shift that patients and clinicians can make.
As you are struggling to identify body parts, another interesting phenomenon occurs. In an attempt to find a specific body part (a face, for example) the brain starts knocking on many neighbors' doors asking if they have seen the face. The neighbors of the face are the jaw, hand, arm, and neck. The end result is the whole neighborhood is alerted and woken up. What started as face pain has now spread to neighboring areas and you may now experience face pain and also jaw, neck, arm, and hand pain. This is completely normal. It does not mean you have increased injuries.	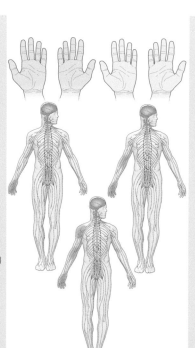	Patients often associate spreading pain with progressive and increased tissue damage. The 'nosy neighbor' metaphor explains spreading sensitization due to the nervous system (alarm system) being connected and spreading hyperalgesia and allodynia. Recognizing that spreading pain is normal and can be explained may additionally help allay fears.

Story/metaphor	Image	Rationale
If smudged and blurred body maps result in pain, the question you should ask us today in the clinic should be: 'How do we turn blurry or smudged body parts sharp and crisp again?'	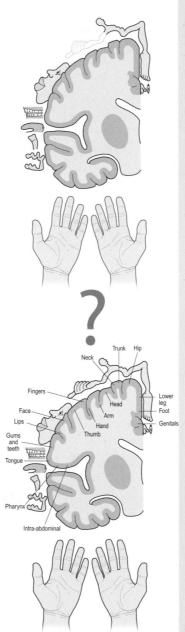	Ultimately, the PNE metaphor used should bring the patient back to the care plan, in this case specifically to graded motor imagery (GMI).

Story/metaphor	Image	Rationale
Movement! When body parts are used and exercised frequently, the body maps gain focus and become well defined. As you move the body part, you are exercising the body map. You are doing brain exercises! As the maps get sharper and sharper, pain decreases. Movement, touch, and exercise are essential for recovery. Therapy exercises may sometimes seem boring or silly, but it is crucial that you keep doing them to help remap the brain.	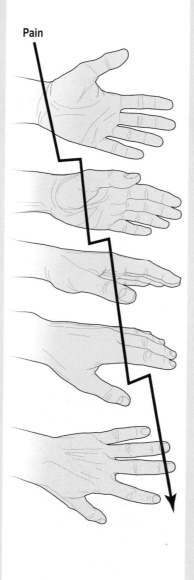 Pain	In physical therapy movement-based strategies are key to recovery. By linking movement and mapping and repeating the message the learning experience is reinforced. Adding touch allows patients to potentially reconceptualize hands-on treatments such as manual therapy.

Story/metaphor	Image	Rationale
What if movement or even the thought of movement makes your pain worse? There are now a series of brain exercises we can have you perform where the brain maps are exercised and strengthened, without you actually moving. For example, imaging movements, positions or tasks help exercise the maps, even without doing the actual movements. We are going to take you through a series of these brain exercises to sharpen the map, which will calm down the alarm system and ultimately your pain, allowing you to recover. As the alarm system calms, we can slowly over time increase regular movements, manual treatments, exercises, and daily tasks.	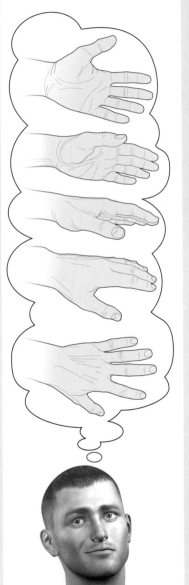	In many patients, movement or even the thought of movement is associated with fear and pain. GMI allows a series of virtual body exercises to occur in the absence of the actual movement. This explanation allows patients to ease their fear of having to move as they can go through a series of virtual exercises with no physical movement. It is important for patients to know that these exercises may in fact ease or even eliminate their pain, that they are not mainstream treatments, and that neuroplasticity changes occur via significant repetition.

Story/metaphor	Image	Rationale
What does this have to do with you and your face or face pain? The same process occurs in people struggling with pain anywhere in the body, including the face. With decreased movement and use the alarm system is ramped up by the brain. Once the alarm is set off in or around the face, it may trigger the neighboring alarm in the jaw, neck, and even shoulder.	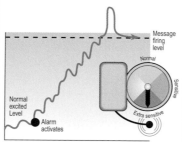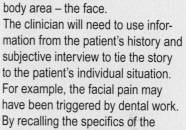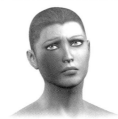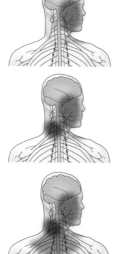	Once the initial concept is described via the hand (nonpainful part), then it should be applied to the affected body area – the face. The clinician will need to use information from the patient's history and subjective interview to tie the story to the patient's individual situation. For example, the facial pain may have been triggered by dental work. By recalling the specifics of the dental work and how it resulted in a sensitive alarm, the patient will see it is not 'just a nice story' but it pertains to him and his situation. Note: All figures in Appendix 18.1 are the copyright of Adriaan Louw and are redrawn with permission.

Appendix 18.1 continued

Chapter 19

Pain psychology, behavior, and the body

Richard Ohrbach, César Fernández-de-las-Peñas

Introduction

In this concluding chapter, we wish to provide an integrated perspective for the goals of this book – to describe various complementary types of treatments for TMDs – within the broader biopsychosocial context which is the currently dominant paradigm for understanding pain, ranging from acute to chronic. The epidemiology of TMD pain clearly highlights the importance of multiple risk determinants, including psychosocial factors, health status, and comorbid pain disorders, for TMD onset and, based on available evidence, for transition to pain chronicity. Current evidence strongly supports the central importance of this broad matrix of multiple risk determinants for muscle pain disorders; in contrast, far less is known about the factors that lead to clinically significant mechanical problems of the joint, exemplified by painful clicking and locking of the temporomandibular joints. While we presently understand little about etiologic mechanisms for TMJ mechanical problems, most of the mechanical problems and degenerative problems within the TMJ remain stable over a period of at least eight years (Schiffman et al., 2017). Mechanical problems are more challenging for both the patient and the clinician when pain is a strong accompanying symptom, which again links the above broad matrix of determinants to the difficult mechanical problems.

Pain and the understanding of the patient with pain, the complex mosaic of factors within which pain emerges and persists, and clinical decision making and integration of treatments targeting different levels of the body are the focus of this chapter. We wish to highlight that while each individual chapter in this book has focused on a given treatment appropriate to a particular conception of disease within the TMD rubric, current treatment models for chronic pain are pointing to the importance of treatments simultaneously targeting multiple levels of the person.

The nature of pain

Tissue damage is regarded as the proximal basis for activation of nociception, giving rise to either inflammatory or nociceptive pain (Woolf, 2004). The IASP definition of pain – an unpleasant sensory and emotional experience associated with actual or potential tissue damage, or described in terms of such damage (IASP, 2017) – highlights the importance of actual or putative tissue damage as a necessary basis for pain based on peripheral input within the somatic or visceral tissues of the body. Tissue damage may be initiated by disease or by injury, and whether the tissue damage is observable or potential is often unclear both clinically and by imaging, but other information (for example from the patient history) can often provide assurances regarding the probability of some type of tissue damage. When disease is suspected to be the cause of the reported pain, the disease must be identified; following identification, its treatment is primary for addressing the symptoms of pain. When the presence of the suspected disease is not confirmed, the clinical situation becomes more complex, and the clinician must maintain an index of suspicion regarding a latent disease not yet severe enough in its manifestation for detection but currently severe enough to produce symptoms (for example nociception and pain) and therefore must monitor the patient for disease progression such that it can be identified, must consider alternative hypotheses (that is differential diagnosis) for the symptom of pain, and meanwhile must also consider palliative treatments for the symptoms and avoiding the risk of doing harm to the patient. In addition, the clinician must also consider whether the pain, particularly if

Chapter 19

persistent, is of the type considered functional pain (Woolf, 2004), in that the direction of treatment will necessarily change.

Regional injury is also a cause of nociception and, like disease, it is also complex (Wall, 1979). Observable tissue damage does not necessarily correlate with extent of reported pain (Melzack, 1993; Melzack & Wall, 1965; Roelofs & Spinhoven, 2007). And injury may occur without observable tissue damage and yet produce pain. Moreover, observed tissue damage (accompanied by pain) may be followed by observed resolution of the tissue damage, yet with persistence of pain beyond the healing phase. If the pain persists beyond the time of usual healing, such pain is generally regarded as 'chronic' (IASP, 2017) though the full meaning of that term is increasingly questioned (Dunn et al., 2008; Von Korff & Dunn, 2008). Winding through these various scenarios of injury is a clear conundrum: while we are sure of the presence of injury when we can observe it (visually or with instruments), other situations exist, likely at equal if not greater incidence, where we cannot observe the presence of patient-reported injury. Because pain, as defined, is an 'unpleasant experience ... described in terms of such [tissue] damage,' the clinician is willing to make an inferential leap and assume that some type of tissue damage must have occurred, even if only at a micro level, if the description of the pain symptoms is '...in terms of such [tissue] damage.' Currently our best available evidence indicates that injury, while sufficient on its own to produce nociception, also contributes to pain disorder onset within a matrix of multiple risk determinants (Sharma et al. [in press]) and certainly persistence of pain after the initial period of healing appears to be a function of this same broad matrix of factors and not solely due to the prior injury. 'Healing' from an injury is a somewhat elusive concept. This uncertainty about whether 'healing' has truly occurred within the specified 'time of usual healing' is surely a fundamental assumption behind many physical treatments for the body, shown to be effective and as described in this book.

The relationship between pain and a proximal bodily cause has rumbled through the history of science (Melzack & Wall, 1965; Perry, 1993; Wordsworth, 2012), with medicine catching on later. When pain occurs without proximal bodily cause, the practice of medicine and the literature of medicine are filled with stories regarding clinical certainty, linked to clinicians' belief systems and specialty affiliations, of a particular physical cause surely responsible for the patient's pain. Such causes are then treated within that particular belief system, for example within the domain of TMD: stress alleviation by the psychologist, TMJ disc replacement by the surgeon, occlusion reshaping by the dentist or by the orthodontist, postural realignment by the physical therapist, and so on. Note that all of these example 'causes' could easily coexist in the same patient, yet attribution to cause of the symptoms has classically been filtered by the specialty window. When the putative cause has been more obscure, clinician certainty has assigned causation to any irregularity found in the body, fueled by the belief that surely that irregularity must be the cause. After all, the patient's pain is real. Therefore, when all such possibilities are pursued and exhausted but the patient still reports that the pain remains (and often, worse for all of the treatments), the exasperated clinician points to mental health problems as the cause. 'My treatment was perfect, so therefore you must be crazy' has been said by more than one clinician to a patient with pain persisting despite such treatments. And, the allegation of being crazy is merely window dressing for the clinician's belief that the pain is probably not so real.

This type of clinical situation is entirely avoidable at this stage in our understanding of pain. Abundant evidence indicates that pain is not tied to a peripheral stimulus but can be maintained by the brain (Melzack, 1993; Melzack, 1971), and consequently the evaluation of the body for physical cause requires simultaneous evaluation of the person for understanding the role of psychosocial factors and behaviors which are inextricably part of the fabric of pain.

Hence, the IASP definition: 'Pain is an unpleasant sensory and emotional experience …' The emotional aspect of pain experience is merely the experienced layer of multiple parallel processes (Apkarian et al., 2009). Therefore, the full spectrum of body and person must be considered in the evaluation, differential diagnosis, and direction of treatment. The individual with a painful intermittently locking TMJ, who is simultaneously embroiled in difficult life circumstances which coincide with symptom onset and progression, may not need direct treatment of the probable disc displacement, but rather needs direct treatment to the way in which life turmoil is translated into bodily reaction. The reported pain in this example patient is influenced by both tissue characteristics within the TMJ as well as by psychosocial processes, but perhaps the emotional turmoil and its psychophysiologic manifestations are the more important factors for a given patient.

The complex mosaic of risk determinants

The two major themes, historically, about TMD etiology have been structural factors (for example occlusion and TMJ disc position as the two most dominant) and psychological factors (for example stress and depression as perhaps the two most often used). Many studies on etiology have been conducted, but with few exceptions, for example (LeResche et al., 2007), most such research has been cross-sectional in design and more often using individuals with chronic TMD as the sample of individuals, by convenience. These study design elements have seriously limited the understanding of etiological factors. A comprehensive prospective study of the first onset of lifetime TMD – OPPERA (Orofacial Pain Prospective Evaluation and Risk Assessment) – has yielded particular insights (Bair et al., 2013; Slade et al., 2013b), indicating that a complex array of factors create vulnerability for the individual to develop TMD; these factors include gender, age, psychosocial status, health status, presence of other comorbid

pain disorders, alterations in pain processing, and characteristics associated with the masticatory system itself. These factors are referred to as risk determinants due to their probabilistic contribution to potential disease onset; 'etiology' and 'causation' are not appropriate concepts for these types of disorders (Rothman & Greenland, 2005).

This complex array of factors is perhaps best summarized as follows (Slade et al., 2016). The annual incidence of first-onset lifetime TMD is approximately 4 per cent (Slade et al., 2013a), but behind that statistic is a substantial extent of symptom flux, such that at any time, many individuals have TMD pain but at or below the threshold level suggestive of a disorder (Slade et al., 2013c); the implications of this symptom flux on the timing of pain disorder onset are enormous, intersecting with the below factors in their contribution to pain disorder onset. Gender does not significantly predict who will posteriorly develop TMD (Slade et al., 2013a), yet gender is substantially associated with individuals who transition to chronic pain and remain chronic. And, as is well known, females with chronic TMD are far more likely to pursue treatment (Drangsholt & LeResche, 1999). Somatic symptoms, of both the body and the facial region, are perhaps the most important psychosocial predictor of TMD incidence; this includes the presence of comorbid pain disorders (Fillingim et al., 2013; Sanders et al., 2013b). While regional pain sensitivity has been hypothesized to lead to pain disorder onset, the evidence suggests that development of the disorder precedes the development of regional pain sensitivity (Slade et al., 2014). Genetic associations with chronic TMD (Smith et al., 2011) are largely not observed as predictors of first-onset TMD but instead point to intermediate phenotypes (Smith et al., 2013); these intermittent phenotypes require more research to better understand what they represent. Yet, the COMT (catechol-O-methyltransferase) genotype modifies the effects of stress on pain sensitivity and on TMD incidence (Slade et al., 2015). Waking oral parafunction, assumed by many to cause TMD and to have good experimental and field evidence (Glaros, 2008; Glaros et al., 2016), is a potent predictor of first-onset TMD (Ohrbach et al., 2013). Interestingly, TMD onset is predicted by prior TMJ sounds and interference in TMJ functioning, but only as determined by self-report and not on the basis of examination-derived information (Ohrbach et al., 2013). Finally, disrupted sleep and sleep-disordered breathing worsen over time for those subjects who subsequently develop TMD (Sanders et al., 2016; Sanders et al., 2013a). Collectively, it is fair at this time to regard TMD as a complex disease. And, complex disease implies comprehensive treatment to address its many simultaneous levels.

The above list represents a complex array of findings, with some of them unique to the OPPERA study and many of them replicating and confirming the previously published findings of other smaller studies. The complex pattern of findings can be simplified, which is important for clinical application. A cluster-model approach selected the following variables (domains): mechanical, pressure, and heat parameters (QST); coping, personality, mood, stress, physical symptoms, anxiety, and depression (psychosocial); sleep quality and number of other conditions (health status); and number of body sites tender to palpation (clinical). This approach led to identification of three clusters of individuals at risk for developing TMD: adaptive, pain-sensitive, and global symptoms as the group with the most severe premorbid profile (Bair et al., 2016); this research is moving forward to develop a simpler set of variables to measure for cluster identification. These groups are similar in their hierarchic structure to previously identified clusters of adaptive copers, interpersonally distressed, and dysfunctional, based on a specific self-report questionnaire (Turk & Rudy, 1990).

Measures assessing the status of the body, either by self-report (for example, history of TMJ noise; bodily symptom counts) or by physical means (for example thermal QST, clinical palpation), rely at least on interoception if not also nociception for integration of the bodily state into the central nervous system representation of the body (Craig, 2002; Craig, 2003). Interoceptive signals represent powerful predictors of TMD onset and these same signals are part of a fear–avoidance process (Leeuw et al., 2007), wherein the individual either confronts pain initiated by, say, injury and recovers, or interprets the pain from a fear perspective and then becomes deconditioned through avoidance of functioning and also develops symptoms of depression which contribute to further pain amplification, thereby reinforcing a vicious cycle process of how an injury can heal yet pain can persist beyond the time of healing. Interoception, as a mechanism, and information to a patient (for example neuroscience education – see below) also provide insights into why behavioral change is an important part of how change in bodily process is centrally represented (Meulders & Vlaeyen, 2012). Behavioral change is simultaneously represented by change in movement patterns. Because peripheral treatments to the body not only alter the tissue but also potentially alter the interoceptive experience of that part of the body, peripheral treatments become an instrumental way to effect the desired behavioral changes which include how tissues are used. In this way, peripheral treatments can alter the trajectory of TMD as a complex disease, but the potential for peripheral treatments to effect change in behavior is greatly enhanced by additional treatments at other levels of the person.

Clinical decision making and integration of treatments

It seems clear that pain in individuals with a TMD is a complex process. Consequently, the current textbook provides many therapeutic management strategies according to different perspectives regarding sources of nociception, how nociception is maintained, and the role of behavior and mood. Current clinical and scientific evidence demonstrate that management of patients with TMD must be multimodal which usually requires the participation of several health care professionals, for example dentists, orthodontists, medical doctors, physical therapists, and/or psychologists, since each type of provider is limited to different components of treatment required by the biopsychosocial paradigm within the complexity of a disorder such as TMD. In fact, we suggest that the complementary therapies in this book be viewed as stepping stones to an eventual full set of therapeutic interventions within the framework of personalized medicine: tailoring the treatments for the patient's point of view. These treatments would include: specific passive and active strategies (as those shown in this textbook), active listening and empathy from the clinician, and proper addressing of the psychosocial issues (for example depression, anxiety, or catastrophizing), if needed, based on the clinical findings during the history and examination and the patient presentation. The promise and advantages of personalized medicine are, however, constrained by how we make clinical decisions and how evidence is used in tailoring a set of treatments for a given individual. Each component treatment must have some efficacy for some part of the complex disease process.

Patient-centered care involves shared decision making with mutual respect between clinicians and patients. Patient beliefs, therapeutic preferences, and expectations must be assessed by the clinician in order to understand the values of the particular patient since those values can condition the therapeutic process. Educating the patient about their complaint and the full scope of associated problems is an important part of compassionate care. That full scope includes addressing the disease mechanisms explained in lay person language (for example neuroscience pain education) as well as explaining the rationale for proposed treatments. In such scenarios, clinicians should consider potential neurophysiologic and cognitive mechanisms underlying the effects (positive and negative) of any intervention that they will apply on a particular individual. All physical treatments of conscious patients have cognitive

components; the most well-known is of course the placebo effect in which expectation (on the part of both patient and provider) plays a known and substantial role (Carvalho et al., 2016; Marchant, 2016; Story et al., 2016; Wager & Atlas, 2015). Addressing both neurophysiologic and cognitive mechanisms, putative though they may be, is particularly important in patients with chronic pain since it is helpful to encourage patients to choose among various treatment options after proper explanation of the benefits and risks of each therapeutic approach. Asking the patient to participate in clinical and therapeutic decision processes allows them to take responsibility for the management of their condition, which is highly relevant when the pain is chronic.

Therefore, the challenge facing clinicians is how to determine a particular treatment approach for a patient with TMD, as each patient is likely to be somewhat different in his or her individual clinical presentation and associated factors. For choosing a multimodal therapeutic approach, clinicians should determine if the clinical pattern of the patient has a peripheral input or central input dominance. If a clinician identifies that the pain in an individual with TMD seems to be mediated primarily by peripheral nociception, specific treatment of the affected tissue (the disc, the joint, or muscle), and application of exercises and functional activities should be encouraged. For instance, in a patient where the pain is mostly located in the teeth after a muscle overload, proper treatment of surrounding affected tissues can be crucial to prevent the development of chronic symptoms. In a patient with acute symptoms located around the TMJ after an injury, proper management of the joint and disc may be effective, noting that simple injury is probably less common than injury occurring in a more complex context of simultaneous multiple risk determinants (Sharma et al. [in press]). If a clinician identifies that the patient's TMD pain seems to be primarily mediated by alterations in central nociceptive processing, a multimodal pharmacological, physical and cognitive

Chapter 19

approach should be encouraged. In this situation, patients should be also educated in optimizing normal functional movements and undertaking active and specific exercises, in combination with proper complementary therapies.

TMD, as a field, has never had a shortage of proposed treatments. The field has had a shortage of evidence regarding the efficacy of those treatments, and that situation remains at the time of the publication of this chapter. The current approach to clinical treatment matching is largely one of a trial-and-error strategy of using one treatment at a time, with up to 50 per cent of individuals experiencing little to no benefit (List & Axelsson, 2010; Michelotti et al., 2004). Self-care strategies are often utilized, but typically one at a time, and their individual failure rate is high (Story et al., 2016). Patients give up, clinicians become discouraged, and treatment adherence is compromised (Merskey, 2012; Ohrbach & List, 2013; Velly & Fricton, 2011). Two reasons for this dismal situation are poor recognition that TMD is a complex disease (at least until recently) and most advocated treatments emerged from specialty or training bias, not from a sufficient understanding of pain physiology and psychology.

Systematic reviews are considered, within the Oxford hierarchy of evidence (Phillips et al., 2011), to be the highest form of evidence for development of clinical decisions, with individual randomized clinical trials (RCTs) providing evidence that has a lower level of confidence for its general applicability. Designing effective RCTs and implementing them is very challenging, and consequently the clinician is often working without adequate evidence for making clinical decisions about which treatment(s) to provide a given patient. A systematic review of 30 systematic reviews regarding treatments for TMDs indicates that most patients with TMD pain without behavioral or psychological involvement, benefit from simple treatments, whereas those patients with TMD pain and major behavioral or psychological disturbances

are in need of a combined therapeutic approach (List & Axelsson, 2010). The combined approach is, of course, where our clinical decision-making becomes very difficult, in that RCTs generally focus on only one treatment, not combinations of treatments, and for a given patient population that may or may not represent the patient in the consulting room. Consequently, RCTs often provide little assistance to the clinician, and systematic reviews provide insight into general patterns about treatments (as illustrated above). Even within these limitations, currently available information can inform us that assigning a given patient into a basic framework – for example, with versus without behavioral or psychological involvement, and acute versus chronic pain – helps clinicians better understand how to begin to tailor treatments. And, to understand that treatments with consistently negative outcomes (for example occlusal treatments [Fricton, 2006]) are to be avoided in favor of more useful and evidence-based models regarding what kind of treatment will be more likely to be helpful.

An important step for managing the chronic pain patient is the active participation of the patient in the therapeutic process. Many health care professions commonly apply passive approaches to the patient, but the patient must be actively integrated into the process. One of the most powerful strategies targeting both peripheral and central nociceptive pain processes is through self-care (Durham et al., 2016; Gatchel et al., 2006; Lorig & Holman, 2003). Patients must be educated that their involvement in their own treatment by way of integrating therapeutic exercise and other forms of self-care into their lifestyle patterns is essential, such that the new behaviors become habits. However, clinicians should be aware that individuals with central sensitization, such as those with TMD pain, can exhibit an abnormal pain response to exercise, and the potential response can be the opposite of what is intended and expected, leading to an aggravation of the symptoms. Therefore, continuous interaction between the clinicians and the patient, with repeat reassessment for symptom change, therapeutic engagement by the patient in terms of adherence, and titrating initial self-care treatments is crucial during treatment in order to maximize the tailoring of the interventions to a particular patient.

Conclusion

The epidemiology of TMD remains informative in this concluding paragraph for this book. Multiple risk determinants contribute, in various combinations, to the different stages of TMD pain: initial onset, transition to chronicity, and persistence. We know less about the putative etiology of TMJ conditions. Available evidence indicates that both peripheral and central factors, again in differing extents, contribute to the pain of most individuals with TMD. Better targeted treatments and, in particular, integration of treatments combine to form an essential next step to address the many factors involved in each individual patient. Treatment decisions need to emerge from comprehensive history, reliable examinations and other tests, and shared decision-making with the patient. This book describes a variety of treatments, each with compelling evidence for clinical consideration, and when integrated into a comprehensive treatment approach tailored to such findings, we believe that treatment outcomes for TMDs will improve.

References

Apkarian AV, Baliki MN, Geha PY. Towards a theory of chronic pain. Prog Neurobiol 2009; 87: 81–97.

Bair E, Brownstein NC, Ohrbach R et al. Study protocol, sample characteristics and loss-to-follow-up: the OPPERA prospective cohort study. J Pain 2013; 14: T2–19.

Bair E, Gaynor S, Slade GD et al. Identification of clusters of individuals relevant to temporomandibular disorders and other chronic pain conditions: The OPPERA Study. Pain 2016; 157: 1266–1278.

Carvalho C, Caetano JM, Cunha L, Rebouta P, Kaptchuk TJ, Kirsch I. Open-label placebo treatment in chronic low back pain: a randomized controlled trial. Pain 2016; 157: 2766–2772.

Craig AD. How do you feel? Interoception: the sense of the physiological condition of the body. Nat Rev Neurosci 2002; 3: 655–666.

Craig AD. A new view of pain as a homeostatic emotion. Trends Neurosci 2003; 26: 303–307.

Drangsholt M, LeResche L. Epidemiology of temporomandibular disorders. In: Crombie IK, Croft PR, Linton SJ, LeResche L,

Von Korff M, (eds). Epidemiology of Pain. Seattle: IASP Press; 1999, pp. 203–233.

Dunn KM, Croft PR, Main CJ, Von KM. A prognostic approach to defining chronic pain: replication in a UK primary care low back pain population. Pain 2008; 135: 48–54.

Durham J, Al-Baghdadi M, Baad-Hansen L et al. Self-management programmes in temporomandibular disorders: results from an international Delphi process. J Oral Rehabil 2016; 43: 929–936.

Fillingim RB, Ohrbach R, Greenspan JD et al. Psychosocial factors associated with development of TMD: the OPPERA prospective cohort study. J Pain 2013; 14: T75–90.

Fricton J. Current evidence providing clarity in management of temporomandibular disorders: summary of a systematic review of randomized clinical trials for intra-oral appliances and occlusal therapies. J Evidence Based Dental Pract 2006; 6: 48–52.

Gatchel RJ, Stowell AW, WIldenstein L, Riggs R, Ellis EI. Efficacy of an early intervention for patients with acute temporomandibular disorder-related pain: a one-year outcome study. JADA 2006; 137: 339–347.

Glaros AG. Temporomandibular disorders and facial pain: a psychophysiological perspective. Appl Psychophysiol Biofeedback 2008; 33: 161–171.

Glaros AG, Marszalek JM, Williams KB. Longitudinal multilevel modeling of facial pain, muscle tension, and stress. J Dent Res 2016; 95: 416–422.

IASP – International Association for the Study of Pain. IASP Taxonomy. IASP; 2017. Available: https://www.iasp-pain.org/Taxonomy [Nov 22, 2017].

Leeuw M, Goossens ME, Linton SJ, Crombez G, Boersma K, Vlaeyen JW. The fear-avoidance model of musculoskeletal pain: current state of scientific evidence. J Behav Med 2007; 30: 77–94.

LeResche L, Mancl LA, Drangsholt MT, Huang G, Von Korff M. Predictors of onset of facial pain and temporomandibular disorders in early adolescence. Pain 2007; 129: 269–278.

List T, Axelsson S. Management of TMD: evidence from systematic reviews and meta-analyses. J Oral Rehabil 2010; 6: 430–451.

Lorig KR, Holman H. Self-management education: history, definition, outcomes, and mechanisms. Annals Behavior Med 2003; 26: 1–7.

Chapter 19

Marchant J. Placebos: Honest fakery. Nature 2016; 535: S14–S5.

Melzack R. Phantom limb pain: implications for treatment of pathologic pain. Anesthesiology 1971; 35 :409–419.

Melzack R. Pain and the brain. APS Journal 1993; 2: 172–174.

Melzack R, Wall PD. Pain mechanisms: a new theory. Science 1965; 150: 971–979.

Merskey H. Introduction. In Giamberardino MA, Jensen TS (eds). Pain Comorbidities: Understanding and Treating the Complex Patient. Seattle: IASP Press; 2012, pp. 1–20.

Meulders A, Vlaeyen JWS. Reduction of fear of movement-related pain and pain-related anxiety: an associative learning approach using a voluntary movement paradigm. Pain 2012; 153: 1504–1513.

Michelotti A, Steenks MH, Farella M, Parisini F, Cimino R, Martina R. The additional value of a home physical therapy regimen versus patient education only for the treatment of myofascial pain of the jaw muscles: short-term results of a randomized clinical trial. J Orofac Pain 2004; 18: 114–125.

Ohrbach R, List T. Predicting treatment responsiveness: somatic and psychologic factors. In Greene CS, Laskin DM. (eds). Treatment of TMDS: Bridging the Gap between Advances in Research and Clinical Patient Management. Chicago: Quintessence; 2013, pp. 91–98.

Ohrbach R, Bair E, Fillingim RB et al. Clinical orofacial characteristics associated with risk of first-onset TMD: the OPPERA prospective cohort study. J Pain 2013; 14: T33–T50.

Perry HT. Stop! Look and listen. J Orofacial Pain 1993; 7: 233.

Phillips B, Ball C, Badenoch D, Straus S, Haynes B, Dawes M. Oxford Centre for evidence-based medicine levels of evidence (May 2001). BJU international 2011; 107: 870.

Roelofs K, Spinhoven P. Trauma and medically unexplained symptoms: towards an integration of cognitive and neuro-biological accounts. Clin Psychol Rev 2007; 27: 798–820.

Rothman KJ, Greenland S. Causation and causal inference in epidemiology. Am J Public Health 2005; 95: S144–S50.

Sanders AE, Essick GK, Fillingim R et al. Sleep apnea symptoms and risk of temporomandibular disorder: OPPERA cohort. J Dental Res 2013a; 92: S70–S77.

Sanders AE, Slade GD, Bair E et al. General health status and incidence of first-onset temporomandibular disorder: the OPPERA prospective cohort study. J Pain 2013b; 14: T51–62.

Sanders AE, Akinkugbe AA, Bair E et al. Subjective sleep quality deteriorates before development of painful temporomandibular disorder. J Pain 2016; 17: 669–677.

Schiffman EL, Ahmad M, Hollender L et al. Longitudinal stability of common TMJ structural disorders. J Dent Res 2017; 96: 270–276.

Sharma S, Ohrbach R, Häggman-Henrikson B. The role of trauma and whiplash injury in TMD. In Connelly ST, Tartaglia GM, Silva R (eds). Contemporary Management of TemporoMandibular Disorders: Current Concepts and Emerging Opportunities. Berlin: Springer-Nature [In press].

Slade GD, Bair E, Greenspan JD et al. Signs and symptoms of first-onset TMD and socio-demographic predictors of its development: the OPPERA prospective cohort study. J Pain 2013a; 14: T20–32.

Slade GD, Fillingim RB, Sanders AE et al. Summary of findings from the OPPERA prospective cohort study of incidence of first-onset temporomandibular disorder: implications and future directions. J Pain 2013b; 14: T116-T24.

Slade G, Sanders A, Bair E et al. Preclinical episodes of orofacial pain symptoms and their association with healthcare behaviors in the OPPERA prospective cohort study. Pain 2013c; 154: 750–760.

Slade GD, Sanders AE, Ohrbach R et al. Pressure pain thresholds fluctuate with, but do not usefully predict, the clinical course of painful temporomandibular disorder. Pain 2014; 155: 2134–2143.

Slade G, Sanders A, Ohrbach R et al. COMT diplotype amplifies effect of stress on risk of temporomandibular pain. J Dental Res 2015; 94: 1187–1195.

Slade GD, Ohrbach R, Greenspan JD et al. Painful temporomandibular disorder: Decade of discovery from OPPERA studies. J Dental Res 2016; 95: 1084–1092.

Smith S, Maixner D, Greenspan JD et al. Case-control association study of TMD reveals genetic risk factors. J Pain 2011; 12: T92-T101.

Smith SB, Mir E, Bair E, Slade GD et al. Genetic variants associated with development of TMD and its intermediate phenotypes: the genetic architecture of TMD in the OPPERA prospective cohort study. J Pain 2013; 14: T91-T101.

Story WP, Durham J, Al-Baghdadi M, Steele J, Araujo-Soares V. Self-management in temporomandibular disorders: a systematic review of behavioural components. J Oral Rehabil 2016; 43: 759–770.

Turk DC, Rudy TE. The robustness of an empirically derived taxonomy of chronic pain patients. Pain 1990; 43: 27–35.

Velly AM, Fricton J. The impact of comorbid conditions on treatment of temporomandibular disorder. JADA 2011; 142: 170–172.

Von Korff M, Dunn KM. Chronic pain reconsidered. Pain 2008; 138: 267–276.

Wager TD, Atlas LY. The neuroscience of placebo effects: connecting context, learning and health. Nat Rev Neurosci 2015; 16: 403–418.

Wall PD. On the relation of injury to pain. Pain 1979; 6: 253–264.

Woolf CJ. Pain: moving from symptom control toward mechanism-specific pharmacologic management. Annals Internal Med 2004; 140: 441–451.

Wordsworth H. The history of 'biopsychosocial' pain – A tale of gladiators, war, papal doctrine and a wrestler; 2012.

INDEX

Note: Page number followed by f and t indicates figure and table respectively.

INDEX

INDEX

INDEX